Spine
Core
Knowledge
in Orthopaedics

SPINE CORE KNOWLEDGE IN ORTHOPAEDICS

ALEXANDER R. VACCARO, M.D.

Professor of Orthopaedic Surgery,
Thomas Jefferson University and
the Rothman Institute,
Philadelphia, PA

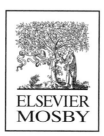

ELSEVIER
MOSBY

ELSEVIER
MOSBY

The Curtis Center
170 S Independence Mall W 300 E
Philadelphia, Pennsylvania 19106

Permissions may be sought directly from Elsevier Inc. Right Department in Philadelphia, USA: phone: (+1) 215 238 7869, fax: (+1) 215 238 2239, email: healthpermissions@elsevier.com. You may also complete your request online via the Elsevier homepage (http://www.elsevier.com), by selecting "Customer Support" and then "Obtaining Permissions."

Notice

Medicine is an ever-changing field. Standard safety precautions must be followed, but as new research and clinical experience broaden our knowledge, changes in treatment and drug therapy may become necessary or appropriate. Readers are advised to check the most current product information provided by the manufacturer of each drug to be administered to verify the recommended dose, the method and duration of administration, and contraindications. It is the responsibility of the treating physician, relying on experience and knowledge of the patient, to determine dosages and the best treatment for each individual patient. Neither the Publisher not the editor assume any liability for any injury and/or damage to persons or property arising from this publication.

The Publisher

Library of Congress Cataloging-in-Publication Data
Spine : core knowledge in orthopaedics / [edited by] Alexander R. Vaccaro.– 1st ed.
    p. ; cm.
  ISBN 0-323-02731-8
   1. Spine–Diseases–Treatment. 2. Spine–Pathophysiology. 3. Spine–Surgery. 4. Orthopedics. I. Vaccaro, Alexander R.
  [DNLM: 1. Spinal Diseases–Handbooks. 2. Spine–surgery–Handbooks, 3. Back Pain–therapy–Handbooks. 4. Orthopedic Procedures–Handbooks. WE 39 S757 2005]
RD768.S674 2005
616.7¢306–dc22
                                                                      2004059217

Printed in the United States of America

Last digit is the print number: 9 8 7 6 5 4 3 2 1

Contributors

TODD J. ALBERT,
M.D., Professor and Vice Chairman, Department of Orthopaedics, Thomas Jefferson University Medical College and the Rothman Institute, Philadelphia, PA

HOWARD S. AN,
M.D., The Morton International Professor of Orthopaedic Surgery, Director of Spine Fellowship Program, Rush Medical College, Director of Spine Surgery, Rush University Medical Center, Chicago, IL

LUKE S. AUSTIN,
Medical Student, Thomas Jefferson University, Philadelphia, PA

ROBERT J. BANCO,
M.D., Boston Spine Group, New England Baptist Hospital, Boston, MA

JOHN M. BEINER,
M.D., B.S., Attending Surgeon, Connecticut Orthopaedic Specialists, Hospital of Saint Raphael; Clinical Instructor, Department of Orthopaedics, Yale University School of Medicine, New Haven, CT.

CHRISTOPHER M. BONO,
M.D., Attending Orthopaedic Surgeon, Boston University Medical Center; Assistant Professor of Orthopaedic Surgery, Boston University School of Medicine, Boston, MA

EUGENE J. CARRAGEE,
M.D., Director, Orthopaedic Spine Center; Professor, Department of Orthopaedic Surgery, Stanford University School of Medicine, Stanford, CA

MATTHEW D. EICHENBAUM,
M.D., Spine Research Fellow, Department of Orthopaedic Surgery, Thomas Jefferson University, Philadelphia, PA

JEFFREY S. FISCHGRUND,
M.D., Spine Surgeon, William Beaumont Hospital, Royal Oak, MI

MARC D. FISICARO,
B.A., Medical Student, Jefferson Medical College, Thomas Jefferson University, Philadelphia, PA

MITCHELL K. FREEDMAN,
D.O., Director of Physical Rehabilitation and Pain Management, The Rothman Institute; Clinical Instructor, Thomas Jefferson University Hospital, Philadelphia, PA.

GUY W. FRIED,
M.D., Medical Director of Outpatient Services, Incontinence Program, and Respiratory Care Program, Magee Rehabilitation Hospital; Clinical Assistant Professor, Thomas Jefferson University Hospital, Philadelphia, PA

STEVEN R. GARFIN,
M.D., Professor and Chair, Department of Orthopaedics, University of California San Diego, San Diego, CA

JONATHAN N. GRAUER,
M.D., Assistant Professor, Co-Director Orthopaedic Spine Surgery, Yale-New Haven Hospital; Assistant Professor, Department of Orthopaedics, Yale University School of Medicine, New Haven, CT

JAMES S. HARROP,
M.D., Assistant Professor of Neurosurgery, Department of Neurosurgery, Thomas Jefferson University, Philadelphia, PA

VICTOR M. HAYES,
M.D., Chief Resident, Long Island Jewish Medical Center, Long Island, NY

HARRY N. HERKOWITZ,
M.D., Chairman, Department of Orthopaedic Surgery, William Beaumont Hospital, Royal Oak, MI

ALAN S. HILIBRAND,
M.D., Associate Professor of Orthopaedic Surgery, Director of Education, Thomas Jefferson University, the Rothman Institute, Philadelphia, PA

LOUIS G. JENIS,
M.D., Boston Spine Group, New England Baptist Hospital, Boston, MA

DAVID H. KIM,
M.D., Orthopaedic Spine Surgeon, The Boston Spine Group, Boston, MA

DMITRIY KONDRACHOV,
M.D., Chief Resident, Long Island Jewish Medical Center, Long Island, NY

BRIAN K. KWON,
M.D., Orthopaedic Spine Fellow, Department of Orthopaedic Surgery, Thomas Jefferson University and the Rothman Institute, Philadelphia, PA; Clinical Instructor, Combine Neurosurgical and Orthopaedic Spine Program, University of British Columbia; and Gowan and Michele Guest Neuroscience Canada Foundation/CIHR Research Fellow, International Collaboration on Repair Discoveries, University of British Columbia, Vancouver, Canada

ERIC LEVICOFF,
M.D., Orthopaedic Surgery Resident, University of Pittsburgh Medical Center, Pittsburgh, PA

RAFAEL LEVIN,
M.D., M.Sc. Comprehensive Spine Care, Emerson, NJ

ROBERTO LUGO,
M.D., Medical Student, Yale University School of Medicine, New Haven, CT

JENNIFER MALONE,
R.N., Department of Neurosurgery, Thomas Jefferson University, Philadelphia, PA

REBECCA S. OVSIOWITZ,
M.D., Thomas Jefferson University, Philadelphia, PA

KEVIN F. RAND,
M.D., Boston Spine Group, New England Baptist Hospital, Boston, MA

MATTHEW ROSEN,
B.A., Thomas Jefferson University College of Medicine, Philadelphia, PA

ARJUN SAXENA,
B.S., Thomas Jefferson Medical College, Philadelphia, PA

DILIP K. SENGUPTA,
M.D., Dr. Med; Assistant Professor, Department of Orthopaedics, Staff Spine Surgeon, Spine Center, Dartmouth-Hitchcock Medical Center, Lebanon, NH

BILAL SHAFI,
M.D., M.S., Surgical Resident, Hospital of University of Pennsylvania, Philadelphia, PA

ASHWINI D. SHARAN,
M.D., Assistant Professor of Neurosurgery, Department of Neurosurgery, Thomas Jefferson University, Philadelphia, PA

FARHAN N. SIDDIQI,
M.D., Chief Resident, Long Island Jewish Medical Center, Long Island, NY

JEFF S. SILBER,
M.D., Assistant Professor, Department of Orthopaedic Surgery, Long Island Jewish Medical Center, North Shore University Hospital Center, Long Island, NY; Albert Einstein University Hospital, Bronx, NY

MARCO T. SILVA,
M.D., Department of Neurosurgery, Jefferson Medical College, Thomas Jefferson University, Philadelphia, PA

KERN SINGH,
M.D., Assistant Professor, Department of Orthopedic Surgery, Rush University Medical Center, Chicago, IL

DANIEL J. SUCATO,
M.D., M.S., Assistant Professor, Department of Orthopaedic Surgery, University of Texas Southwestern Medical Center; Staff Orthopaedic Surgeon, Texas Scottish Rite Hospital for Children, Dallas, TX

KEVIN P. SULLIVAN,
M.D., MetroWest Medical Center, Framingham, MA; Nashoba Valley Medical Center, Ayer, MA; The Boston Spine Group, Southboro, MA

PRIYA SWAMY,
M.D., Thomas Jefferson University, Philadelphia, PA

SCOTT G. TROMANHAUSER,
M.D., Boston Spine Group, New England Baptist Hospital, Boston, MA

EERIC TRUUMEES,
M.D., Attending Spine Surgeon, William Beaumont Hospital, Royal Oak, MI; Adjunct Faculty, Bioengineering Center, Wayne State University, Detroit, MI

ALEXANDER R. VACCARO,
M.D., Professor of Orthopaedic Surgery, Thomas Jefferson University and the Rothman Institute, Philadelphia, PA

BRADY T. VIBERT,
M.D., Resident, Orthopaedic Surgery, William Beaumont Hospital, Royal Oak, MI

Preface

"The great aim of education is not knowledge but action"
Herbert Spencer

Our understanding of spinal disease is increasing at an expediential rate, in part due to the progress of imaging technology (MRI, CT imaging), diagnostic injections and advances in implant technology. The most learned spinal surgeon is challenged just to keep up with the myriad of published contemporary spine journals and books.

Common to all medical disciplines is a core foundation of knowledge i.e. anatomy, physiology and the nature history of the disorder, which must be understood in order to embark on new frontiers in research and medical treatment. *A Resident and Fellows Guide to the Fundamentals of Spine Surgery* was written to provide a resident, fellow, or even an established spinal surgeon with a simple and general, but complete overview of the basics of spinal surgery. This book is a wonderful asset for a medical student on a spinal surgery rotation or spine fellow at the commencement of their fellowship. The bulleted format of the text and accompanying text boxes and illustrations allow for a rapid review of information in a short period of time providing a foundation for learning that would normally take hours to accomplish with a standard text format. Established spinal surgeons will enjoy an easy to digest and timely review of the basics of spinal surgery which is often necessary on a periodic basis as one moves further from their formal training. Lastly, nurses, physician assistants, spinal care physicians (chiropractors, anesthesiologists, physiatrists) and hospital administrators may also use this book to become familiar with a review of commonly used terminologies and frequently performed spinal procedures.

The overall structure of the book is designed to be a high yield, efficient source of clinical information. The book is organized by medical relevance and conceptual difficulty. Within each chapter are numerous algorithms, pictures, grafts and drawings that highlight the most important clinical pearls of each subject matter and organize the information in a logical way to facilitate learning and recall. The annotated references at the end of each chapter serve as a source for those who would like to expand on the topics found in each chapter.

We hope that you enjoy reading this book as much as we enjoyed editing it and we hope that it serves as a useful tool until the next edited version is available.

Alexander R. Vaccaro, M.D.
Marc Fisicaro

Contents

Introduction

This book is designed to function as a pocket aid or reference for medical and graduate students, residents, and those in the beginning of their fellowship training interested in spinal medicine. A general but complete overview of topics commonly encountered in clinical spinal medicine is presented, intended to focus and supplement daily readings and round discussions. Students will find this text useful initially in building a foundation of the core principles of spinal care. Spine fellows and even attending physicians will find this book useful as a quick, on-the-spot review of contemporary treatment principles of commonly encountered spinal disorders.

The design of this text allows you to quickly scan a topic of interest to acquire useful information while on rounds or before entering the operating arena. The book is written in an informal bulleted format with a plethora of outlines, pictures, charts, and graphs. The student or fellow on rounds can refer to any pertinent topic being discussed that day and assimilate the most important facts regarding a particular topic while actively participating in clinical rounds.

The book begins with a basic overview of spinal anatomy, surgical approaches, and physical examination of the spine. As you progress through the book, the topics become more focused on specific but common spinal disorders, such as primary and metastatic tumors of the spine, spinal trauma, and spondylolisthesis. For the seasoned spinal care physician, the book is a wonderful review of specific pathologies that can be read in a short period and can be used for teaching students, residents, ancillary personnel, and spine fellows.

This book is a must for any physician or physician in training who wishes to review on a yearly basis the basics and, if necessary, the details of a particular spinal pathology to maintain a well-rounded understanding of the principles of spinal care.

CHAPTER 1

Basic Anatomy of the Cervical, Thoracic, Lumbar, and Sacral Spine

Marc D. Fisicaro★, Jonathan N. Grauer §, John M. Beiner †, Brian K. Kwon ‡, and
Alexander R. Vaccaro ‖

★B.A., Medical Student, Jefferson Medical College, Thomas Jefferson University,
Philadelphia, PA
§M.D., Assistant Professor, Co-Director Orthopaedic Spine Surgery, Yale-New Haven
Hospital; Assistant Professor, Yale School of Medicine, New Haven, CT
†M.D., B.S., Attending Surgeon, Connecticut Orthopaedic Specialists, Hospital of
Saint Raphael; Clinical Instructor, Department of Orthopaedics, Yale University School
of Medicine, New Haven, CT.
‡M.D., Professor of Orthopaedic Surgery, Jefferson Medical College, Thomas Jefferson
University, Philadelphia, PA
‖ M.D., Orthopaedic Spine Fellow, Department of Orthopaedic Surgery, Thomas Jefferson
University and the Rothman Institute, Philadelphia, PA; Clinical Instructor, Combine
Neurosurgical and Orthopaedic Spine Program, University of British Columbia; and Gown
and Michele Guest Neuroscience Canada Foundation/CIHR Research Fellow, International
Collaboration on Repair Discoveries, University of British Columbia, Vancouver, Canada

Introduction

- A thorough understanding of spinal anatomy is crucial for a comprehensive evaluation of a patient with spinal disorders (Moore 1999, An 1998, Frymoyer et al. 2001, Rothman et al. 1999, Hoppenfeld et al. 1994).
- The primary roles of the spine are maintaining stability, protecting the neural elements, and allowing range of motion. Specifically adapted anatomic features facilitate these functions.
- The vertebra is the structural building block of the spine, with specific morphologic and functional roles based on the vertebra's position in the spinal column. The intervertebral disks, ligaments, and muscles add stability and control.
- The spinal cord travels within, and is protected by, the spine. Paired nerve roots exit at each spinal level.

Bony Vertebral Column

- The vertebral column consists of 33 vertebrae—7 cervical, 12 thoracic, 5 lumbar, 5 sacral, and 4 coccygeal

(Fig. 1–1). The 24 cervical through lumbar vertebrae are mobile.

- The vertebral column has four distinct curves—cervical lordosis, lumbar lordosis, thoracic kyphosis, and sacral kyphosis. In stance, the sagittal vertical axis passes through the odontoid, posterior to the cervical vertebrae, through the C7-T1 intervertebral disk, anterior to the thoracic vertebrae, through the T12-L1 intervertebral disk, posterior to the lumbar vertebrae, through the L5-S1 intervertebral disk, and anterior to the sacrum.
- The primary curves are those of the kyphotic thoracic and sacral regions. These form during the fetal period. The secondary curves are those of the lordotic cervical and lumbar regions. These are initiated during the late fetal period but do not become significant until after birth when the spinal column begins to bear the weight of the body and head. Primary curves are caused by the wedge-shaped nature of involved vertebrae, whereas secondary curves are caused by differences in the anterior and posterior dimensions of the intervertebral disks.

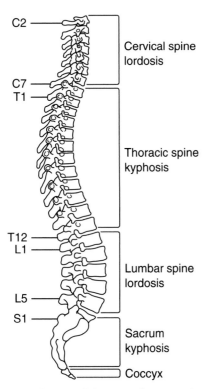

Figure 1–1: Lateral view of the spine demonstrating the normal spinal curvatures.

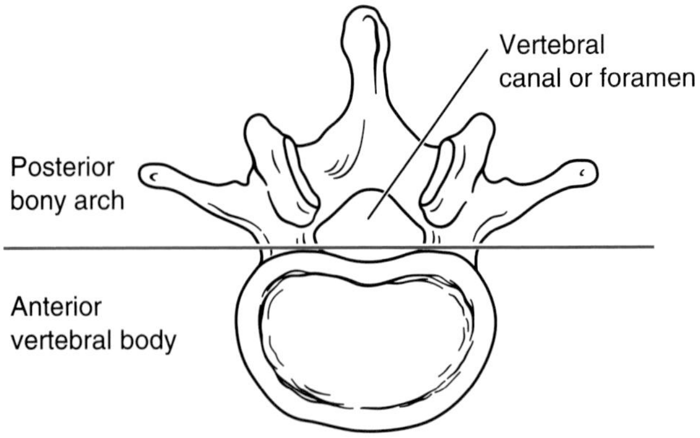

- Each vertebra consists of an anterior body and a posterior bony arch (Fig. 1–2). Together these surround the vertebral canal or foramen. Lateral spaces between the posterior arches of adjacent vertebrae form the foramen through which the spinal nerve roots pass (Fig. 1–3).
- The posterior vertebral arch consists of the pedicles, laminae, spinous processes, facet joints, and transverse processes. The pedicles and laminae form the borders of the vertebral canal with the posterior border of the vertebral body. The spinous and transverse processes are sites of attachment of supporting ligaments and muscles. Of note, the posterior arches include the thickest cortex of the vertebra (Doherty et al. 1994).
- The superior articular process is the portion of the posterior elements that articulates with the supra-adjacent vertebra. The inferior articular process articulates with the subadjacent vertebra. The orientation of the articular

Figure 1–3: Borders of the intervertebral foramen through which the spinal nerve roots pass.

Figure 1–2: Anatomic configuration of a lumbar vertebra.

processes changes when one moves down the vertebral column. The bony region between the two articular processes of an individual vertebra is termed the pars interarticularis.
- The vertebral bodies of the lumbar spine support an average of 80% of the axial load experienced by the spinal column; the facet joints support the other 20%.

Specific Vertebral Anatomy

Atlas (C1)

- The atlas is the first cervical vertebra (Fig. 1–4). This is a ring-like structure that does not have an anterior body or a posterior spinous process. There is an anterior and a much longer posterior arch.
- The posterior arch has a groove along its superior border where the vertebral artery passes in its tortuous path toward the foramen magnum of the skull.
- The superior articular facets are saucer-like and form the atlanto-occipital articulation with the occipital condyles. Because of the orientation of these facets, the majority of cervical flexion and extension of the upper cervical spine is possible in this region.
- The inferior articular facets are flatter, more circular, and contribute to the atlantoaxial articulation with the second cervical vertebra, or axis. The remainder of this articulation is through the unique relationship of the

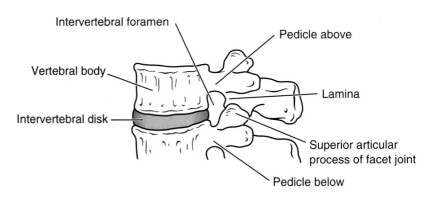

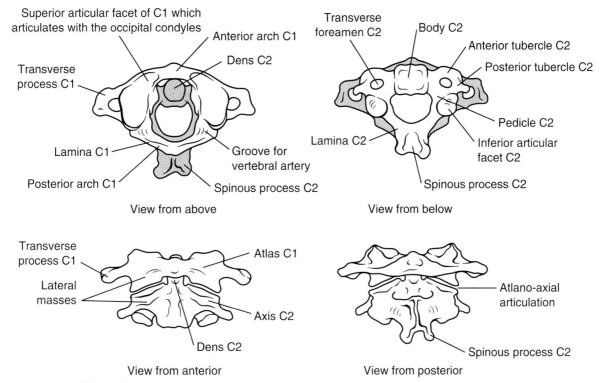

Figure 1–4: C1 and C2 vertebrae.

posterior border of the anterior arch of the atlas and the dens.

- The transverse processes of the atlas are longer and larger than those of the other cervical vertebrae. Within the transverse processes is the transverse foramina through which the vertebral artery passes.

Axis (C2)

- The axis is the second cervical vertebra (Fig. 1–4). This includes the dens, or odontoid, which projects superiorly from the anterior vertebral body to articulate with the atlas.
- The atlas contacts the axis through the posterior facet joints and the anterior atlantodens articulation. A synovial joint is present between the anterior arch of C1 and the dens and transverse ligament that bonds the odontoid to the anterior C1 arch. The majority of upper cervical rotation occurs at the atlantoaxial joint.
- The transverse ligament is a stout ligament that runs from one side of the atlas to the other and holds the dens

against the posterior surface of the anterior C1 arch (Fig. 1–5). Extensions of this ligament superiorly and inferiorly create the cruciform ligament.
- The dens is further stabilized by the alar ligaments that connect the odontoid tip to the occipital condyles. The apical ligament, at the tip of the dens, is a remnant of the notochord.
- The C2-C3 articulation is anatomically similar to the rest of the subaxial cervical levels.
- The C2 pedicle is relatively large and projects 30 degrees medially and 20 degrees superiorly (Xu et al. 1995).
- The C2 spinous process is large, bifid, and often palpable. This serves as the site of attachment for several muscles.
- The transverse processes of this vertebra are similar in morphology, but smaller, than those of the other cervical vertebrae. The vertebral artery passes through the transverse processes in the transverse foramen.

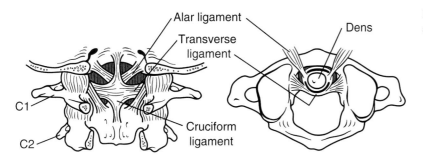

Figure 1–5: Ligaments specific to the atlantoaxial articulation.

Subaxial Cervical Spine (C3-C7)

- The C3-C6 vertebral bodies are small in relationship to their vertebral canals (Fig. 1–6). The canal, triangular in shape, has the greatest cross-sectional area at C2.
- The superior surfaces, or endplates, of the cervical vertebrae are concave. The inferior endplates are convex. As such, the lateral aspects of the superior endplates curve superiorly to approach the supra-adjacent vertebrae to form what is known as the uncovertebral joints, or the joints of Luschka.
- The facets gradually become steeper and more sagittally oriented as one descends the cervical levels. The bony regions between the cervical facets, called the lateral masses, are just lateral to the laminae.
- The spinous processes are short and bifid.
- Similar to the atlas and axis, the vertebral artery travels within the transverse foramina of the transverse processes. This divides the transverse processes into the anterior and posterior tubercles.
- Between the two tubercles of the transverse processes is the groove on which the exiting nerve roots pass after exiting the intervertebral foramen.
- The seventh cervical vertebra (vertebra prominens) is a transitional vertebra and has several unique characteristics.
- The inferior surface of C7 is larger than its superior surface. The lateral masses of C7 are taller and shallower than those of the other subaxial cervical vertebrae. The pedicles also begin to enlarge as one goes caudally from this level.
- The C7 spinous process is long, nonbifid, and almost horizontal. This serves as a site of attachment for the ligamentum nuchae.
- The transverse processes of C7 do have transverse foramina, but the vertebral arteries rarely (5% of cases) pass through this vertebra. Rather, the vertebral artery usually joins the spinal column at C6.

Thoracic Spine

- The thoracic vertebrae are intermediate in size between the cervical and lumbar vertebrae (Fig. 1–7). Their size increases as one moves down the spinal column.
- The defining characteristic of thoracic vertebrae is their intimate relationship with the ribs (Vollmer et al. 1997). A rib articulates at the junction of the vertebral body and pedicle (superior costal facet) of its named vertebra and the vertebra above (inferior costal facet). The rib also articulates with the transverse costal facet of the transverse process of its named vertebra. These relations of the rib and the vertebrae are supported by accessory ligaments that make the thoracic spine mechanically stiffer than the cervical and lumbar spine.
- Anteriorly, the thoracic vertebral bodies are relatively heart shaped. Sometimes, the left side of the vertebrae has a depression secondary to the descending aorta.
- The pedicles of the thoracic vertebrae are oval in cross section. These have been reported to be 10 mm in height and 4.5 mm in width at T4 and 14 mm height and 7.8 mm in width at T12 (Vaccaro et al. 1995). As with the pedicles of the lumbar spine, the walls are thicker medially than laterally.
- The spinal canal has less free space for the spinal cord than the cervical and lumbar regions.
- Posteriorly, the thoracic vertebrae have long, slender spinous processes that point downward and overlap the vertebral arches of the inferior vertebra.
- The transverse processes are posteriorly angulated, leaving room for the ribs to pass anterior to them.

Lumbar Spine

- The lumbar vertebrae are stouter than those of the other spinal regions because they bear the greatest weight (Fig. 1–8).
- Anteriorly, the lumbar vertebral bodies are kidney shaped. Their bodies are wider transversely than they are deep anteroposteriorly, and both of these dimensions exceed their height.

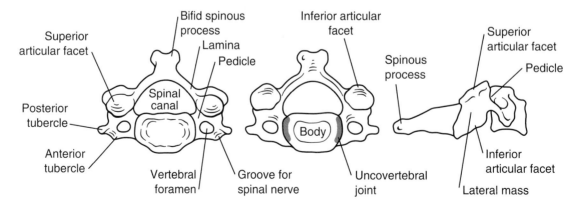

C4 view from above   View from below   Lateral view

Figure 1–6: C4 as a representative subaxial vertebra.

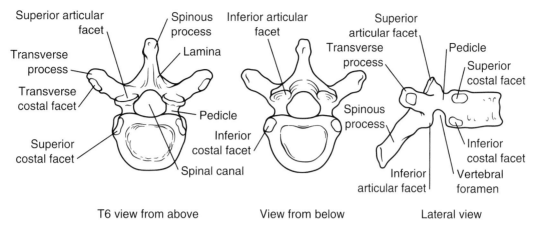

Figure 1–7: T6 as a representative thoracic vertebra.

- The pedicles are short and large and arise from the upper part of the vertebral body. Based on posterior landmarks, a pedicle is located behind the facet of the named vertebra and the supra-adjacent vertebra. In the cephalad–caudad direction, it is in the midline of the associated transverse process. In the medial–lateral direction, the medial aspect of the pedicle is in line with the lateral aspect of the pars interarticularis.
- At L1, the transverse pedicular diameter is approximately 9 mm with a medial angle of 12 degrees (Zindrick et al. 1987). The height-to-width ratio at L1-L4 is approximately 1:8, but this decreases to 1:1 at L5 (Panjabi et al. 1992). L1 and L2 are transitional vertebrae similar to the thoracic vertebrae (Panjabi et al. 1992).
- The lumbar facets are in a relative sagittal orientation. As such, axial rotation is limited. The exception is the L5-S1 facet, which is more coronal and resists anteroposterior translation (An 1998). The pars interarticularis is more defined in this region of the spine than in the cervical or thoracic region.

- The nerve roots pass under the lateral recess of the pedicles/articular facets and through the intervertebral foramina. These foramina are bordered by the pedicles above and below, the vertebral body and intervertebral disk anteriorly, and the lamina and facets posteriorly (Fig. 1–3).
- The spinous processes are broad and tall within the lumbar spine.
- The transverse process of L5 is often much smaller than the transverse processes of the other lumbar vertebrae. The L5 transverse process is the site of attachment of the iliolumbar ligament. As with the other lumbar transverse processes, L5 often has an irregular accessory process on the medial aspect of the transverse process near where it joins the rest of the posterior bony arch and a mammillary process at the prominence of the facet joint.

Sacrum

- The sacrum is composed of five fused vertebrae and is a large, wedge-shaped bone (Fig. 1–9).

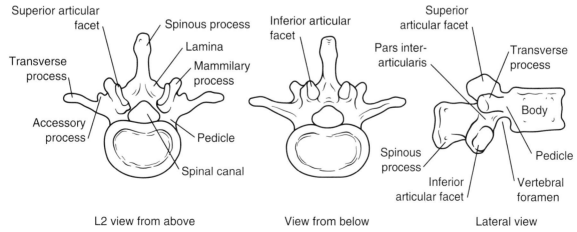

Figure 1–8: L2 as a representative lumbar vertebra.

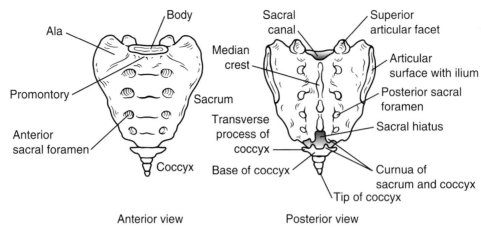

Figure 1–9: Sacrum and coccyx.

- The functions of the sacrum are to provide strength and stability to the pelvis and to transmit the weight of the body from the vertebral column to the pelvic girdle through articulation with the ilea (the sacroiliac joints).
- The spine has an acute angle at L5-S1, which is called the sacrovertebral angle.
- The promontory is the superior flare of the sacrum that articulates with L5. The transverse lines are the residual of the divisions of the sacral vertebrae. The alae are the two lateral wings that extend laterally to the sacroiliac joints. These are derived from fused transverse processes of the sacral vertebrae. The median sacral crest is formed by the fused sacral spinous processes.
- The sacrum has four pairs of anterior and posterior foramina through which the ventral and dorsal primary rami exit. The anterior sacral foramina are larger than the posterior foramina (Esses et al. 1991).
- The sacral hiatus is formed by the absence of the laminae and spinous process of S5. The sacral hiatus is the termination of the sacral canal. This contains the fatty connective tissue, the filum terminale, the S5 nerves, and the coccygeal nerves.
- The sacral cornu is formed by the pedicles of the fifth sacral vertebra. They project inferiorly on each side of the hiatus.

Coccyx

- The coccyx, colloquially called the "tail bone", is the terminal portion of the spinal column. It consists of four fused rudimentary vertebrae.
- The primary role of the coccyx in the human is to serve as a site of attachment for muscles of the pelvic floor.
- The coccygeal cornua are proximal extensions of the coccyx. The tip of the coccyx is usually flexed forward.

Intervertebral Disks

- Intervertebral disks are located between the vertebral bodies of C2-C3 through L5-S1. The disks are located between the vertebral endplates covered with hyaline cartilage and supported by subchondral bone.
- Analogous to the menisci of the knee, the intervertebral disk is a relatively avascular structure with only the outermost layers receiving nutrients from peripheral vascularization. The central portions of the disk receive nutrients through diffusion from the vertebral endplates.
- The nucleus pulposus is the inner portion of the disk (Fig. 1–10). This mucoid portion of the disk is

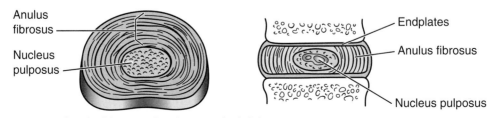

Figure 1–10: Transverse and sagittal images of an intervertebral disk.

predominantly made of type II collagen and is a remnant of the primitive notochord. The nucleus acts at a cushion to axial loads.

- The anulus fibrosus is the outer portion of the disk. This multilayered, fibrocartilaginous structure is predominantly made of type I collagen. A lattice is made with overlapping sheets running in opposite directions to give the anulus increased strength, especially in rotation. The anulus is thickest anteriorly and thinnest posterolaterally.
- The anulus absorbs the radially directed forces from the nucleus and converts these to hoop stresses at the periphery of the disk, where they are firmly attached to the vertebral endplates.
- The outermost portions of the anulus are continuous with the anterior and posterior longitudinal ligaments.
- The intervertebral disks contribute {1/4} of the length to the spinal column, but this is a dynamic measure. When in the horizontal position, nutrients and fluid enter the disk, increasing height. With prolonged stance, nutrients and fluids exit the disk, decreasing height.

Ligaments of the Vertebral Column

Anterior Longitudinal Ligament

- The anterior longitudinal ligament runs along the anterior aspect of the vertebral column (Fig. 1–11). It begins at the anterior border of the anterior margin of the foramen magnum (basion) as the anterior occipital membrane and ends on the anterior surface of the sacrum.
- As the ligament descends, it widens, and it is thickest opposite the disk spaces. The deepest fibers of this

ligament are found at only one level. The intermediate fibers span two or three levels. The most superficial fibers span four or five levels.

- The functions of the anterior longitudinal ligament are to prevent hyperextension and to support the anulus fibrosus anteriorly.

Posterior Longitudinal Ligament

- The posterior longitudinal ligament runs along the posterior aspect of the vertebral column (Fig. 1–11). It begins along the posterior border of the basion as the tectorial membrane, continues within the spinal canal, and ends on the posterior surface of the sacrum.
- The posterior longitudinal ligament is narrow over the middle of the vertebral bodies and expands over the disks and vertebral endplates (Fig. 1–12). The lateral expansions are thin, and the central portion of the ligament is thick.
- The posterior longitudinal ligament is double layered—its superficial layer is adjacent to the dura and contributes to the enveloping connective tissue underlying neural elements. The deep layers connect to the anulus fibrosus centrally and blend into the intervertebral foramen laterally.
- The functions of the posterior longitudinal ligament are to prevent hyperflexion and to support the posterior aspects of the anterior vertebral column.

Ligamentum Flavum

- The ligamentum flavum, or the yellow ligament, is a thick, segmental ligament that runs between the lamina of adjacent vertebrae (Fig. 1–11). It begins on the undersurface of the inferior border of the lamina and courses down to the leading superior edge of the lamina (Fig. 1–12).
- There are gaps at the midline of the ligamentum flavum to allow the veins to exit.

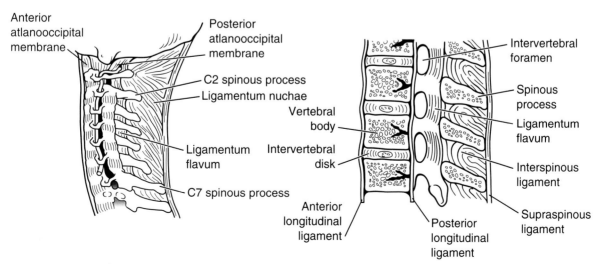

Figure 1–11: Ligaments of the spinal column.

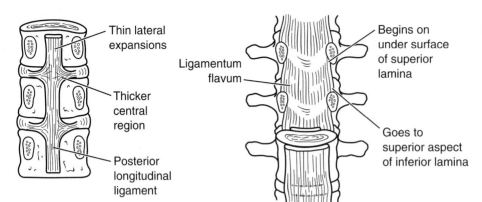

Figure 1–12: Posterior longitudinal ligament and ligamentum flavum.

- The function of the ligamentum flavum is to maintain upright posture. It helps to preserve the normal curvature of the spine and to straighten the column after it has been flexed. However, the elasticity of the ligamentum flavum decreases with age, and this may be associated with hypertrophy and buckling.

Supraspinous Ligament

- The supraspinous ligament is a midline structure that runs over the posterior aspect of the spinous processes (Fig. 1–11). The cervical expansion of this ligament is called the ligamentum nuchae.
- The nuchal portion of this ligament extends from the seventh cervical spinous process to the external occipital protuberance. It is attached to the posterior tubercle of the atlas and to the spinous processes of the other cervical vertebrae.
- The primary purpose of this ligament is to act as a tension band in preventing hyperflexion. It also acts as a site of attachment for the fascial coverings of the medial spinal muscles.

Additional Spinal Ligaments

- The interspinous ligaments connect adjacent spinous processes. As with the supraspinous ligament, this contributes to the posterior tension band preventing hyperflexion.
- Intertransverse ligaments connect adjacent transverse processes. These help to limit lateral bending and act as a border between anterior and posterior structures, particularly in the lumbar spine.
- Denticulate ligaments are fine intradural ligaments that attach neural elements to overlying covering membranes.

Muscles of the Vertebral Column
Posterior Muscles

- The extrinsic posterior muscles of the back include the trapezius and latissimus dorsi, the serratus posterior superior, and the serratus posterior inferior.
- The intrinsic posterior spinal muscles are located under the more superficial extrinsic musculature. The intrinsic spinal muscles extend, rotate, and laterally bend the vertebral column. As a rule, superficial spinal muscles are longer than deeper spinal muscles. Many of these muscles are named in subdivisions based on the site of insertion of portions of the muscle.
- The intrinsic posterior muscles are divided into superficial, intermediate, and deep layers (Fig. 1–13, Table 1–1). These are innervated by the dorsal ramus of the spinal nerves.
- The superficial layer consists of the splenius capitis and the splenius cervicis muscles.
- The muscles of the intermediate layer are also known as the erector spinae muscles. This layer is composed of: (1) the iliocostalis, subdivided into the cervicis, thoracis, and lumborum portions; (2) the longissimus, subdivided into the capitis, cervicis, and thoracic portions; and (3) the smaller spinalis muscle group, subdivided into the capitis, cervicis, and thoracis portions.
- The muscles of the deep layer are also known as the transversospinalis muscles. This layer is composed of: (1) the semispinalis, subdivided into the capitis, cervicis, and thoracis portions; (2) the multifidus; (3) the rotators; and (4) the short rotators (the interspinales and intertransversarii muscles).
- The muscles of the upper cervical spine make up the suboccipital triangle (Fig. 1–13, Table 1–1). The suboccipital triangle is bound medially by the rectus capitis posterior, laterally by the obliquus capitis superior, and inferiorly by the obliquus capitis inferior. The roof is formed by the semispinalis capitis and longissimus capitis. The posterior arch of the atlas and posterior atlanto-occipital membrane form the floor of the triangle. Within the triangle are the vertebral artery and suboccipital nerve and vessels. All of the muscles are innervated by the suboccipital nerve.

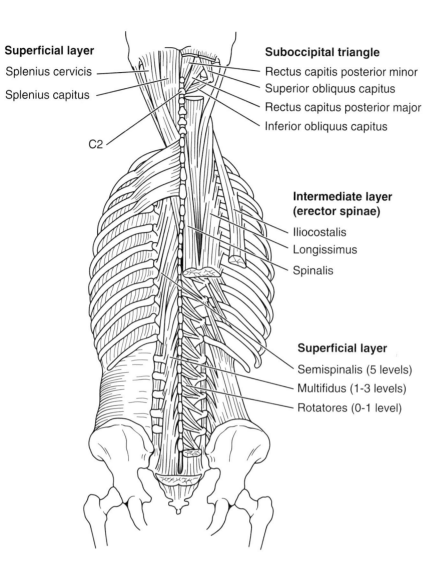

Figure 1–13: Posterior intrinsic spinal muscles.

Superficial layer
Splenius cervicis
Splenius capitus

C2

Suboccipital triangle
Rectus capitis posterior minor
Superior obliquus capitus
Rectus capitus posterior major
Inferior obliquus capitus

Intermediate layer (erector spinae)
Iliocostalis
Longissimus
Spinalis

Superficial layer
Semispinalis (5 levels)
Multifidus (1-3 levels)
Rotatores (0-1 level)

Anterior Spinal Muscles

- Anterior muscles that flex, laterally bend, and rotate the spine generally act a greater distance from the vertebral column than the posterior muscles.
- The sternocleidomastoid, scalene muscles, longus colli, and longus capitis act on the cervical spine.
- The abdominal, psoas, and quadratus lumorum muscles act on the thoracolumbar spine.

Blood Supply and Venous Drainage

- The arterial blood supply of the spine is predominantly from segmental vessels that originate from the vertebral arteries, aorta, and iliac vessels (Fig. 1–14). Not only are these important for the bony spine, but they also are crucial for the functioning of the spinal cord.

- Segmental vessels have dorsal branches that divide into anterior and posterior radicular arteries when they enter the intervertebral foramen. These form a single anterior spinal artery and a pair of posterior spinal arteries, respectively.
- The artery of Adamkiewicz is a particularly large radicular vessel that generally arises in the left thoracolumbar region and is considered to contribute significantly to the anterior vascular supply of the spinal cord at this level.
- The vertebral artery deserves specific mention. This is a branch off the subclavian artery that, as discussed in preceding sections, usually enters the transverse foramen of the cervical vertebra at C6, gives off segmental branches when it ascends the cervical spine, and then curves medially, after passing through C1, to within 1.5 cm of midline in the adult before entering the foramen magnum.

Table 1–1: Posterior Spine Muscles

	MUSCLE	ORIGIN	INSERTION	PRIMARY FUNCTIONS
Superficial	Splenius capitis	Ligamentum nuchae, spinous processes	Mastoid process, occipital nuchal line	Extension, lateral bending, rotation
	Splenius cervicis	Same	Posterior tubercles C1-C3	Same
Intermediate (erector spinae)	Iliocostalis	Iliac crests, sacrum, spinous processes	Ribs, cervical transverse processes	Extension, lateral bending
	Longissimus	Same	Ribs, transverse processes, mastoid process	Same
	Spinalis	Same	Spinous processes, skull	Same
Deep layer (transversospinalis and short rotators)	Semispinalis	Transverse processes	Spinous processes of vertebrae 5-6 levels above	Extension, rotation
	Multifidus	Sacrum, ilium, transverse processes	Spinous processes of vertebrae 1-3 levels above	Stabilizing effect
	Rotators	Transverse processes	Spinous processes of vertebrae 1-2 levels above	Extension, rotation
	Interspinales	Spinous processes	Spinous process of adjacent vertebra	Extension
	Intertransversarii	Transverse process	Transverse process of adjacent vertebrae	Lateral bending
Suboccipital muscles	Rectus capitis posterior major	C2 spinous process	Lateral portion of nuchal line of skull	Extension, rotation of head
	Rectus capitis posterior minor	Posterior tubercle of atlas	Medial portion of nuchal line of skull	Same
	Superior obliquus capitis	Transverse process of C1	Lateral portion of nuchal line of skull	Same
	Inferior obliquus capitis	Spinous process of C2	Transverse process of C1	Same

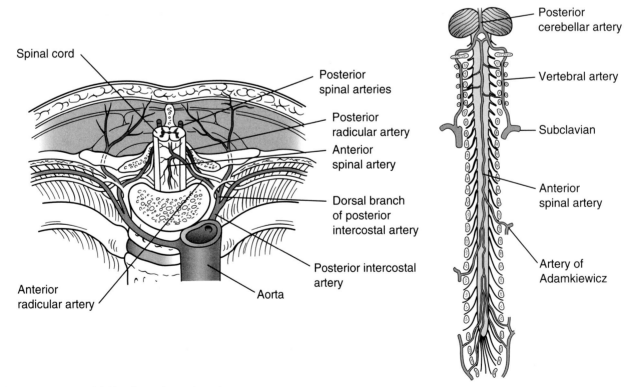

Figure 1–14: Arterial blood supply to the spine.

- The spinal veins form plexuses within the vertebral bodies and around the epidural space (Fig. 1–15).

Neuroanatomy

- There are 31 pairs of spinal nerves—8 cervical, 12 thoracic, 5 lumbar, 5 sacral, and 1 coccygeal (Fig. 1–16). The first seven cervical nerves leave the vertebral canal above their named vertebrae. The eighth cervical and the remainder of the spinal nerves exit the vertebral canal below their named vertebrae.
- The dorsal and ventral rootlets coalesce to form the dorsal and ventral roots, respectively (Fig. 1–17). The dorsal root has the cell bodies of the entering sensory neurons (dorsal root ganglion) medial to its union with the motor neurons of the ventral root. The dorsal and ventral roots form the spinal nerve that divides into the dorsal and ventral primary rami after developing sympathetic branches.
- The dorsal primary ramus innervates the skin and deep muscles of the back. The ventral primary ramus forms the plexi, intercostals, and subcostal nerves.
- The spinal cord is shorter than the vertebral column; it usually ends at L1 or L2. The spinal cord has cervical and lumbar enlargements because the nerves branch out to the upper and lower extremities, and it terminates in the conus medullaris. Nerve roots continue more distally in the cauda equine until the thecal sac terminates in the filum terminale (Fig. 1–16).
- The spinal cord is covered by three layers of meninges—the dura, the arachnoid, and the pia mater, from peripheral to central (Figs. 1–17 and 1–18). Together these form the thecal sac.
- The pia is closely related to the spinal cord and therefore cannot be dissected from it. It is relatively

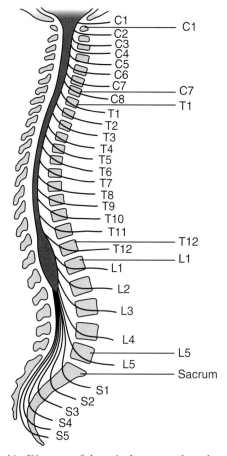

Figure 1–16: Diagram of the spinal nerves when they exit the vertebral column.

thick and gives rise to a longitudinal projection on each side called the denticulate ligament. These ligaments anchor the spinal cord to the arachnoid and, through it, to the dura.

- The arachnoid is a transparent layer that connects to the pia by web-like trabeculations. Under it is the subarachnoid space, which is filled with cerebrospinal fluid. This space extends down to S2. There is a large subarachnoid space between L1 and S2 called the lumbar cistern.
- The dura is the tough, fibrous, outer covering of the spinal cord. Between the dura and the arachnoid is a potential space, called the subdural space, that also extends to S2. The epidural space is outside the dura and contains the internal venous plexus and epidural fat.
- The internal morphology of the spinal cord consists of central gray matter, which is predominantly cell bodies, surrounded by peripheral white matter, which is predominantly axons that make up specific neural tracts (Fig. 1–17 and Table 1–2).

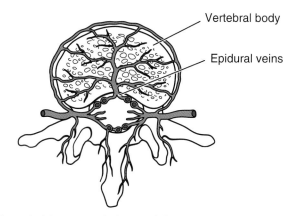

Figure 1–15: Venous drainage of the spine.

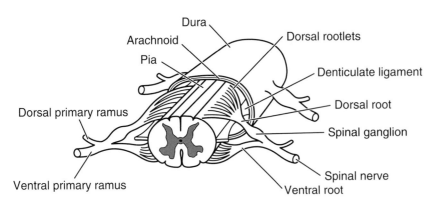

Figure 1–17: Spinal root and nerve anatomy.

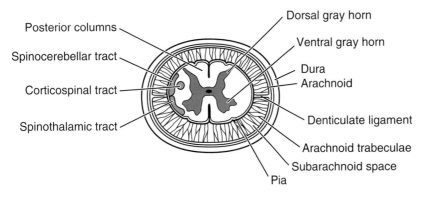

Figure 1–18: Spinal supra-adjacent cord anatomy.

Table 1–2:	Spinal Tracts	
NAME OF TRACT	INFORMATION TRANSMITTED	DECUSSATION
Posterior columns	Light touch, vibration, proprioception	Caudal medulla
Spinocerebellar	Unconscious proprioception	No decussation
Corticospinal	Voluntary movement	Caudal medulla
Spinothalamic	Pain, temperature	At level of spinal cord entry

References

An HS, ed. (1998) Principles and Techniques of Spine Surgery, Baltimore: Williams and Wilkins.
    A reference textbook with well-prepared illustrations.

Doherty BJ, Heggeness MH. (1994) Quantitative anatomy of the atlas. Spine 19(22): 2497-2500.
    The authors establish the range and variability of external dimensions of the atlas using cadaveric specimens.

Esses SI, Botsford DJ, Huler RJ et al. (1991) Surgical anatomy of the sacrum: A guide for rational screw fixation. Spine 16(6 Suppl.): S283-S288.
    The authors studied prepared cadaveric specimens to allow safe screw placement.

Frymoyer JW, Ducker TB, Hadler NM et al., eds. (1991) The Adult Spine: Principles and Practice, 2nd edition. New York: Raven Press.
    A reference spine textbook with well-prepared sections on spinal anatomy.

Hoppenfeld S, deBoer P. (1994) Surgical Exposures in Orthopaedics: The Anatomic Approach. Philadelphia: Lippincott-Raven.
    Unlike anatomy texts, this book highlights the anatomy seen during specific surgical approaches.

Moore K. (1999) Clinically Oriented Anatomy, 4th edition. Philadelphia: Lippincott Williams & Wilkins.
    A complete, well-illustrated basic anatomy textbook presented with clinical correlations. This book is a popular medical school textbook.

Panjabi MM, Goel V, Oxland T et al. (1992) Human lumbar vertebrae: A three-dimensional anatomy. Spine 17(3): 299-306.

The authors used prepared cadaveric specimens to study various surface dimensions of the lumbar vertebrae.

Rothman R, Simeone FE, eds. (1999) The Spine, 4th edition. Philadelphia: W.B. Saunders.

A comprehensive spine textbook that covers spinal anatomy, physical examination, myriad spinal disorders, and their nonoperative and operative treatment.

Vaccaro AR, Rizzolo SJ, Allerdyce TJ et al. (1995) Placement of pedicle screws in the thoracic spine. J Bone Joint Surg 77A: 1193-1199.

The authors studied the morphology of thoracic vertebrae using 17 prepared cadaveric specimens.

Vollmer DG, Banister WM. (1997) Thoracolumbar spinal anatomy. Neurosurg Clin N Am 8(4): 443-453.

The authors reviewed the anatomy of the thoracolumbar spine relevant to disorders of the region.

Xu R, Naudaud MC, Ebraheim NA et al. (1995) Morphology of the second cervical vertebra and the posterior projection of the C2 pedicle axis. Spine 20: 259-263.

The authors studied 50 dried C2 vertebrae to assess their structural features.

Zindrick MR, Wiltse LL, Doornick A et al. (1987) Analysis of the morphometric characteristics of the thoracic and lumbar pedicles. Spine 12: 160-166.

The authors measured pedicles of T1-L5 using CT scan and roentgenograms.

Physical Examination of the Spine

Jennifer Malone★, James S. Harrop §, Ashwini D. Sharan §, Matthew D. Eichenbaum †, and Alexander R. Vaccaro ‡

★ R.N., Department of Neurosurgery, Thomas Jefferson University, Philadelphia, PA
§ M.D., Assistant Professor of Neurosurgery, Department of Neurosurgery, Thomas Jefferson University, Philadelphia, PA
† M.D., Spine Research Fellow, Department of Orthopaedic Surgery, Thomas Jefferson University, Philadelphia, PA
‡ M.D., Professor of Orthopaedic Surgery, Thomas Jefferson University and the Rothman Institute, Philadelphia, PA

Introduction

- The spine is a complex biomechanical structure that does the following:
  - Protects the neural structures
  - Allows an upright posture
  - Aids in respiration and ambulation
- Unfortunately, these requirements place a great strain on the spine and may promote accelerated aging or symptomatic degeneration.

Anatomy of the Spinal Column

- The vertebral spinal column does the following:
  - Supports the cranium and trunk
  - Allows movement
  - Protects the spinal cord
  - Absorbs stresses produced by walking, running, and lifting
- The vertebral spinal column consists of 33 vertebrae with 23 intervening fibrocartilage intervertebral disks supported by numerous ligaments and paraspinal muscles.
- The spinal column is divided into five regions consisting of the following:
  - 7 cervical vertebrae
  - 12 thoracic vertebrae
  - 5 lumbar vertebrae
  - 5 sacral vertebrae
  - 3 to 4 coccygeal vertebrae
- Spinal ligaments include the following:
  - The anterior longitudinal ligament
  - The posterior longitudinal ligament
  - The ligamentum flavum
  - Interspinous ligaments
  - Numerous smaller ligaments

Muscles of the Back

Superficial Extrinsic Back Muscles

- The following muscles connect the upper limbs to the trunk and control limb movements:
  - Trapezius
  - Latissimus dorsi
  - Levator scapulae
  - Rhomboid major
  - Rhomboid minor

Intermediate Extrinsic Back Muscles

- The following superficial respiratory muscles are deep to the rhomboids and latissimus:
  - Serratus posterior superior
  - Serratus posterior inferior

Superficial Intrinsic Back Muscles (Fig. 2–1)

- Splenius capitis
- Splenius cervicis

Intermediate Intrinsic Back Muscles—The Erector Spinae (Fig. 2–1)

- The following muscles are massive and strong and function as the chief extensors of the vertebral column:
  - Iliocostalis—Lateral column
  - Longissimus—Intermediate column
  - Spinalis—Medial column

Deep Intrinsic Back Muscles—The Transversospinal Muscle Group (Fig. 2–1)

- The following muscles are deep to the erector spinae and obliquely disposed:
  - Semispinalis—Superficial layer
  - Multifidus—Intermediate layer
  - Rotators—Deepest layer

Minor Deep Intrinsic Back Muscles

- Interspinales
- Intertransversarii
- Levatores costarum

Prevertebral (Deep) Muscles of the Neck (Fig. 2–2)

Anterior Vertebral Muscles

- The following muscles are deep to the anterior cervical triangle and are anterior flexors of the head and neck:
  - Longus colli
  - Longus capitis
  - Rectus capitis anterior
  - Rectus capitis lateralis

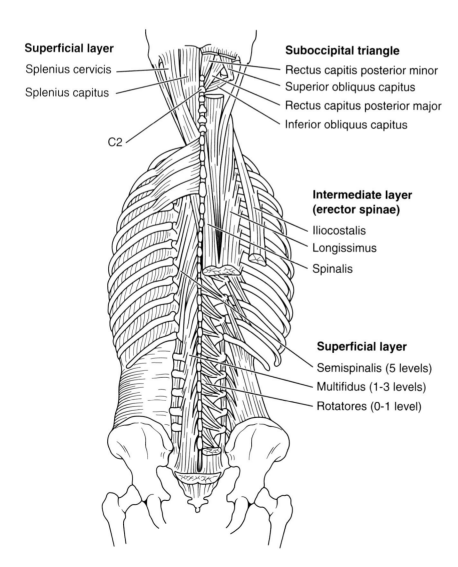

Superficial layer
Splenius cervicis
Splenius capitus
C2

Suboccipital triangle
Rectus capitis posterior minor
Superior obliquus capitus
Rectus capitis posterior major
Inferior obliquus capitus

Intermediate layer (erector spinae)
Iliocostalis
Longissimus
Spinalis

Superficial layer
Semispinalis (5 levels)
Multifidus (1-3 levels)
Rotatores (0-1 level)

Figure 2–1: Superficial, intermediate, and deep back musculature.

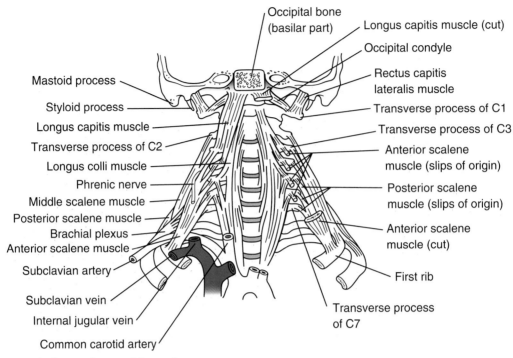

Figure 2–2: Prevertebral musculature of the neck.

Lateral Vertebral Group

- The muscles of this group are deep to the posterior cervical triangle and are rotators and lateral flexors of the neck:
  - Splenius capitis
  - Posterior scalene
  - Middle scalene
  - Anterior scalene

Coronal and Sagittal Spinal Alignment

- The vertebral column has four major curves (Fig. 2–3):
  - Cervical
  - Thoracic
  - Lumbar
  - Sacrococcygeal or pelvic
- The thoracic and sacrococcygeal curves are referred to as primary curves because they retain the kyphotic curvature from embryogenesis, as seen in the fetus.
- The cervical and lumbar spines are secondary curves. They develop or adapt a lordotic structure as a result of postural changes to accommodate sitting and ambulation.
- There is a large degree of variability in what is considered the "normal" sagittal curvature of the cervical, thoracic, and lumbar spine. (Table 2–1)

Table 2–1: Curvature of the Spine	
CURVATURE	**NORMAL CURVATURE**
Cervical lordosis	20 to 40 degrees
Thoracic kyphosis	20 to 45 degrees
Lumbar lordosis	40 to 60 degrees
Sacral kyphosis	Sacrum fused in a kyphotic curve

- Overall, the spine should support the head over the pelvis, a state referred to as being in coronal and sagittal balance or alignment.
- The length of the cervical spinal canal measured in the sagittal plane during flexion (kyphotic posture) is greater than the length during extension (lordotic posture).
- The normal cervical lordosis allows the neural elements to traverse the spinal canal through a shorter course without ventral compression.
- The lordotic cervical curvature might also protect against neural injury because axial loads are dispersed dorsally onto the facet joints and large articular pillars rather than onto the vertebral body.
- The flexibility of the cervical spine allows it to compensate for misalignment of the thoracic and lumbar spine.
- An increased lordotic cervical posture is observed in the setting of exaggerated thoracic kyphosis.

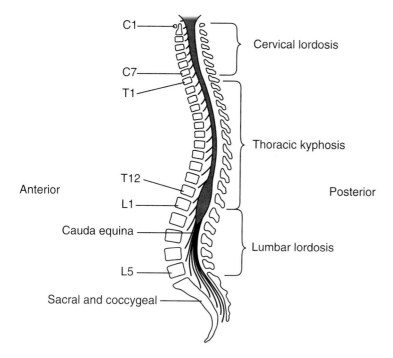

Figure 2–3: Spinal cord (lateral view).

- A plumb line dropped from C7 should fall and cross the posterior vertebra line or body walls at the L5-S1 interspace.
- Variability in sagittal alignment is influenced by age and gender; females have a greater degree of thoracic kyphosis than males, and older people have a greater degree of thoracic kyphosis than younger people.
- There is also a significant degree of variability in spinal alignment on a segmental basis, particularly at the transitional regions of the lordotic cervical and lumbar spine.
- Normal thoracic kyphosis has been reported to be between 20 and 45 degrees.

Spinal Curvatures

Flattening of the Lumbar Curve (Fig. 2–4)

- The most common cause of loss of lumbar lordosis is degenerative disk disease.
- Secondary causes include lumbar compression fractures or iatrogenic flatback posture from distraction instrumentation placed in the posterior lumbar spine.
- Younger patients may assume a flattened lumbar posture in the setting of an acute muscle spasm or a symptomatic acute herniated disk.

Exaggerated Lumbar Lordosis

- An exaggeration of the normal lumbar lordotic curve can develop to compensate for the protuberant abdomen of pregnancy or marked obesity.
- It may also develop as a compensation for exaggerated thoracic kyphosis or contractures of the hips.
- Superficially, a deep midline furrow may be seen between the lumbar paravertebral muscles on a posterior examination of a patient with increased lumbar lordosis.

Thoracic Kyphosis (Fig. 2–5)

- An increase in thoracic kyphosis is seen with aging and in the setting of multiple thoracic vertebral compression fractures.
- In adolescent patients, thoracic kyphosis may be secondary to Scheuermann's disease.

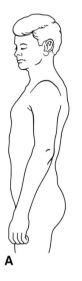
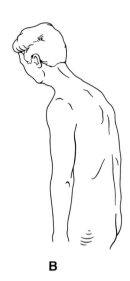
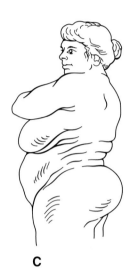

Figure 2–4: Spinal curvatures. **Normal spinal curvature (A), flattening of the lumbar curve (B), and lumbar lordosis (C).**

A   B   C

Gibbus (Fig. 2–5)

- A gibbus is a prominent thoracic bony ridge caused by a severe kyphotic angle.
- It most often occurs as a result of an angular deformity caused by a collapsed vertebra.

Scoliosis

- Scoliosis is a lateral curvature of the spine (Fig. 2–6).
- The body normally attempts to compensate for coronal plane curves by developing secondary coronal curves. A plumb line dropped from C7 or T1 should pass through the gluteal cleft.
- Scoliosis may be structural or functional.

Structural Scoliosis

- Structural scoliosis typically is associated with a rotation of the vertebrae upon each other, and the rib cage is accordingly deformed.
- This deformity is best seen when the patient flexes forward.
- On the side of the thoracic convexity, the ribs bulge posteriorly and are widely separated.
- On the opposite side (concavity), they are displaced anteriorly and are close together.

Functional Scoliosis

- Functional scoliosis compensates for other abnormalities such as unequal leg lengths.
- It involves neither fixed vertebral rotation nor fixed thoracic deformity.
- The scoliosis resolves with correction of the primary process.

List (Fig. 2–6)

- List is a lateral tilt of the spine.
- A plumb line dropped from the spinous process of T1 falls to one side of the gluteal cleft.
- Causes include a symptomatic herniated disk and painful spasms of the paravertebral muscles.

Surface Landmarks

- Surface landmarks help orient the examiner to certain vertebral levels.
- The spinous processes of C7 and T1 are typically large and prominent, making them readily palpable at the base of the neck.
- The interspace between T7 and T8 is typically at the level of the inferior angle of the scapula.

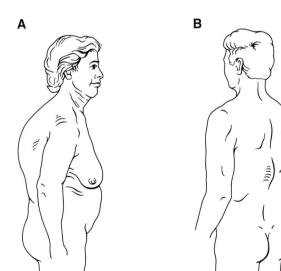

A   B

Figure 2–5: Thoracic kyphosis (A) and gibbus deformity (B).

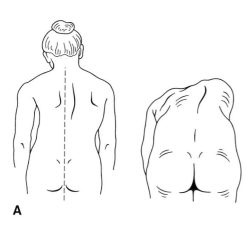

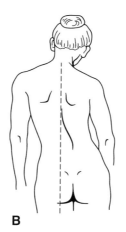

Figure 2–6: Scoliosis (A) and list (B).

A　　　　　　　　　　　　　　　　　　**B**

- An imaginary line connecting the highest point on each iliac crest crosses the L4 body.
- An imaginary line connecting the two dimples found over the posterior superior iliac spine indicates the level of S1.

Techniques of Examination— Inspection

- Examination of the spine begins with inspecting and observing the patient's static and dynamic posture and gait when they enter the room.
  - Drape or gown patients to expose the entire neck and back for complete inspection.
  - Patients should be observed in their natural standing position with the feet together and the arms hanging at the sides. The head should be midline in the same plane as the sacrum, and the shoulders and pelvis should be level.
  - Neck stiffness, the splinting of an extremity, or an uncomfortable writhing in the sitting position all may reveal underlying spinal pathology.
- Examination of the skin should be performed to observe any pigmented or raised lesions. The presence of cafe-au-lait spots or neurofibromas may suggest a neurocutaneous syndrome such as neurofibromatosis.
- The posterior midline should be examined to evaluate cutaneous midline rosy spots, tufts of hair, or dimples. These observations may indicate a failure of midline skeletal fusion during embryogenesis and possibly may suggest an occult spinal dysraphism.
- Gait is a complex process relying on the input and output of information from all aspects of the neuraxis; it is also dependent on the structural properties of the spinal column.
  - Examination of gait involves observation of cadence, ease of movement, arm swing, and overall steadiness.

- Patients are asked to walk at their usual pace across the room or down the hall, turn, and return to the starting position.
- The examiner should observe posture, balance, swinging of the arms, and movements of the legs.
1. Balance should be easily maintained.
2. The arms should freely swing at the patient's sides.
3. Turns should be accomplished smoothly and without difficulty.

- A gait that lacks coordination, with reeling and instability, is referred to as ataxic and may be caused by cerebellar disease or loss of proprioception.
- Patients are asked to walk heel-to-toe in a straight line (also called tandem walking).

Range of Motion of the Spine (Figs. 2–7 and 2–8)

- Range of motion consists of the following:
  - Flexion
  - Extension
  - Lateral bending to the right and left
  - Rotation to the right and left
- Approximately 50% of cervical flexion and extension occurs between the occiput and C1, and 50% of rotation occurs between C1 and C2.

Atrophy

- Atrophy is the loss of the muscle bulk or mass and definition.
- It has multiple etiologies.
- It is most commonly caused by a loss of anterior horn cells from neural compression.
- Myopathies are typically present with proximal muscle wasting.
- Fasciculations are spontaneous discharges of individual muscles fibers and are seen as twitches under the skin.

Figure 2–7: Range of motion of the spine. **Extension and lateral bending.**

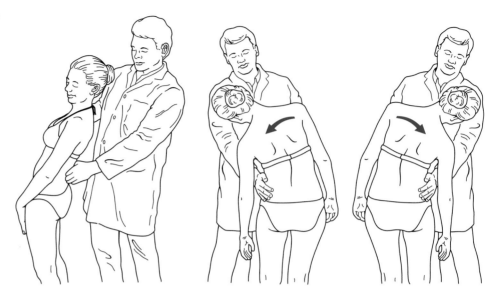

Techniques of Examination— Palpation

- Palpation of each spinal vertebra and muscle follows inspection.
- Tenderness may suggest a bruise, a fracture, or a dislocation if preceded by trauma; the presence of an underlying infection; or arthritis.
- In the cervical spine, palpation may elicit discomfort from the posterior facet joints, located about one inch lateral to the spinous processes of C2-C7. These joints lie deep to the trapezius muscle and may not be palpable unless the neck muscles are relaxed.
- In the lumbar spine, the examiner may palpate for any vertebral "step-offs" to determine the presence of vertebral translocation or spondylolisthesis. Working caudally, palpation over the sacroiliac joint—often identified by the dimple overlying the posterior superior iliac spine—may reveal tenderness resulting from sacroiliac joint pathology, a common cause of low back pain.
- Palpation of the paravertebral musculature is essential. Muscles in spasm may feel firm and knotted. Spasms may be the result of bony, ligamentous, or muscle sprain or injury and are not necessarily helpful in the localization of a causative process.

Motor Examination

- The motor examination begins proximally and proceeds distally.

Figure 2–8: Rotation.

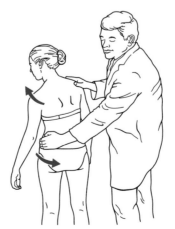 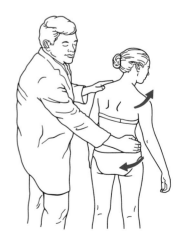

Motor Examination of the Upper Extremities (Fig. 2–9)

- The deltoid muscles should be examined with the arms held at a 90-degree angle to the torso.
- The biceps muscles are tested by flexion at the elbows with the hands fully supinated.
- The wrist extensors are tested by applying tension to the wrist while the patient attempts to extend the wrist.
- The triceps muscles are tested with the arms held against the body with the elbows flexed. The patient then attempts to extend at the elbows against resistance.
- The intrinsic hand muscles are tested with finger flexion or by spreading of the fingers.

Motor Examination of the Lower Extremities (Fig. 2–10)

- The iliopsoas muscle is tested by applying downward force against hip flexion.
- The quadriceps muscles are tested by applying force against knee extension.
- The anterior tibialis muscles are tested by applying force against active ankle dorsiflexion.
- The extensor hallucis longus muscles are tested by applying force against active toe dorsiflexion.
- The gastrocnemii muscles are tested by applying force against active ankle plantar flexion.

Muscle Tests

- The motor examination is designed to detect muscle weakness in a pattern that localizes the level of pathology or dysfunction (central nervous system, spinal cord, peripheral nerve, or muscle) and provides a reproducible means of assessing strength (Tables 2–2 and 2–3).
- The tone of the muscle is defined as the degree of tension of the muscle at rest.
- Spasticity is increased muscle tone or a resistance to motion.
- Muscles should be noted for stiffness, elasticity, rigidity, cogwheeling, and the presence of postural tremor.

Sensory Examination

- The sensory examination is the most subjective portion of the neurologic or spinal evaluation (Table 2–4). There are four distinct sensations with defined anatomic pathways in the spinal cord.
- Pain perception may be tested with the sharp portion of a safety pin.
- Light touch may be tested with a cotton swab.
- Temperature may be tested with two test tubes containing either a hot or a cold solution.
- Proprioception examination begins distally at the distal phalanx or great toe and proceeds proximally to each larger joint. Testing is specifically conducted to assess

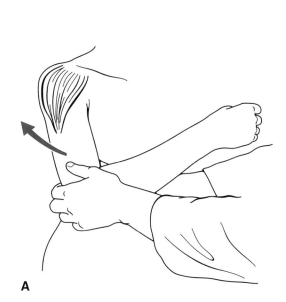

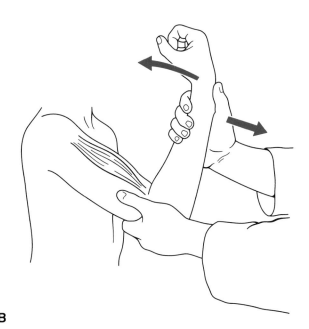

A   **B**

Figure 2–9: Muscle tests of the upper extremities. A, Shoulder abduction, deltoid—C5. B, Biceps—C5, C6.

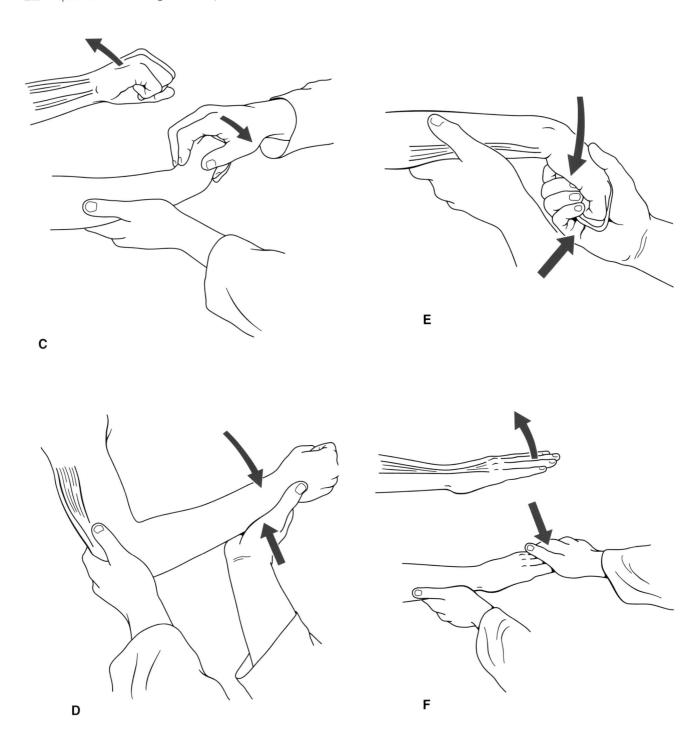

Figure 2–9: Cont'd C, Wrist extension—C6. D, Triceps—C7. E, Wrist flexion—C7, C8. F, Finger extension—C7.

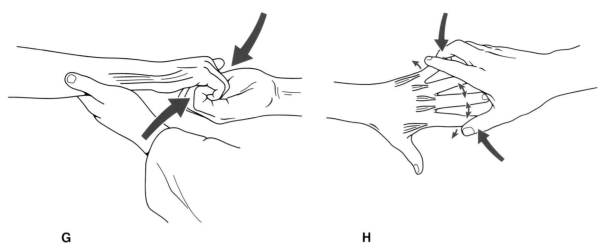

G   **H**

Figure 2–9: Cont'd **G, Finger flexion—C8. H, Finger abduction—adduction,** T1.

whether the patient can reliably detect excursion of the joint and position sense.
* The aim of sensory testing is to identify whether there is a dermatomal pattern of sensory dysfunction, which would suggest spinal root pathology; a peripheral nerve disorder; or possibly a glove or stocking distribution deficit, which would suggest a neuropathy.

Localizing Dermatomes (Fig. 2–11)

C6—Thumb
C7—Middle digit
C8—Fifth digit
T4—Nipple
T10—Umbilicus
L1—Inguinal ligament

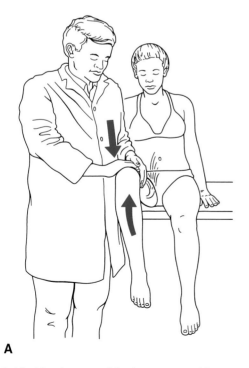

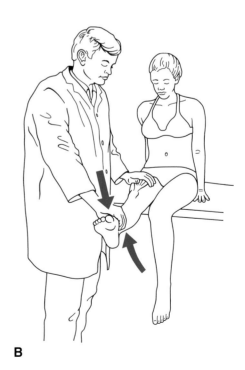

A   **B**

Figure 2–10: Muscle tests of the lower extremities. **A, Iliopsoas—L2, L3. B, Quadriceps—L3, L4.**

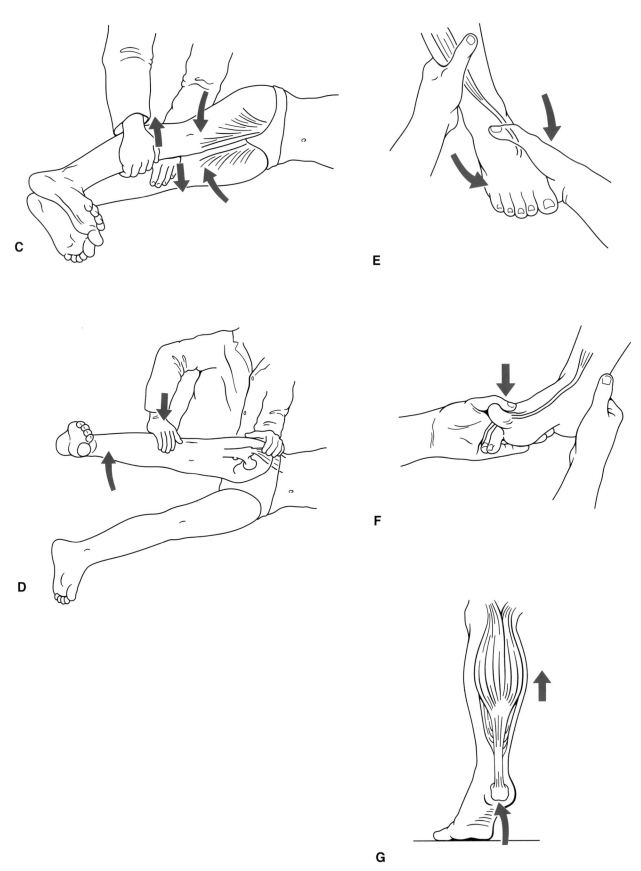

Figure 2–10: Cont'd C, Hip adductors—L2, L3. D, Hip abductors—L4, L5, S1. E, Tibialis anterior—L4. F, Extensor hallucis longus—L5. G, Gastrocnemius or soleus—L5, S1.

Table 2–2:　Motor Function Grading

MOTOR FUNCTION	DESCRIPTION	GRADE
Absent	Total paralysis	0
Trace	Palpable or visible contraction	1
Poor	Active movement through the range of motion with gravity eliminated	2
Fair	Active movement through the range of motion against gravity	3
Good	Active movement through the range of motion against resistance	4
Normal	Normal strength	5

Table 2–3:　Spinal Nerve Innervation

SPINAL SEGMENT	MUSCLE	FUNCTION
C3-C5	Diaphragm	Inspiration
C5, C6	Biceps brachii brachialis	Elbow flexors
C6, C7	Extensor carpi radialis longus and brevis	Wrist extensors
C7, C8	Triceps brachii	Elbow extensors
C8, T1	Interossei thenar group	Hand intrinsics
L2, L3	Iliopsoas	Hip flexion
L2, L3	Adductor longus and brevis	Hip adductors
L3, L4	Quadriceps	Knee extensors
L4, L5	Tibialis anterior	Ankle dorsiflexors
L4-S1	Gluteus medius	Hip abductors
L5-S1	Extensor hallucis longus	Great toe extensor
S1, S2	Gastrocnemius soleus	Ankle plantarflexors
S2-S4	Sphincter ani externus	Anal sphincter

Table 2–4:　Spinal Nerve Innervation

ROOT	MUSCLES	REFLEX	SENSATION
C5	Deltoid, biceps	Biceps	Lateral arm *Axillary nerve*
C6	Biceps, wrist extensors	Brachioradialis	Lateral forearm *Musculocutaneous nerve*
C7	Triceps, wrist extensors, finger extensors	Triceps	Middle finger *Median nerve*
C8	Hand intrinsics, finger flexors		Medial forearm *Median antebrachial cutaneous nerve*
T1, T2	Hand intrinsics		Medial arm *Median brachial cutaneous nerve*
T2-T12	Intercostals, rectus abdominus	Beevor's sign—Abnormal	T2—Clavicle, axilla T3—Axilla T4-T6—Nipple line to inferior xiphoid process T7-T9—Xiphoid process to inferior umbilicus *Ventral and lateral cutaneous branches of intercostal nerves* *Upper lateral cutaneous nerve of arms* T10, T11—Umbilicus T12—Groin *Lateral cutaneous branches of subcostal and iliohypogastric nerves* *Femoral branch of the genitofemoral nerve* *Ilioinguinal nerve*
T12, L1-L3	Iliopsoas (hip flexion)	Patellar tendon reflex (supplied by L2-L4)	T12—Groin L1-L3—Anterior thigh between the inguinal ligament and the knee *Ilioinguinal nerve* *Lateral, anterior, medial femoral cutaneous nerves of the thigh* *Obturator nerve*
L4	Tibialis anterior	Patellar tendon	Medial leg *Saphenous nerve*
L5	Extensor hallucis longus		Lateral leg and dorsum of the foot *Lateral cutaneous nerve of the calf* *Medial plantar nerve*
S1	Peroneus longus and brevis	Achilles tendon	Lateral foot *Lateral plantar nerve*

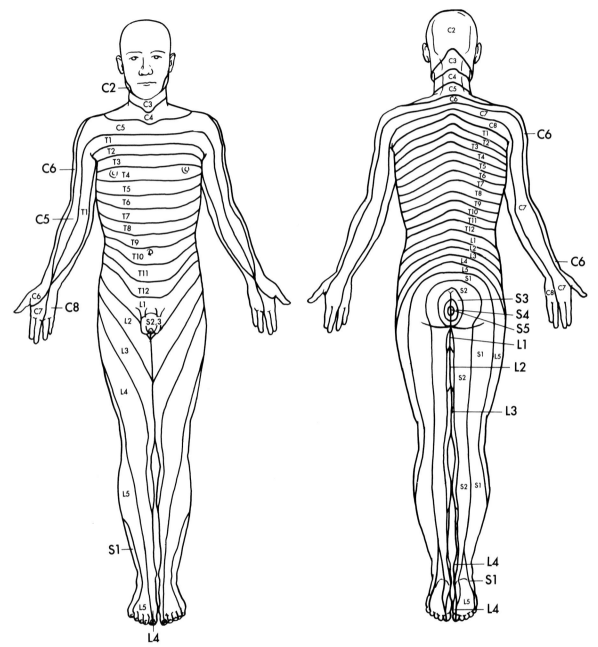

Figure 2–11: Sensory examination points. (**Leventhal 2003.**)

Reflexes

- Reflex testing is an essential part of the examination and provides a means of differentiating between spinal cord and peripheral pathology.
- A simple monosynaptic reflex consists of an afferent input that synapses in the spinal cord and returns to the extremity through an efferent output (Fig. 2–12). Upper motor neurons inhibit the output of the efferent signal; therefore, if reflexes are increased, the examiner should suspect a decrease in upper motor influence.
- Decreased reflexes may imply the loss either of sensory input or of motor neuron or mruscle integration.

- Reflexes are graded from 0 to 4. Hyperactive reflexes are graded 3 or 4 and suggest the presence of spinal cord pathology or upper motor nerve dysfunction.
  - Reflex grading is as follows:
  0—Absence
  1—Diminished
  2—Normal reflex
  3—Hyperactive reflex
  4—Clonus present
- Distracting patients may help elicit reflexes through techniques such as the Jendrassik maneuver (having patients pull their hands apart while the stimulus is being applied).

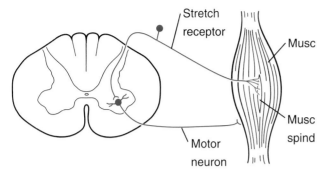

Figure 2–12: A simple monosynaptic reflex.

- The examination of the upper extremity deep tendon reflexes includes tests of the biceps tendon, the brachioradialis, and the triceps tendon reflexes. Reflexes in the lower extremities include the quadriceps reflex (knee jerk) and the gastrocnemius reflex (ankle jerk). In addition, reflexes of the hamstring muscles (biceps femoris) can be tested.

Upper Extremity

- Triceps reflex—Forearm extension
- Biceps reflex—Elbow flexion
- Brachioradialis reflex
  - Tap distal radius → Lateral wrist flexion and partial supination of the forearm

Lower Extremity

- Patellar reflex—Contraction of quadriceps (strongest muscles in body) and extension of the leg
- Suprapatellar reflex—Above the knee; same response
- Achilles reflex—Causes plantar-flexion of foot

Upper Extremity Long Tract Reflexes

- Hoffman's reflex—Triggered by taking the middle finger, flicking the distal phalanx from the palm, and observing a pincer movement between the thumb and the index finger (Fig. 2–13).
- Trömner sign—Elicited by elevating the middle finger from the rest of the hand and flicking the distal phalanx toward the palm, again looking for the pincher movement between the thumb and the index finger.
- These two reflexes may not necessarily be signs of pathology; rather, they may be indications of brisk muscle stretch reflexes. Asymmetry may be significant and may herald the presence of a central nervous dysfunction or a significant cervical cord compression, especially in an elderly patient.

Nerve Root Tension Signs

- Spurling's sign—This extends the neck with concurrent lateral bending and an axial load on the head. This is a positive sign if the maneuver reproduces the patient's pain in a radicular nature; this is suggestive of a cervical radiculopathy (Fig. 2–14).
- Lasègue's sign (straight leg raise)—Flexing the leg at the hip reproduces the patient's radicular pain in the leg and not the back. Pain should be reproduced with less than 60 degrees of flexion to be positive. This is highly suggestive of nerve root irritation, typically by a herniated lumbar disk (**Fig.** 2–15).
- Bowstring sign—After reproducing the patient's pain and obtaining a positive Lasègue's sign, the knee is flexed. This is positive if the patient's pain resolves with flexion at the knee. If the pain persists, this is suggestive of hip pathology.
- Cram test—The cram test is similar to the Lasègue's sign. The patient is supine; the leg is flexed at the hip and then

Figure 2–13: Hoffmann's reflex.

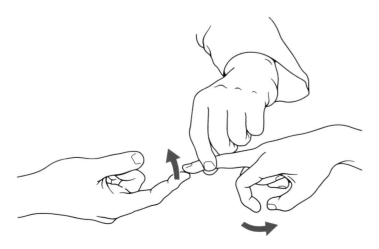

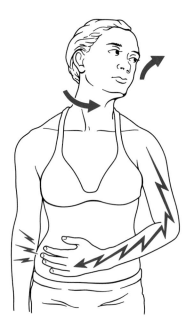

Figure 2–14: Spurling's sign.

Pathologic Long Tract Signs

- Babinski's sign (extensor plantar reflex)—This is elicited by applying a gentle stimulus to the lateral aspect of the sole starting over the heel and extending toward the base of the little toe. A positive Babinski's sign refers to the initial dorsiflexion of the great toe upward and the spreading of the other toes; it is indicative of corticospinal tract dysfunction (Fig. 2–17).
- Crossed adductor's sign—This stimulates the patellar reflex and causes the contralateral thigh adductors to contract. This is suggestive of an upper motor lesion.
- Chaddock's sign—This is tested by laterally abducting the little toe briskly and allowing it to slap back against the other toes, looking for dorsiflexion of the great toe, or flicking the third or fourth toe down rapidly, again looking for great toe dorsiflexion.
- Clonus—This is a rhythmic, nonvoluntary movement of muscle with stimulation.
- Lhermitte's sign—Flexion of the neck causes an electric shock-like sensation to shoot down the spine. This originally was described with multiple sclerosis and believed to be the result of posterior column dysfunction. It may be seen in patients with severe cervical cord compression from stenosis or a disk herniation (Fig. 2–18).

Superficial Reflexes

- The following are cutaneous abdominal reflexes:
  - Superficial abdominal reflex—This reflex is elicited by scratching from the abdominal margins toward the umbilicus and observing a quivering motion of the abdominal muscles.

extended at the knee. It is positive if it reproduces the patient's pain.
- Frajersztajn's sign (contralateral straight leg raise)—flexing the leg at the hip with an extended knee of the asymptomatic leg reproduces the pain in the contralateral leg (Fig. 2–16).
- Femoral stretch sign—The patient is placed prone and the leg is straightened and extended at the hip. This places tension on the femoral nerve (L2-L4) and may suggest an upper lumbar radiculopathy.

Figure 2–15: Lasègue's sign.

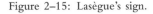
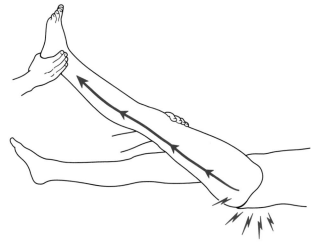

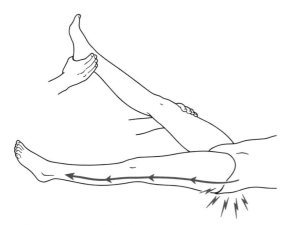

Figure 2–16: Frajersztajn's sign.

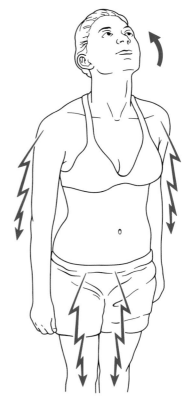

Figure 2–18: Lhermitte's sign.

- Deep abdominal reflex—This is elicited by tapping over the anterior rectus abdominal muscle sheath and observing a contraction of the abdominal muscles.
- Beevor's sign—Patients perform a quarter sit-up with the arms crossed behind the head. The examiner should be watching the navel. Beevor's sign is considered positive if the navel moves up, down, or to either side. A positive Beevor's sign occurs if the lower abdominal musculature (controlled by the spinal cord below T9) is weaker than the upper abdominal musculature (Fig. 2–19).

- Cremasteric reflex (in males)—This is elicited by stroking the thigh (the genitofemoral nerve) and observing the ascent of the ipsilateral testicle (Fig. 2–20).
- Anal wink reflex—Contraction of the external anal sphincter follows application of a sharp stimulus. This test is used to determine the end of spinal shock in the context of spinal cord injury (Fig. 2–21).

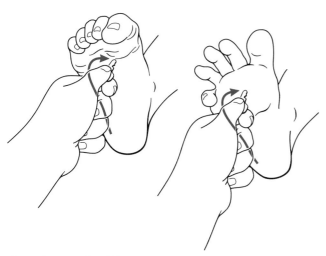

Figure 2–17: Babinski's sign.

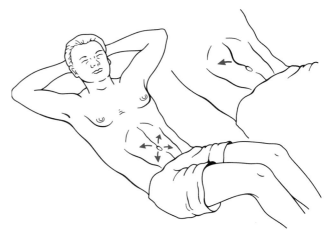

Figure 2–19: Beevor's sign.

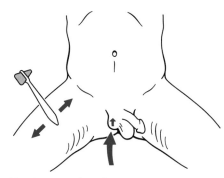

Figure 2–20: Cremasteric reflex.

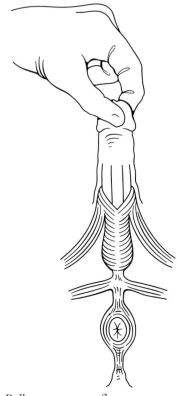

Figure 2–22: Bulbocavernosus reflex.

- Bulbocavernosus reflex—The anal sphincter is contracted by compressing the glans penis. This test is used in the setting of spinal cord injury to identify the end of spinal shock (Fig. 2–22).

Spinal Syndromes

- Syndromes are collections of signs and symptoms that occur consistently when a lesion is present in a particular anatomic region. Spinal cord syndromes therefore indicate the location of a lesion but do not indicate a specific cause. The syndromes described in this section usually occur as a result of trauma.

Central Cord Syndrome

- Central cord syndrome (Fig. 2–23) occurs in the cervical level and usually results from hyperextension

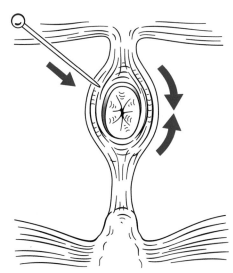

Figure 2–21: Anal wink reflex.

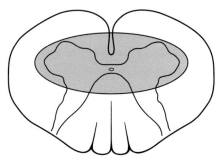

Figure 2–23: Spinal cord injury pattern in central cord syndrome.

injuries of the spinal cord. It typically occurs in an elderly stenotic, spondylotic cervical canal without associated fractures.

- The hands are usually more severely compromised than the legs.
- If the lesion or injury is minimal, the patient may only have loss of pain and temperature because of an interruption of the spinothalamic fibers crossing the midline.
- More significant injuries impair upper motor function because of the medial location of upper limb fibers in the lateral corticospinal tracts.

Brown-Séquard's Syndrome

- Brown-Séquard's syndrome (Fig. 2–24) results from a hemisection injury of the spinal cord.
- It is manifested as ipsilateral loss or diminished appreciation or function of voluntary motor control, conscious proprioception, and discriminative touch below the level of the lesion.
- Contralateral loss or diminished appreciation or function of the sensations of pain and temperature may occur below the level of the lesion.

Dissociated Sensory Loss

- This is a band of sensory loss with normal sensation below the area.
- Decussating fibers located along the central canal (pain and temperature) are impaired, resulting in a decrease or a loss of pain or temperature sensation.
- Position, touch, and vibratory sensations are not impaired.
- Dissociated sensory loss is typically caused by intramedullary lesions such as primary neoplasms or syringomyelia.

Anterior Cord Syndrome

- Anterior cord syndrome (Fig. 2–25) occurs from damage to the ventral portion of the spinal cord with interruption of the ascending spinothalamic tracts and descending motor tracts.
- There is a loss of pain and temperature sensation along with a loss of motor control.
- The tracts conveying proprioception and discriminative touch information are located in the posterior cord; these functions are spared.
- These lesions may be caused by thrombosis of the anterior spinal artery and resultant spinal infarction.

Foix-Alajouanine Syndrome

- This rapid loss of spinal cord function is caused by venous engorgement and ischemic infarction of the spinal cord.
- The results are caused by obstructed venous outflow, typically as a result of an arteriovenous malformation.
- This typically affects the lower thoracic level, the lumbosacral level, or both.
  - Gray matter (as compared with white matter) structures are more severely involved.
  - Masses of enlarged, tortuous, and thick-walled subarachnoid veins are observed overlying the surface of the cord (primarily on the posterior aspect).
  - Smaller blood vessels with thickened fibrotic walls also are present within the affected spinal cord segments.
  - The enlarged, abnormal veins are associated with a dural arteriovenous shunt, which is associated with the reflux of arterial blood into the venous drainage of the cord.
- This increases venous pressure in the affected regions of the spinal cord, possibly leading to ischemic injury.

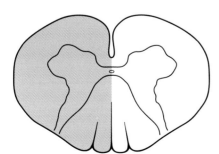

Figure 2–24: Spinal cord injury pattern in Brown-Séquard's syndrome.

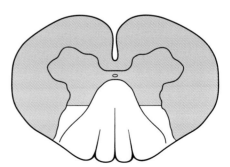

Figure 2–25: Spinal cord injury pattern in anterior cord syndrome.

- Patients show increasing unilateral and/or bilateral extremity weakness and numbness or tingling in the lower extremities, which may be symmetric.
- Symptoms begin as a heavy feeling in the legs after brief exertion. The feeling improves with rest.
- Symptoms gradually worsen over months, and the patient may have difficulty standing for long periods.
- Urinary and fecal incontinence eventually appear.
- Complaints of nonradiating lower back pain in the lumbosacral or coccygeal regions are common.
- Weakness or numbness eventually can progress to the upper extremities.

References

Bickley, LS. (1999) Bates' Guide to Physical Examination and History Taking, 7th edition. Philadelphia: Lippincott Williams & Wilkins.

> This textbook provides a solid foundation for learning physical examination and history taking. With numerous illustrations and photographs, this edition highlights procedures, interpretations, and common abnormalities throughout the physical examination.

Bondurant FJ, Cotler HB et al. (1990) Acute spinal cord injury: A study using physical examination and magnetic resonance imaging. Spine 15: 161-168.

> A preliminary report from a study conducted at the University of Texas Medical School in Houston shows a clear relationship between the appearance of spinal cord injuries, as identifiable on an MRI, and the postinjury neurologic recovery.

Cailliet R. (1988) Low Back Pain Syndrome, 4th edition. Philadelphia: FA Davis.

> This book explains low back pain syndrome; it focuses on functional anatomy, lumbar spine diseases, clinical diagnosis, and comprehensive therapeutic approaches in treatment.

Chadwick PR. (1984) Examination, assessment, and treatment of the lumbar spine. Physiotherapy 70: 2-10.

> One in a series of articles elucidating a standard approach to evaluation and management of lumbar spine pathology.

Cipriano JJ. (1991) Photographic Manual of Regional Orthopaedic and Neurological Tests, 2nd edition. Baltimore: Williams & Wilkins.

> Extensively photographed atlas with definitions illustrating the key points of a thorough neurologic and musculoskeletal examination.

Hoppenfeld S. (1976) Physical Examination of the Spine and Extremities. Norwalk, CT: Appleton-Century-Crofts.

> This functional guidebook allows the rapid assimilation of the basic knowledge essential to physical examination of the spine and extremities.

Hoppenfeld S. (1977) Orthopaedic Neurology: A Diagnostic Guide to Neurologic Levels. Philadelphia: JB Lippincott and Co.

> A concise, well-diagrammed text that systematically explains the characteristics and clinical correlates of a complete spine and extremity neurological examination.

Leventhal MR. (2003) Fractures, dislocations, and fracture-dislocations of spine. In: Campbell's Operative Orthopaedics (Canale ST, ed.), 10th edition. Philadelphia: Mosby.

Lucas JT, Ducker TB. (1979) Motor classification of spinal cord injuries with mobility, morbidity, and recovery indices. Am Surgeon 45: 151.

> This article presents a new motor classification for patients with spinal cord injuries that provides statistically discrete subdivisions, which can be mathematically summarized and more accurately analyzed.

Marino RJ, ed. (2000) International Standards for Neurological Classification of Spinal Cord Injury. Chicago: American Spinal Injury Association.

> This booklet summarizes and standardizes evaluation and recording of spinal cord injuries.

Moore KL, Dalley AF. (1999) Clinically Oriented Anatomy, 4th edition. Philadelphia: Lippincott Williams & Wilkins.

> An updated version of a popular medical student anatomy textbook. Organized by organ systems within anatomic regions, this text includes numerous clinical correlates and surface anatomy pearls.

Netter FH. (1997) Atlas of Clinically Oriented Anatomy, 2nd edition. East Hanover, NJ: Novartis.

> One-volume collection of normal anatomic renditions covering the entire human body.

Rengachary SS. (1996) Examination of the motor and sensory systems and reflexes. In: Neurosurgery (Wilkins RH et al., eds.), 2nd edition. New York: McGraw-Hill.

> Chapter in a textbook that explains, in detail, a systematic examination of the motor system; muscle contour and abnormal movements; motor tone, strength and coordination; and assessment of reflex activity.

Rengachary SS. (1996) Gait and station: Examination of coordination. In: Neurosurgery (Wilkins RH et al., eds.), 2nd edition. New York: McGraw-Hill.

> Chapter in a textbook that describes the examination and assessment of gait with common gait disturbances seen in clinical practice.

Singer KP, Jones TJ, Breidahl PD. (1990) A comparison of radiographic and computer-assisted measurements of thoracic and thoracolumbar sagittal curvature. Skeletal Radiol 19: 21-26.

> Report from a study of 286 radiographs comparing the Cobb technique with a computer-aided digitizer to measure sagittal plane curve characteristics of the thoracolumbar spine.

Snider RK, ed. (1997) Essentials of musculoskeletal care. Rosemont, IL: American Academy of Orthopedic Surgeons, American Academy of Pediatrics.

> The spine section includes a concise review of the vertebral levels associated with specific neurologic symptoms or findings and illustrations that may help clinicians to distinguish psychogenic from mechanical symptoms.

Williams PL, Bannister LH et al., eds. (1995) Gray's Anatomy, 38th edition. Churchill-Livingstone.

> The first revision of the British version of the classic anatomy reference since 1989; it shows the effects advances in molecular biology and imaging have had on medicine in its illustrations and commentaries.

Surgical Approaches to the Spine

Kern Singh⋆, Howard S. An §, and Alexander R. Vaccaro †

⋆ M.D., Assistant Professor, Department of Orthopedic Surgery, Rush University Medical Center, Chicago, IL
§ M.D., The Morton International Professor of Orthopedic Surgery, Director of Spine Fellowship Program, Rush Medical College, Director of Spine Surgery, Rush University Medical Center, Chicago, IL
† M.D., Professor of Orthopaedic Surgery, Thomas Jefferson University and the Rothman Institute, Philadelphia, PA

Introduction

- A thorough knowledge of human anatomy is paramount in performing any surgical procedure (Box 3–1).
- The intimate association of muscular, osteoligamentous, and neurovascular structures in the cervical spine requires a precise understanding of their relationships to safely and efficiently navigate these structures during any surgical procedure.
- The cervical spine can be approached surgically from the anterior or posterior depending on the location of pathology.

Anterior Cervical Spine Procedures

Transoral Approach

- The transoral approach to the spine allows midline surgical exposure of the arch of the atlas to the C2-C3 intervertebral disk.
- The exposure may be increased in a cephalad direction by dividing the soft and hard palate to allow access to the foramen magnum and the lower half of the clivus and sphenoid sinus.
- The transoral approach allows excellent midline access but is limited laterally by the vertebral arteries within the spine (Box 3–2).

Technique

- The patient is placed in the supine position.
- The key surgical landmark is the anterior tubercle of the atlas to which the anterior longitudinal ligament and longus coli muscles are attached.
- The vertebral arteries are at least 20 mm from the midline bilaterally.
- A transoral tongue retractor is inserted, exposing the posterior oropharynx.
- The palatal retractors are inserted to elevate the soft palate and expose the anterior rim of the foramen magnum, the atlas, and the axis.
- The area of incision is infiltrated with 1:200,000 epinephrine.
- A midline 3-cm vertical incision centered on the anterior tubercle of the atlas is made through the pharyngeal mucosa and muscle (Fig. 3–1).
- A pharyngeal retractor is inserted, converting the vertical incision into a hexagon to expose the tubercle of the atlas, the anterior longitudinal ligament, and the longus colli muscles.
- The origins of the anterior longitudinal ligament and the longus colli muscles are divided with a Bovie and elevated in a subperiosteal fashion to expose the arch of the atlas (Fig. 3–2).
- To achieve good wound healing, the pharyngeal mucosa and muscle should be closed carefully in two layers using

Box 3–1:	Anatomic Landmarks of the Cervical Spine

- Arch of the atlas—Hard palate
- C2-C3—Lower border of the mandible
- C3—Hyoid bone
- C4-C5—Thyroid cartilage
- C6—Cricoid cartilage
- C6—Carotid tubercle

Box 3–2:	Indications for the Transoral Approach

- Irreducible atlantoaxial subluxation
- Midline anterior extradural or intradural spinal cord compression
- Midbasilar artery aneurysms

interrupted 3-0 absorbable sutures, one layer for muscle and one for mucosa.

Anterior Retropharyngeal Approach

- The anterior retropharyngeal approach to the upper cervical spine allows visualization from the clivus to C3.
- This approach may be extended inferiorly to expose the middle and lower cervical spine (Box 3–3).

Technique

- A modified transverse submandibular incision is made (Fig. 3–3).
- An incision is made through the skin, the subcutaneous tissue, and the platysma.

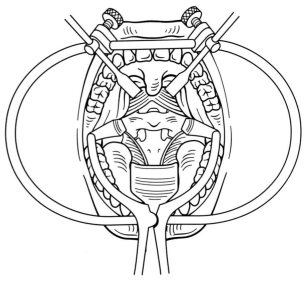

Figure 3–2: The arch of the atlas has been exposed. The anterior longitudinal ligament and longus colli muscles have been divided and retracted.

- The mandibular branch of the facial nerve is identified (Fig. 3–4).
- It is important to use bipolar cautery on the retromandibular and facial veins to avoid inadvertent injury to the mandibular branch of the facial nerve.
- If the mandibular branch of the facial nerve is injured, the patient will have a noticeable droop of the ipsilateral

Box 3–3:	Indications for the Anterior Retropharyngeal Approach

- Decompression and stabilization of fixed atlantoaxial subluxation
- Anterior upper cervical vertebral debridement or decompression

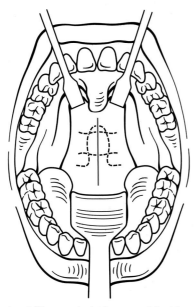

Figure 3–1: A midline vertical pharyngeal incision made during a transoral approach.

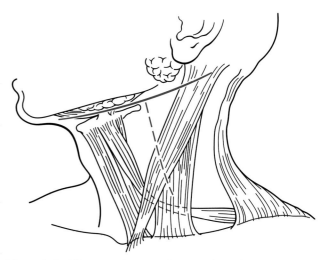

Figure 3–3: The retropharyngeal approach to the upper cervical spine. A submandibular incision is illustrated with an optional vertical extension to the subaxial cervical spine.

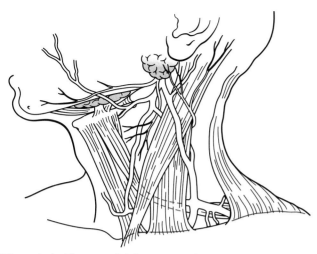

Figure 3–4: The superficial neurovascular structures in the anterolateral neck.

aspect of the mouth secondary to denervation of the orbicularis oris muscle.

- The common facial vein is usually continuous with the retromandibular vein. The mandibular branch of the facial nerve usually crosses the retromandibular vein superficially and superiorly and is superficial to the anterior facial vein.
- The submandibular gland is displaced and the digastric muscle is divided (Fig. 3–5).
- The facial, lingual, and superior thyroid vessels, with the exception of the superior thyroid artery, are isolated, ligated, and divided.
- The superior laryngeal nerve may run close to the superior thyroid artery.

- After the superficial layer of the deep cervical fascia is incised along the anterior border of the sternocleidomastoid, the superior thyroid artery and vein are ligated.
- The hypoglossal and superior laryngeal nerves are mobilized.
- Branches of the carotid artery and internal jugular vein are ligated to allow retraction of the carotid sheath posteriorly and laterally when the pharynx is mobilized medially.
- The submandibular gland may be resected if necessary (its duct being sutured to prevent salivary fistula formation).
- The posterior belly of the digastric and stylohyoid muscles is tagged with suture for later repair.
- Care must be taken not to retract near the origin of the posterior belly of the digastric and stylohyoid muscles to avoid neuropraxic injury to the facial nerve.
- Division of the posterior belly of the digastric and stylohyoid muscles allows mobilization of the hyoid bone anteriorly and medially, thus allowing mobilization of the pharynx.
- The hypoglossal nerve is mobilized from the base of the skull to the posterior border of the mylohyoid bone, where it is then retracted superiorly for the remainder of the case.
- The dissection continues within the retropharyngeal space between the carotid sheath laterally and the pharynx, larynx, and esophagus medially.
- The alar and prevertebral fascia are split longitudinally to expose the longus colli muscles that run longitudinally on the anterior lateral aspects of the spine (Fig. 3–6).

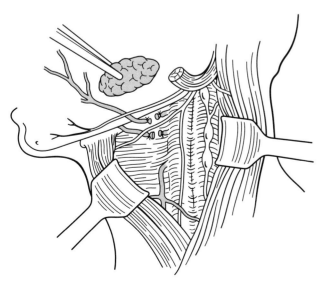

Figure 3–5: The neck after the submandibular gland has been resected and the digastric muscle has been divided.

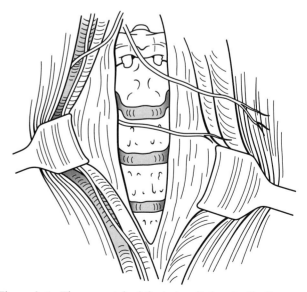

Figure 3–6: The prevertebral fascia is split longitudinally between the longus colli muscles, exposing the anterior atlas and the C2 body.

Smith-Robinson Approach to the Subaxial Spine

- The most common anterior approach to the subaxial (middle, lower) cervical spine is the Smith-Robinson approach (Box 3–4).

Technique

- The patient is positioned supine with a bump placed in the interscapular region.
- Extending the neck and slightly rotating the head toward the contralateral shoulder helps to provide greater ease of exposure to the spinal elements.
- A transverse incision is used in most cases, but an oblique incision may be used for exposure of multiple levels.
- A right- or left-sided approach may be selected.
- If the surgeon extends the approach below the level of C5, a left-sided approach is theoretically safer in avoiding inadvertent injury to the recurrent laryngeal nerve.
- A transverse incision in line with the skin crease is made from the midline to the anterior aspect of the sternocleidomastoid muscle (Fig. 3–7).
- The skin and subcutaneous tissues are undermined slightly and the platysma is divided (Fig. 3–8).
- Retraction of the platysma exposes the sternocleidomastoid muscle laterally and the strap muscles medially.
- The sternocleidomastoid muscle is retracted laterally with the carotid sheath (enclosing the common carotid artery, internal jugular vein, and vagus nerve) (Fig. 3–9).
- Carefully palpate the carotid sheath retracted laterally with the sternocleidomastoid.
- The sternohyoid and sternothyroid strap muscles (with the trachea and esophagus) are retracted medially, allowing blunt dissection through the pretracheal fascia.
- The prevertebral fascia and longus colli muscles are exposed (Box 3–5).
- The prevertebral fascia is divided longitudinally to expose the disk and vertebral body (Fig. 3–10).

Posterior Cervical Approach

- The posterior cervical approach is commonly used to perform a laminectomy, foraminotomy, or laminaplasty with or without a fusion (Box 3–6).

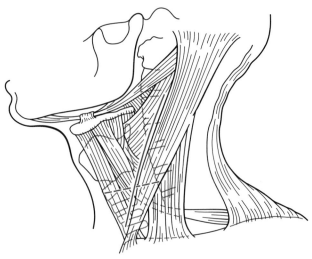

Figure 3–7: The Smith-Robinson approach to the subaxial cervical spine. **A transverse and oblique incision is illustrated.**

- The bony spinous processes are palpable posteriorly with noted large, spinous processes at C2, C7, and T1.
- The C2 and C7 spinous processes are large and the C3-C6 spinous processes are usually bifid.
- A direct midline interfascial, internervous approach is used to expose the posterior vertebrae (Fig. 3–11, Box 3–7).
- The ligamentum nuchae, a fibroelastic septum with few elastic fibers, originates from the occiput and inserts onto the C7 spinous process.
- The supraspinous ligaments are in continuity with the ligamentum nuchae and spinous processes posteriorly, and they blend with the interspinous ligaments anterior to them.
- The course of the vertebral artery (Fig. 3–12) along the posterior superior arch of C1 makes it prone to injury if

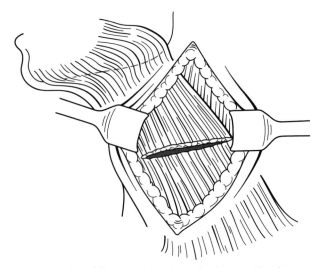

Figure 3–8: An oblique incision is made through the skin, followed by a horizontal incision through the underlying platysma.

Box 3–4:	**Indications for the Smith-Robinson Approach to the Subaxial Cervical Spine**

- Anterior cervical discectomy and fusion
- Anterior cervical corpectomy and fusion

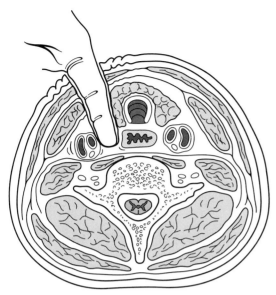

Figure 3–9: Blunt finger dissection is used to divide the pretracheal fascia while palpating and retracting the carotid sheath laterally.

Box 3–5: Smith-Robinson Approach

- The superior thyroid artery is encountered above C4 and the inferior thyroid artery is encountered below C6. These vessels should be identified and ligated as necessary.
- The thoracic duct may be exposed in surgical approaches below the C7 level during a left-sided approach.

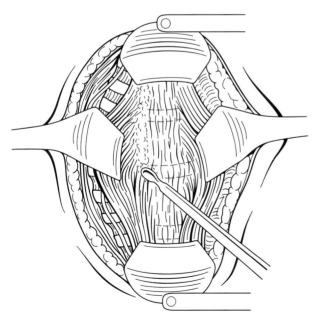

Figure 3–10: The longus colli muscles are mobilized laterally with the aid of a curette.

Box 3–6: Indications for the Posterior Cervical Approach

- Decompress spinal cord or nerve root
- Excision of herniated disks
- Fusion of cervical vertebrae

dissection in the adult is performed more than 1.5 cm from the midline of the C1 posterior tubercle. (The distance is only 1 cm in the child).
- The artery enters the operative field when it passes from the transverse foramen of the atlas, immediately behind the atlanto-occipital joint, and pierces the lateral angle of the posterior atlanto-occipital membrane. It is vulnerable in this region during surgical exposures (Fig. 3–13).
- The C1 nerve is also referred to as the suboccipital nerve, and the C2 nerve is referred to as the greater occipital nerve.
- The posterior cervical musculature is elevated in a subperiosteal manner with care taken not to disturb the surrounding facet capsules.

Anterior Exposures of the Cervicothoracic Junction

- Anterior exposure of the cervicothoracic junction (C7-T2) is a challenging surgical exercise because of the overlying clavicle and sternum and the proximity of the great vessels.
- Three methods with various modifications of anterior approaches to the cervicothoracic junction have been described:
  1. High transthoracic
  2. Manubrium or sternal splitting partial resection
  3. Low cervical and high transthoracic

High Transthoracic

- A periscapular J-shaped incision is made approximately 2.5 cm medial to the superior angle of the scapula and continued down around its inferior angle (Fig. 3–14).
- Dissection continues in the line of the incision through the subcutaneous fat to the level of the superficial muscles of the back.
- The trapezius is divided close to the spinous processes and parallel to the direction of the skin incision to avoid injuring the spinal accessory nerve (CN XI).
- The latissimus dorsi is divided as medially as possible to allow adequate retraction of the scapula and to avoid injuring the thoracodorsal nerve.
- The rhomboid major muscle is divided near its insertion onto the scapula.

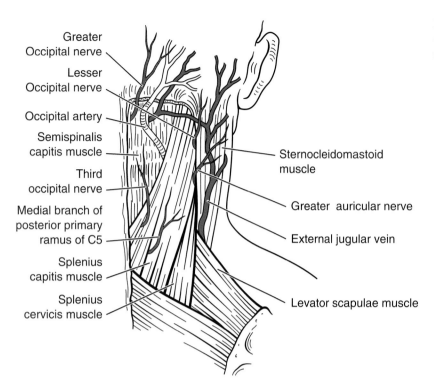

Greater
Occipital nerve

Lesser
Occipital nerve

Occipital artery

Semispinalis
capitis muscle

Third
occipital nerve

Medial branch of
posterior primary
ramus of C5

Splenius
capitis muscle

Splenius
cervicis muscle

Sternocleidomastoid
muscle

Greater auricular nerve

External jugular vein

Levator scapulae muscle

Figure 3–11: The posterior aspect of the cervical spine. **Depicted are the superficial nerves and musculature.**

- Lying inferiorly and laterally, the serratus anterior muscle is divided as caudally as possible to avoid injuring its nerve supply, the long thoracic nerve (Fig. 3–15).
- The scapula can be retracted superolaterally after protecting its medial surface with a saline-soaked sponge.
- The periosteum of the third rib is incised along its longitudinal axis and sharply dissected with the use of an elevator.
- The rib can be divided posteriorly 1-2 cm from its attachment to the transverse process and anteriorly at its junction with the costal cartilage (Fig. 3–16).
- Exposure through the pleural cavity involves making an incision through the parietal pleura and retracting the dome of the lung inferiorly to expose the anterior surface of the spine.
- The parietal pleura overlying the upper thoracic vertebrae are carefully incised to avoid injuring the superior intercostal vein, artery, and the sympathetic trunk and ganglion (Fig. 3–17).

Box 3–7: Posterior Paracervical Muscular Layers

- Superficial layer—Trapezius
- Intermediate layer—Splenius capitis
- Deep layer—Semispinalis capitis (superficial), semispinalis cervicis (intermediate), and multifidus (deep)

Sternal Splitting Approach to the Cervicothoracic Junction

- An oblique incision is made along the anterior border of the sternocleidomastoid muscle and courses inferiorly over the midline of the manubrium and sternum (Fig. 3–18).
- Dissection continues through the subcutaneous tissue and platysma in line with the skin incision.
- The deep cervical fascia (which invests the anterior border of the sternocleidomastoid) is divided sharply, allowing the sternocleidomastoid muscle to be retracted laterally.
- While protecting the carotid sheath laterally, the pretracheal fascia is divided sharply by spreading it with the blunt tips of a forceps, allowing the carotid sheath to be taken laterally and the strap muscles of the neck and the underlying trachea or esophagus to be retracted medially.
- This allows exposure of the prevertebral fascia, which invests the longus colli muscles on both sides of the cervical spine.
- The soft tissue aponeurosis investing the superior border of the sternal notch is released, and blunt finger dissection is used to clear the underlying retrosternal adipose tissue from the undersurface of the manubrium.
- The muscular aponeurotic soft tissue attachments to the inferior xiphoid process are released sharply and the retrosternal fatty tissue is separated from its undersurface.
- A sternotomy is performed (Fig. 3–19).

Figure 3–12: The coursing of the vertebral artery and greater occipital nerve in relation to the posterior midline.

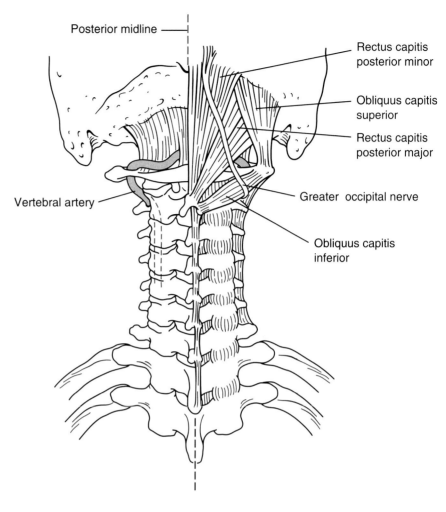

Posterior midline

Rectus capitis posterior minor

Obliquus capitis superior

Rectus capitis posterior major

Greater occipital nerve

Obliquus capitis inferior

Vertebral artery

Figure 3–13: The various muscular layers of the posterior cervical spine.

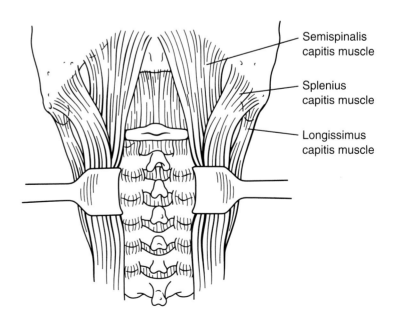

Semispinalis capitis muscle

Splenius capitis muscle

Longissimus capitis muscle

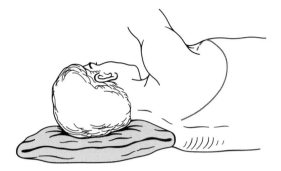

Figure 3–14: The incision for the transthoracic approach to the upper thoracic spine. The trapezius muscle is divided close to the spinous processes and parallel to the skin.

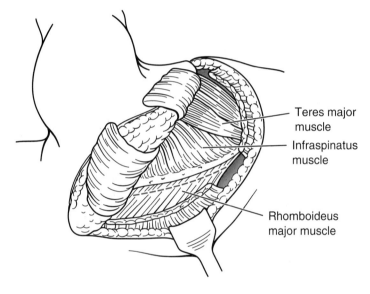

Figure 3–15: The rhomboid major is divided near its insertion and the serratus anterior muscle is divided as caudally as possible.

Teres major muscle

Infraspinatus muscle

Rhomboideus major muscle

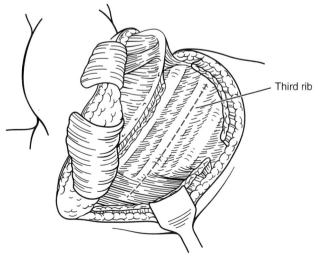

Figure 3–16: The scapula can then be retracted superolaterally, and the periosteum can be incised.

Third rib

Figure 3–17: Retractors are positioned and the upper thoracic spine is exposed.

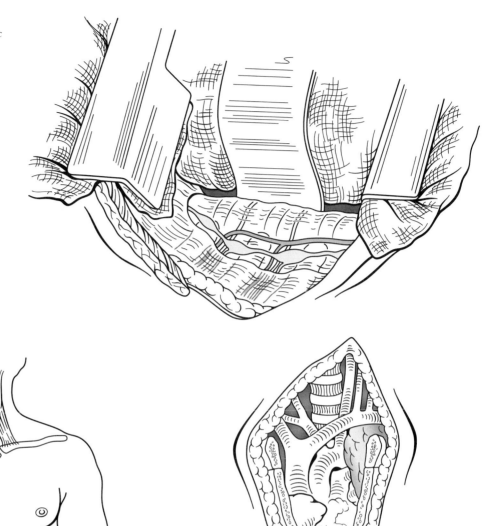

Figure 3–18: The incision for the sternal splitting approach.

Figure 3–19: The omohyoid is divided along with the traversing inferior thyroid artery. The sternotomy is performed exposing the cervical spine.

- Dissection is continued from the exposed subaxial cervical spine in a caudal direction through the pretracheal fascia exposing the left innominate or brachiocephalic vein.
- The vein can be ligated with the inferior thyroid artery if necessary.
- To complete exposure of the prevertebral fascia, the esophagus, the trachea, and the brachiocephalic truck are retracted gently to the right using flexible spatulas; the thoracic duct, the cupola of the pleura, and the left common carotid artery are retracted to the left.
- The prevertebral fascia is then divided in the midline to allow sub-periosteal dissection of the vertebral body (Fig. 3–20).

- Variations of this approach are now more popular in which only the manubrium or the proximal portion of the sternum is divided and separated.
- In these modified approaches, a T-shaped incision may be made with the vertical limb overlying the manubrium and upper portion of the sternum and the horizontal limb of the incision overlying the base of the neck approximately 1 cm above the clavicle.
- The medial third of the clavicle may be resected and later replaced for further exposure.
- The sternal and clavicular heads of the sternocleidomastoid muscle on the side of the approach are detached at the level of the manubrium, and the clavicle is retracted.

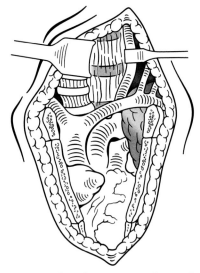

Figure 3–20: To complete the exposure, the esophagus, trachea, and brachiocephalic trunk are gently retracted to the right; the thoracic duct is retracted to the left.

- The strap muscles on the ipsilateral side of the approach are detached from the clavicle and retracted medially.
- The sternal origin of the pectoralis major is stripped laterally off the clavicle (Fig. 3–21).
- The medial half of the clavicle is stripped subperiosteally and its medial third is removed with a Gigli saw.
- The sternoclavicular joint is disarticulated sharply and curetted.
- A rectangular piece of manubrium with its posterior periosteum may be removed using power drill holes and heavy scissors.
- The remainder of the approach is similar to the sternal splitting approach.

Combined Cervical and Thoracic Approach

- An oblique cervical incision is made parallel to the clavicle with division of the platysma in line with the incision, and a high thoracic incision is made around the inferior and medial border of the scapula (Fig. 3–22).
- For the cervical incision, the deep cervical fascia along the anterior medial border of the sternocleidomastoid muscle is incised, allowing rotation and retraction of this muscle laterally to expose its deep surface.

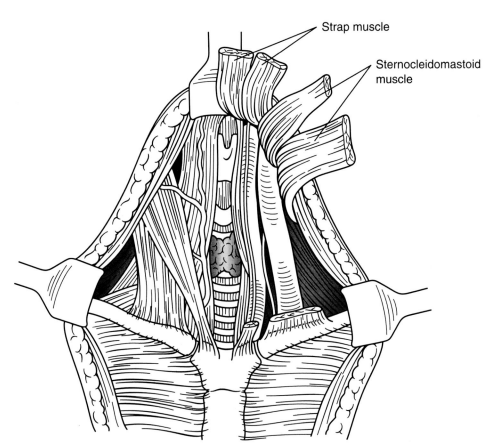

Figure 3–21: The sternal and clavicular heads of the sternocleidomastoid are detached at the level of the manubrium.

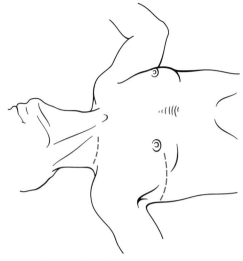

Figure 3–22: The combined cervical and thoracic approach to the cervicothoracic junction.

- The carotid sheath is retracted anteriorly following gentle blunt exposure of its posterior border.
- The inferior thyroid artery is ligated when it courses posterior to the carotid sheath to obtain better exposure.
- The cervical vertebrae covered by the longus colli muscles can be palpated.
- The cervical wound is packed, and the transthoracic approach is continued as described previously.

Posterolateral (Costotransversectomy) Approach to the Thoracic Spine

- The classic posterolateral approach to the thoracic spine was developed for drainage of tuberculous abscesses.
- The major advantage of the posterolateral approach is that it does not involve entering the thoracic cavity (Box 3–8).
- The patient is placed prone on an operating table.
- A linear incision is made over the midline or curvilinear incision about 8 cm lateral to the desired spinous process; the linear incision is 10-13 cm (Fig. 3–23).
- There is no true internervous plane in this approach.
- The approach involves splitting the trapezius muscle and dividing the paraspinal muscles.

Box 3–8:	Indications for the Posterolateral Approach to the Thoracic Spine

- Abscess drainage
- Vertebral body biopsy
- Partial vertebral body resection
- Thoracic disk excision
- Anterolateral decompression of the spinal cord

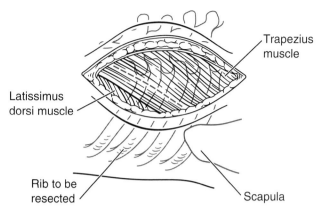

Figure 3–23: Following the skin incision, the trapezius is divided.

- The trapezius is cut parallel with its fibers close to the transverse processes. Deep to it are the paraspinal muscles.
- All muscle attachments are separated from the rib of interest in a subperiosteal manner.
- Dissection is performed laterally along the superior border of the rib and medially along the inferior border.
- The rib is cut 6-8 cm from the midline (Fig. 3–24).
- The retropleural space is carefully entered with digital palpation and dissection removing the parietal pleura from the vertebral body.
- Blunt dissection is used to avoid entering the pleural cavity while exposing the vertebral body and disk space.

Anterior (Transthoracic) Approach to the Thoracic Spine (Box 3–9)

- The patient is placed in the lateral decubitus position and stabilized with a kidney rest or sandbags.
- Although the thoracic vertebrae can be approached from either side, approaching it from the right side is easier because the aortic arch and heart can be avoided.

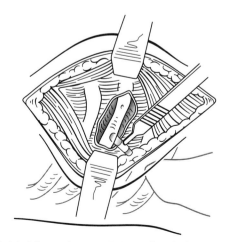

Figure 3–24: The periosteum is incised and elevated off the rib using a periosteal elevator.

Box 3–9:	Indications for the Transthoracic Approach

- Debridement or decompression of the anterior vertebral body and or disk space
- Correction of scoliosis
- Correction of kyphosis
- Osteotomy of the spine
- Biopsy of the spine

- The incision is often started two rib spaces above the vertebral body of interest and curved forward toward the inframammary crease (Fig. 3–25).
- The latissimus dorsi muscle is divided posteriorly in line with the skin incision.
- The serratus anterior muscle is divided in line with the skin incision down to the level of the ribs.
- The thoracic cavity can be entered either through an intercostal space or by resection of one or more ribs (Fig. 3–26).
- Rib resection creates better exposure, and the cut ribs can be used for bone grafting (Fig. 3–27).

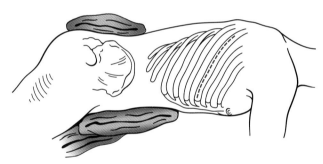

Figure 3–25: The incision used for the transthoracic approach to the spine.

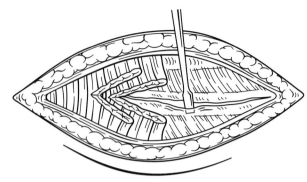

Figure 3–26: The anterior aspect of the latissimus is divided, exposing the underlying rib. The underlying rib is dissected free of the periosteum.

Anterior (Transperitoneal) Approach to the Lumbar Spine

- The anterior transperitoneal approach to the lumbar spine is primarily used for accessing the L5-S1 junction.
- The umbilicus typically lies opposite the L3-L4 disk space, but it may vary depending on the patient's body habitus.
- A longitudinal midline incision is made from just above the umbilicus (2-3 cm), curving gently to the left of the umbilicus and continuing to just above the pubic symphysis (Fig. 3–28).
- Dissection is continued down to the level of the fibrous rectus sheath.
- The rectus sheath is incised longitudinally, beginning in the lower half of the incision, to reveal the two rectus abdominis muscles.
- The muscles are bluntly separated with the surgeon's fingers to expose the underlying peritoneum (Fig. 3–29).
- The peritoneum is carefully incised after making sure no viscera lie beneath it.

Figure 3–27: The overlying rib is resected near its articulation with the costovertebral junction. The parietal pleura are incised and the overlying prevertebral fascia is identified. Shown are the ligated segmental vessels overlying the thoracic vertebrae.

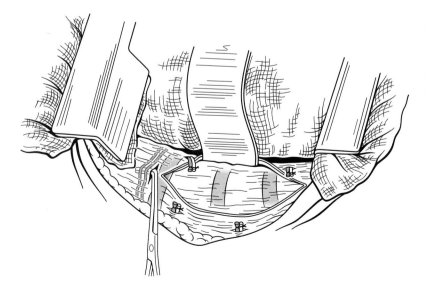

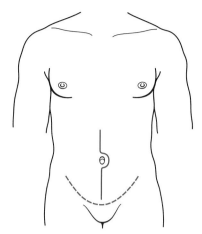

Figure 3–28: The transperitoneal approach incision to the lumbar spine.

- Using a self-retaining Balfour retractor, the rectus abdominis muscles are retracted laterally and the bladder is retracted distally.
- The tissue over the anterior surface of the sacral promontory is often infiltrated with a few milliliters of saline solution to make dissection easier and to allow identification of the presacral parasympathetic nerves.
- The L5-S1 disk space lies below the bifurcation of the aorta; it should be possible to expose it fully without mobilizing any of the great vessels (Fig. 3–30).

Anterolateral (Retroperitoneal) Approach to the Lumbar Spine

- The retroperitoneal approach has several advantages over the transperitoneal approach.

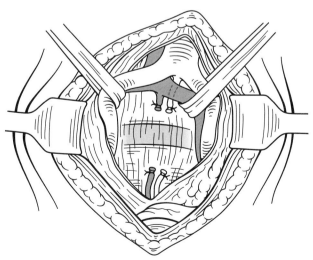

Figure 3–29: The overlying peritoneum is incised with care being taken to avoid damaging the underlying peritoneum. The abdominal viscera are retracted and the underlying vertebral bodies are exposed.

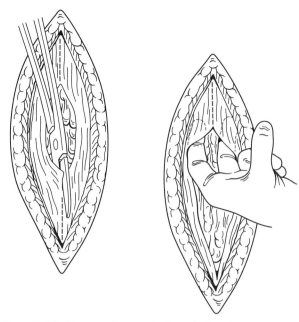

Figure 3–30: The sacral artery is ligated, allowing greater mobilization of the great vessels.

- It provides access to all the vertebrae from L1 to the sacrum and minimizes the potential for a postoperative ileus (Box 3–10).
- Because of the nature of the vascular anatomy of the retroperitoneal space, it is slightly more difficult to reach the L5-S1 space using this approach.
- The patient is placed in a semilateral decubitus position.
- An oblique flank incision is made, extending toward the rectus abdominis muscle and stopping at its lateral border about midway between the umbilicus and the pubic symphysis (Fig. 3–31).
- The three muscles of the abdominal wall (external oblique, internal oblique, transverses abdominis) are divided in line with the skin incision (Fig. 3–32).
- With blunt finger dissection, a plane is developed between the retroperitoneal fat and the fascia that overlies the psoas muscle.
- The peritoneal cavity is gently mobilized and its contents are retracted medially.
- The psoas fascia can now be identified.
- The medial surface of the psoas is followed to the reach the anterior lateral surface of the vertebral bodies (Fig. 3–33).

Box 3–10:	Indications for the Retroperitoneal Approach to the Lumbar Spine

- Debridement or decompression and fusion of the anterior vertebral body and or disk space
- Biopsy of the anterior vertebral body and disk space

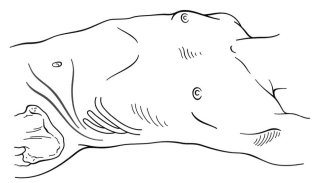

Figure 3–31: Various incisions for the retroperitoneal approach to the lumbar spine.

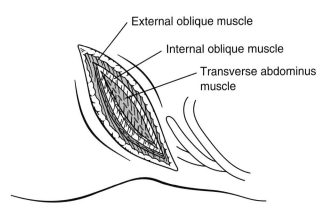

Figure 3–32: The external oblique, the internal oblique, and the transverse abdominus are incised in line with skin.

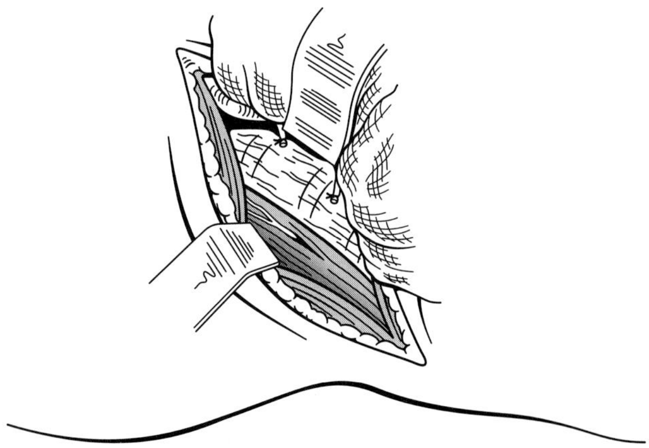

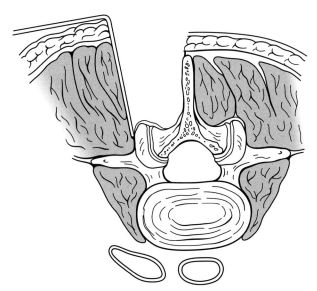

Figure 3–33: Malleable retractors are passed around the vertebral body, exposing the prevertebral fascia.

- The aorta and vena cava are bound to the anterior surfaces of the vertebral bodies by the lumbar arteries and veins.
- Segmental vessels may be identified and ligated as necessary so that the aorta and vena cava can be mobilized and the anterior surface of the vertebral bodies can be exposed.

Posterior Approach to the Thoracic and Lumbar Spine

- The patient is placed in a prone position with the abdomen free of pressure.
- The spinous processes are easily palpable in the midline. The iliac crest is approximately at the level of the L4-L5 interspace.
- A midline longitudinal incision is made over the spinous processes.
- The internervous plane lies between the two paraspinal muscles (erector spinae), each of which receives a segmental nerve supply from the posterior primary rami of the lumbar nerves.
- The paraspinal muscles are elevated in a subperiosteal manner to expose the bony elements.
- Close to the facet joints, in the area between the transverse processes, are the vessels supplying the paraspinal muscles on a segmental basis. These branches of the lumbar vessels often bleed when the dissection is carried out laterally (Fig. 3–34).

Figure 3–34: A transverse diagram depicting the path of the dissection during a posterior lumbar or thoracic approach to the spine.

References

An HS. (1998) Approaches to the cervical spine. In: An Atlas of Surgery of the Spine (An HS et al., eds.). London: Martin-Dunitz.

An illustrative atlas detailing a step-by-step approach to surgical dissection of the human spine with full color photos and cross-sectional illustrations.

An HS. (1999) Surgical exposure and fusion techniques of the spine. In: Spinal Instrumentation (HS An et al., eds.), 2nd edition. Baltimore: Williams and Wilkins.

A thorough description of various exposure and instrumentation techniques commonly employed in the cervical spine with detailed explanations regarding commonly made errors and technical pearls.

An HS. (1998) Surgical exposures and fusion techniques of the spine. In: Principles and Techniques of Spine Surgery (An HS, ed.). Philadelphia: Williams & Wilkins, pp. 31-62.

A comprehensive textbook devoted to various instrumentation systems used in the spine. Also a detailed overview of commonly used surgical approaches in the cervical spine.

An HS, Simpson JM. (1994) Surgery of the Cervical Spine. Philadelphia: Martin Dunitz and Williams and Wilkins.

A detailed description of the surgical approach, the operative management, and the indications for various cervical procedures. The textbook covers a broad spectrum of topics including the indications for operation, the potential complications, and the various instrumentation systems employed in the cervical spine.

Hoppenfeld S, DeBoer P. (1994) Surgical Exposures in Orthopaedics: The Anatomic Approach, 2nd edition. Philadelphia: Lippincott Williams & Wilkins.

The most commonly referenced anatomic textbook to orthopedic surgical procedures. The book highlights the various approaches to the cervical spine.

Robinson RA, Southwick WO. (1960) Surgical approaches of the cervical spine. In: The American Academy of Orthopaedic Surgeons, Instructional Course Lectures, Vol. XVII. New York: Mosby.

The authors' original description of the anterior approach to the cervical spine with a detailed account of the anatomic dissection and potential complications associated with the approach.

Verbiest H. (1969) Anterolateral operations for fractures and dislocations in the middle and lower parts of the cervical spine. JBJS 51A: 1489-1530.

An account of the anterolateral approach to the lower cervical spine in the setting of acute cervical trauma.

Lumbar Degenerative Disk Disease

Understanding the Pain Generator

Eugene J. Carragee

M.D., Director, Orthopaedic Spine Center, Professor, Department of Orthopaedic Surgery, Stanford University School of Medicine, Stanford, CA

Introduction

- Specific definitive anatomic diagnoses for low back pain (LBP) are the exception more than the rule in LBP syndromes.
  - Symptoms resolve in most patients within one week and few have serious persistent symptoms after 6-8 weeks. Because the natural history of nonspecific LBP in most patients is spontaneous resolution, most do not require a formal anatomic diagnosis.
- In a few patients, certain **so-called "red flag" clinical features** may suggest serious underlying conditions such as tumors, infections, or fractures. In those patients, an *early* and *aggressive* evaluation to rule out serious underlying pathology should be performed.
  - However, even in patients with such red-flag clinical variables, serious underlying disease is still uncommon.
- A **thorough diagnostic evaluation is usually recommended** when a patient with nonspecific LBP is unimproved after 6-8 weeks. This evaluation may find either of the following:
  - If clear pathology accounts for symptoms (e.g., tumor, infection, or fracture), proceed to treatment.
  - If a thorough investigation does not disclose such clear pathologic diagnoses (and it usually will not), some clinicians may try to identify what is commonly called the **pain generator** among the otherwise **common degenerative or age-related changes** found in the spine.

Definition of a "Pain Generator"

- For a definitive diagnosis to be clinically relevant, the identified pain generator not only must be capable of causing some discomfort but also should be reasonably felt to be the primary cause of the patient's apparent severe illness.
  - The practical clinic issue is not whether pain may at some time originate from a certain disk or other structure but whether the pathology of that structure can adequately explain the clinical symptoms that caused the patient to seek medical attention.

Two Schools of Thought

- It is not clear that this task—finding the discrete local pain generator that may cause the serious LBP illness in even a minority of patients—can be accomplished.

Multifactorial School

- LBP illness is often multifactorial—including mechanical, psychological, and neurophysiological contributors. It is therefore unreasonable to expect a specific anatomic study to confirm a "diagnosis" for every patient's LBP illness. Even if a pain generator is suspected, it is not clear how can this be reliably confirmed to be the cause of the patient's perceived pain, impairment, and disability in the face of complex social, emotional, and neurophysiological confounders (Allan et al. 1989, Nachemson 1989, Burton et al. 1995).

Single Disabling Pathology School

- The precise identification of the pain generator is central to the spinal evaluation. It is a reasonable expectation of patients, and it determines the choice of treatments aimed at the suspected disk or facet. In this model, the social issues of disability or litigation, psychological distress, and apparent pain intolerance are *secondary* to the crippling effect of a painful but unrecognized spinal structure. These clinicians believe the pain generator in spinal disorders will usually need to be determined by specialized testing such as provocative discography or differential anesthetic blockage (Aprill et al. 1992; Schwarzer, Aprill et al. 1995; Schwarzer, Bogduk 1996).

Scientific Basis

- It is self-evident that an agreed-upon scientific basis for a pain generator that can explain the morbidity of chronic LBP illness is elusive.

Pain Generator
General Usage

- This term describes the pathoanatomic site from which the primary cause of a patient's LBP is thought to originate and implies certain premises that make the term clinically meaningful.

Pathologic Structure

- A supposed pain generator is usually considered a **pathologic structure** and not a physiologic or psychological response.

Example

- The muscle pain from momentarily holding an awkward posture (transient ischemia) is not commonly considered a pain generator, nor is primary psychogenic pain without anatomic cause.

Primary Cause of LBP Illness

- A supposed pain generator is usually considered the primary or sole cause of a patient's illness.

Examples

- When an evaluation turns up a discitis or myeloma, the clinician is reasonably certain that the pain generator causing the severe disabling LBP illness has been identified definitively. The presence of mild arthritic changes at an adjacent segment may also cause some low

back discomfort but would not normally be considered the pain generator causing this patient's serious illness.
- Similarly, the same **mild facet arthrosis** in a patient gravely disabled by the psychiatric illness of a somatization disorder, with a long history of severe diffuse pain attributed to minimal or no local pathology, would not have the facet arthrosis diagnosed as the primary cause of this patient's severe illness.

Pain Generator Theory and Associations with Comorbidities

- Chronic LBP illness associated with only degenerative changes is rarely one dimensional. It is distinctly unusual for a patient to have one site of severe degenerative disease and no changes at other segments or psychosocial comorbidities.
  1. Psychological and social comorbidities are more common in subjects with chronic LBP illness based on degenerative changes than in patients with chronic LBP from other causes.
- Work on zygapophyseal pain, sacroiliac pain, and discogenic pain syndromes shows that 70%-80% of patients coming to evaluation have personal injury or litigation claims (Schwarzer, Aprill et al. 1995; Carragee 2001).
  2. Furthermore, the pain signals from various structures are not simple direct "circuits" from the injured part to the patient's perception. There are common sites associated with back and buttock pain and a neuraxis capable of modulating pain transmission and perception.

Modulation of Pain Perception in LBP

- Many common factors are known to have potential dampening or amplifying effects on the perception of LBP from any specific site. These factors are important in determining the clinical expression of LBP syndromes— as well as in interpreting common diagnostic tests such as provocative discography, diagnostic facet, or sacroiliac joint anesthetic blockade.

Adjacent Tissue Injury

- Significant injury to nearby structures may increase the perception of pain through a local **hyperalgesic effect**. This is a well-known phenomenon, occurring with any tissue damage. Pain perception is amplified by increasing local inflammatory processes or neurologic sensitization in areas not directly injured, such as the area surrounding a burn or a fracture that is sensitive although without any thermal or mechanical injury (Birrell et al. 1991, Siddall et al. 1997).

Local Anesthetic

- Local anesthetic injections, the application of cold packs, and so on, may decrease the perception of pain at local sites and sometimes at distal or proximal sites through uncertain mechanisms (Kibler et al. 1960, North et al. 1996, Siddall et al. 1997).

Tissue Injury in Adjacent or Same Sclerotome

- Tissue injury with the same or adjacent sclerotomal afferents as those of the lower spinal elements may increase LBP sensitivity at a site. This effect is thought to be caused by physiologic and anatomic changes at the level of the dorsal root ganglion or spinal cord ascending tracts. In animal models, single afferent neurons from a diagnosis-related group may innervate three adjacent disks. This effect is important in considering the specificity of discography at sites adjacent to a known pathologic structure (e.g., nonunion, spondylolisthesis, or painful iliac crest bone graft site) (Kawakami et al. 1997, Carragee et al. 1999).

Chronic Pain Syndrome

- Chronic pain syndromes may complicate the evaluation of LBP syndromes. Chronic pain from regional sites near the LBP (chronic pelvic pain, irritable bowel syndrome, or failed hip arthroplasty) or far from the LBP (chronic neck pain, chronic headache, or temporal–mandibular joint syndrome) may increase pain sensitivity at lower spinal elements. This effect may be regional or global and may be related to neurophysiological changes at multiple levels along the neuraxis. Preexisting chronic pain syndromes are also associated with depression, narcotic use, and habituation, which have independent pain perception effects (Burton et al. 1995; Carragee et al. 1999; Carragee, Chen et al. 2000; Carragee, Paragioudakis et al. 2000; Carragee et al. 2002).

Narcotic Analgesia

- Narcotic medications act at multiple levels to decrease pain thresholds, intensity, and affective response (Gracely et al. 1979).

Narcotic Habituation

- Chronic narcotic habituation may decrease pain tolerances in the absence of increased narcotic intake. This effect will decrease endogenous abilities to modulate peripheral nociceptive input. This effect is multifactorial. Chronic narcotic habituation is also associated with depression and sleep disturbances (Gracely et al. 1979).

Depression, Anxiety, and Somatic Distress

- Clinical depression and anxiety disorders may be seen as predisposing factors to chronic LBP syndromes, as reactions to the pain and disability of chronic LBP illness, or both. In these situations, emotional distress will usually decrease the pain threshold and increase the perceived pain intensity and affective response. Theses effects are

likely caused by both central neurochemical changes and systemic effects (Burton 1997, Pincus et al. 2002).

Social Imperatives

- Overriding social imperatives may decrease pain perception or disassociate pain perception and functional loss. A decreased pain perception or even an absence of pain perception despite injury can be seen during some short-term stressful events such a motor vehicle accident, combat, or certain training environments (Allan et al. 1989, Burton et al. 1995, Burton 1997, Carragee 2001, Pincus et al. 2002).

Social Disincentive

- Secondary gain issues may exaggerate pain responses of all types. When the intensity of pain behavior and report is correlated with a real or perceived social benefit or monetary compensation, the measurable pain perception may be increased (Allan et al. 1989, Burton et al. 1995, Burton 1997, Carragee 2001, Pincus et al. 2002).
- When considering the certainty of diagnosis of a possible pain generator implicated in chronic LBP illness, it is necessary to view the preceding confounding factors for contribution to the illness observed.

Examples

- Major acute upper extremity trauma, narcotic administration, and social imperatives at the site of an accident may mask the perception of a significant LBP injury that, absent of these confounders, may manifest as clearly symptomatic and disabling.
- Minor nociceptive input from a disk can be amplified in a patient with multiple chronic pain syndromes, narcotic habituation, depression, and compensation issues (social disincentives). In this case, a common, mild backache pain generator becomes a catastrophic illness by amplification at multiple levels.

Pain Generator and Diagnostic Anaesthetic Injections

- Diagnostic anesthetic blockade of a suspected pain generator site is a frequently used method recommended for establishing a diagnosis in persistent LBP syndromes. A critical evaluation of the scientific basis of this diagnostic method points out the inherent difficulty in evaluating the pain generator in degenerative spinal conditions.
  - **Criteria**—This method is used primarily for suspected facet joint, spondylolysis, and sacroiliac joint pain. The "blocked" structure is assumed to be the primary pain generator if the anesthetic blockage of a structure results in some arbitrary degree of pain relief: 50%, 75%, 100%, etc. (Saal 2002).

- **Incidence**—The incidence of facet joint pain as a cause of serious LBP when derived from these diagnostic blocks is between 15% and 40% in select groups (Schwarzer et al. 1994; Schwarzer, Wang et al. 1995; Saal 2002). However, these estimates are conjectural because none of these studies used a "gold standard" test to establish the validity of these injection blocks in making a diagnosis. One problem is the placebo effect seen with pain interventions.
- **Neurophysiological basis**—However, neurophysiological studies also indicate that anesthetic blockade at one site may affect distal or proximal pain sites and pain perception from distant or regional pathology not in the infiltration site. That is even without a "placebo effect." The injection does not have to block the painful site itself to result in bona fide subjective relief.

Facet Joint Pain

Facet Joint Stimulation or Experimental Pain

- The facet joint, capsule, and surrounding structures can be painful. Stimulation by injection of the facet joint with synovial and capsular distension results in LBP discomfort in asymptomatic volunteers and in patients undergoing diagnostic injections (McCall et al. 1979). There is modest predictability in the location and character of referred pain with saline injections into the facet joints in asymptomatic volunteers but no predictable pattern of referral in LBP patients (Marks et al. 1992, Fukui et al. 1997). Pain "wiring" and perception is altered in symptomatic people in ways poorly understood but likely related to local and central modulation.

Anesthetic Blockade of Experimental Pain

- The experimental pain associated with facet capsule distension appears usually to be blocked by local anesthetic at the medial branches of the primary dorsal rami above and below a facet (Kaplan et al. 1998). But it is unclear whether this applies in the clinical situation.
  - When the clinical features of patients responding to facet blocks were examined, there did not appear to be a clear clinical presentation that correlated with pain relief (Schwarzer, Wang et al. 1995).
  - In addition, a positive response of pain relief to anesthetic facet injections does not appear to correlate with radiographic evidence of facet arthrosis (Revel et al. 1998).

Mechanism of Pain Relief in Clinical Pain

- The failure to identify any reliable clinical pattern or radiological finding associated with pain relief by facet

block demonstrates the problem of having no gold standard in these studies to confirm the diagnostic test.
  - These results may indicate that the painful lesion being locally anaesthetized is simply not detectable by imaging studies and is protean in symptom manifestation.
  - On the other hand, it may indicate that the test does not identify a true clinical entity. The response in many patients may instead be related to the anesthetic effects on collateral or central pain pathways or perception.

Methods to Limit False-Positive Injections

- To address the possibility of placebo or collateral effects and thereby perhaps increase the reliability of results, some authors have advocated additional controls on these blocks (Saal 2002).
  - **Placebo injections**—The use of sham injections limits the placebo response.
  - **Differential block**—The use of short-acting versus long-acting anesthetic agents differentiates true responders from false-positive results.
  - **Small injection quantity**—The careful placement of tiny anesthetic doses on the posterior primary ramus (median branch) innervating the facet joint may decrease the diffusion effects of larger volumes.
  - **Gold standard**—Still, without a gold standard to validate the method, the isolation of a clinically significant pain generator by neuroblock remains controversial.

Therapeutic Trial as a Confirmation of the Test Result

- It may be possible to indirectly support a diagnostic method such as anesthetic facet injections if a certain treatment method was reliably effective.
  - There have been numerous trials using steroid injections and a smaller series of local nerve ablations in subjects diagnosed by these injection techniques. Most of these trials have had equivocal results at best.
  - The best evidence supporting the differential block technique was reported by Dreyfuss et al. (2000). This trial of median branch ablation made the diagnosis of "chronic zygapophyseal joint pain" by differential blocks of short- and long-acting anesthetics. In this study, more than 80% pain relief for more than one hour after a lidocaine injection and more than two hours after bupivacaine injection was used to determine a positive response to median branch block. For patients meeting these criteria, the results were reported as highly successful in pain relief and improved function.
  - The Dreyfuss et al. study still raised serious questions regarding the mechanism of action and the logic of differential blocks of the facet joint as a diagnostic tool to identify the pain generator. For instance, contrary to

pharmacologic expectations and the premise of differential short-acting versus long-acting anesthetics, both lidocaine (short-acting) and bupivacaine (long-acting) anesthetic injections produced the same duration of relief (4–5 hours).

Conclusion

- Although increasingly elaborate methods are being developed to accurately identify the pain generator, no method exists to confirm that this diagnosis is truly the primary source of a patient's illness rather than other spinal processes or the central effects of neurophysiological or psychosocial factors.

Pain Generator and Provocative Discography

- The lumbar disk may be the structure most commonly implicated as the primary cause of disabling chronic LBP illness. This diagnosis is purported to be confirmed by provocative discography alone.
  - Clinical history and physical signs do not correlate with the positive concordant response to disk injection (Schwarzer, Aprill et al. 1995).
  - No finding (e.g., high-intensity zone, or HIZ, lesion; disk desiccation; or Modic changes) or set of findings on magnetic resonance imaging (MRI) are found only in the injection-positive disk (Boden et al. 1990, Jensen et al. 1994, Carragee, Paragioudakis et al. 2000).

Technique

- The technique of provocative discography points out the need for a careful understanding of the pain generator concept in the evaluation of chronic LBP illness.
  - Discography uses the percutaneous pressurization of a disk with a contract dye to determine whether this disk is the source of pain in an individual with chronic LBP illness.
  - The examiner relies on the patient to report the intensity of pain and the similarity of the pain to their usual LBP. Both of these reports are obviously subjective. Furthermore, the stimulation of nociceptive fibers at the disk and the transmission of those signals to form a perception of pain are subject to amplification and down-regulation at multiple levels between the disk and the cortical processing.

Criticism

- The primary criticism of this technique is that many people without significant LBP troubles may report painful disk injections—risking false-positive results.

Specificity

- The specificity of a test refers to the likelihood that a positive result will occur only in a subject with the disease being tested for. In the case of provocative discography, this would be the likelihood that a patient with chronic LBP illness who has a "concordant and painful response to an injection" is suffering from a pain syndrome because of the disk itself.
- **Apparent false-positive tests** have appeared in clinical practice. Block et al. (1996) and Ohnmeiss et al. (1995) independently reported that psychological comorbidities appeared to correlate with the report of severe pain after the injection of morphologically normal disks. Carragee et al. (1997) reported apparent false-positive injections in LBP patients ultimately found to have nondiscogenic causes of LBP, including sacroiliac joint pathology and spinal tumor.

Best Case Scenario

- Walsh et al. in 1990 found the rate of painful injections in healthy young men, paid as "asymptomatic volunteers," was very low. Only 1 in 10 described the pain with injection as "bad," or 3 of 5 on a 5-point scale. This clearly is the best case scenario. These subjects had little or no degenerative changes in their disks. They also had no known risk factors as described in the preceding sections for pain amplification: adjacent tissue injury, regional or generalized pain syndrome, narcotic habituation, depression, anxiety disorder, or social disincentives to health pain modulation (e.g., litigation, sick role support, or financial counterincentives). Despite these study limitations, these data have been cited as having proven a zero or negligible false-positive rate for provocative discography.

False-Positive Discography in Subgroups at Risk

- Because it is unusual for chronic LBP illness patients to have no or few comorbidities, as was the case with the healthy volunteers in the Walsh et al. (1990) study, it is difficult to estimate the risk of a false-positive disk injection. A follow-up study on asymptomatic patients in regards to LBP at the Stanford University School of Medicine looked at patient subgroups with different pain modulation characteristics:
  1. Asymptomatic LBP subjects with degenerative disk changes and without chronic pain processes
  2. Asymptomatic LBP subjects with degenerative disk changes but with a nonlumbar chronic pain process
  3. Asymptomatic LBP subjects with serious psychological somatization issues and chronic nonlumbar pain
- By the Walsh et al. (1990) criteria of positive experiment injections, 10% of group 1, 40% of group 2 (chronic pain), and 75% of group 3 (somatization and chronic pain) were false-positive injections (Carragee, Tanner et al. 2000).

Increased Risk of False-Positive Injections

- Psychological distress
- Chronic pain syndrome and behavior
- Increased somatic awareness
- Anular disruption
- Litigation or worker's compensation dispute

Low Risk for Painful Reporting of Injections

- In a recent study of unblinded medical professionals without LBP who underwent experimental discography, few subjects reported significant pain with injection. This data suggest that social incentive can work both ways, either to magnify or to minimize reported pain depending on circumstances. In this cohort, many of whom had a professional interest in reporting low pain intensity with injections, the pain intensity reports were skewed below the arbitrary 6/10 cutoff of a "positive" test result. Still, most injected disks were painful (55%).

Discography in Subjects with Common Backache

- The difficulty in deciding what is a clinically significant pain generator is further demonstrated in subjects with backache perceived to be below the clinical threshold that usually results in functional loss or a search for medical treatment.
  - In volunteer subjects without clinically irrelevant common backache undergoing experimental discography, concordant and back pain rated "bad" or worse was reproduced in 9 of 25 subjects (36%). Pain intensity with injection was predicted by pre–existing chronic pain conditions (nonlumbar) and psychological distress (Carragee et al. 2002).

Implications

- The disturbing aspect of this data lies in the potential for patients with a bona fide, serious pain generator from a spondylolisthesis or other pathology and a mild backache-only disk. A discographic injection of the mild backache-only disk had a high risk of being positive even though this is not the source of the patient's pain syndrome. That is, the discogram is identifying a clinically irrelevant pain generator—and it should not be considered a pain generator in the usual sense used and defined previously.

Concordancy and the Discographic Pain Generator

- Provocative discography is only considered positive when pain similar to the patient's usual pain in quality and location is elicited on injection. The reliability of the test would be substantially supported only if patients could identify the quality of pain coming from a particular disk and differentially compare that sensation to their usual pain.
  - Data from the evaluation of other provocative tests would indicate that caution should be used in interpreting the "concordant" pain response. In the presence of chronic pain, there is a general, known increased responsiveness to normally innocuous stimuli. Furthermore, there may be hyperalgesia of uninjured tissue in the area surrounding an injury. It is also known that the stimulation of structures near a lesion may mimic the quality and affective component of the patient's usual pain. Even primarily psychogenic pain may be simulated by provocative testing at a specific anatomic stimulation.

Concordancy in Experimental Subjects

- Volunteer subjects were tested who had no history of back pain but who were scheduled to undergo posterior iliac crest bone graft harvesting for nonspinal problems, mainly fracture nonunions or bone tumors. Most patients experience low back and buttock pain for some months after a posterior iliac crest bone graft harvest. This pain has a similar distribution to what is normally considered discogenic lumbar pain. The areas have similar sclerotomal origins and referred pain distributions. Discography was then performed some months after the bone graft harvesting; the subjects were asked to compare the quality and location of disk-injection pain to their usual iliac crest pain (Carragee et al. 1999).

Results

- Twenty-four disks were injected in eight volunteer subjects. The same protocol as the Walsh et al. (1990) study was employed. Of the 14 disk injections causing some pain response, 5 were felt to be "different" (nonconcordant) pains (35.7%), 7 were "similar" (50.0%), and 2 were "exact" pain reproductions (14.3%).

Risk Factors for Reporting False-Positive "Concordant" Pain with Discography

- The presence of *anular disruption* predicted concordant pain reproduction (p < 0.05). Of 10 disks with anular tears, the injection of 7 elicited "similar" or "exact" pain reproduction to the iliac crest pain at bone graft harvest sites. All positive disk injections had anular fissures. Half of the positive disk injections occurred at low pressures (< 20 psi).

Practical Guideline for Discography Use

Best Utility

- **Negative discogram** useful in determining the end of the fusion in deformity or other potentially long fusion
- Positive, **single-level disk** in a subject without risk factors for false-positive injection (e.g., normal psychological profile, no chronic pain behavior or history, and no compensation issues)

Unclear Utility

- Positive **two-level disks** but no risk factors
- **Postoperative disk** but otherwise no risk factors
- **Intermediate (at-risk) psychological profile,** single-level disk pathology

Poor Utility

- Spine with multilevel pathology
- Abnormal or chronic pain behavior
- Abnormal psychometric findings
- Disputed compensation cases

Discography Conclusion

- It is not clear what should be inferred from a report of concordant pain on discography. Test reliability depends on patient risk factors of false-positive testing—psychological factors, social factors, chronic pain behavior, and other modulators of pain perception that act along the neuraxis.

Conclusion

- The concept of a single, stand-alone pain generator, existing independently of the larger clinical picture and diagnosable by simple provocative or anesthetic maneuvers, is outdated given our current understanding of chronic pain syndromes. Although some patients may have such a lesion, it is an unlikely assumption. The pain reported clinically, as well as the pain reported with provocative testing or anesthetic block, occurs within the context of the whole patient. This includes the presence of other pain processes, coping styles, emotional and psychological reserve, drug use, dependence, abuse, and the balance of social imperatives and disincentives to pain reporting and pain behavior.
- Although the neurophysiological literature may be new and interesting, the basic point is quite old. Sir William Osler's dictum that a physician had better know the patient better than the disease has not changed. With respect to the pain generator concept in spinal disorders, it remains imperative.

References

Allan DB, Waddell G. (1989) An historical perspective on low back pain and disability. Acta Orthop Scand Suppl 234: 1-23.

An excellent review of the concepts that have shaped our thinking of LBP through history to the present. The epidemiological evidence of increasing LBP disability throughout the twentieth century, particularly after World War II, is described, as well as social and medical reasons that have contributed to this epidemic of LBP disability.

Aprill C, Bogduk N. (1992) High-intensity zone: A diagnostic sign of painful lumbar disc on magnetic resonance imaging. Br J Radiol 65(773): 361-369.

This report demonstrated that HIZ findings on MRI are frequently seen in subjects with LBP and that on discography these appear to be painful. This is the original description of the HIZ in LBP patients undergoing discography; it was done in the absence of knowledge of how frequently this finding occurs in asymptomatic or minimally symptomatic people.

Birrell G, McQueen D, Iggo A et al. (1991) PGI2-induced activation and sensitization of articular mechanonociceptors. Neurosci Lett 124: 5-8.

Prostaglandin (PGI2) appears to induce a local pain sensitization effect in a rat laboratory model. This report suggests that the effect of PGI2 is specific for the sensory afferent nerves and appears to lower the threshold for nociceptive responses in inflamed joints.

Block A, Vanharanta H, Olhmeiss DD et al. (1996) Discographic pain report: Influence of psychological factors. Spine 21(3): 334-338.

A strong correlation was found between abnormal MMPI scores for hypochondriasis and hysteria scales and reports of significant pain with the injection of morphologically normal disks. The risk of these false-positive discographic injections in subjects with abnormal scores ranged from 40%-60%.

Boden S, Davis D, Dina TS et al. (1990) Abnormal magnetic resonance scans of the lumbar spine in asymptomatic subjects: A prospective investigation. JBJS [Am] 72-A(3): 403-408.

This report found an increasing incidence of abnormal lumbar MRI scans with increasing age in asymptomatic individuals. For asymptomatic subjects over 60, 36% had disk herniation, 21% had spinal stenosis, and approximately 60% had an abnormal MRI finding of some type.

Burton A. (1997) Spine update: Back injury and work loss—biomechanical and psychosocial influences. Spine 22(21): 2575-2580.

This is a review article on the biomechanical and psychosocial influences of back injury. The evidence to date showed that biomechanical and ergonomic factors may be related to the occurrence of a LBP "injury" but that chronic disability and chronic LBP illness appear to be more clearly related to psychosocial influences.

Burton AK, Tillotson KM, Main CJ et al. (1995) Psychosocial predictors of outcome in acute and subchronic low back trouble. Spine 20(24): 2738-2745.

This study found that psychosocial factors had moderately good predictability of progression to longstanding back pain when patients were seen early in an LBP episode.

Carragee E. (2001) Psychological and functional profiles in select subjects with low back pain. Spine J 1: 198-204.

This study of patients with 6 to 18 months of severe back pain found that psychological distress was much more common when the ultimate diagnosis was "discogenic pain" than when it was unstable spondylolisthesis or spinal infection. This study further points out that most patients with severe spinal illness reported in concrete diagnoses do not develop serious psychological distress.

Carragee E, McCormack M, Schilling P et al. (2001) Resilience in occupational low back disability: Back pain, disability, and stress in soldiers undergoing heavy physical training. Proc Int Soc Study Lumbar Spine, Edinburgh, UK.

This study of soldiers undergoing special operations forces training in the U.S. Army demonstrated that factors including unit leadership and cohesion qualities were more important than physical factors in determining soldiers' ability to complete strenuous training associated with reports of significant LBP. The most common reason to fail to complete training on a medical basis was an LBP complaint.

Carragee EJ, Alamin TF, Miller J et al. (2002) Provocative discography in volunteer subjects with mild persistent low back pain (2001 Outstanding Paper Award). Spine J 2: 25-34.

A study of experimental discography in subjects with mild persistent LBP found that these subjects frequently reported significant pain with disk injection and that pain with disk injection in this subgroup was associated with anular disruption and other nonlumbar chronic pain states.

Carragee EJ, Chen Y, Tanner CM et al. (2000) Provocative discography in patients after limited lumbar discectomy: A controlled, randomized study of pain response in symptomatic and asymptomatic subjects. Spine 25(23): 3065-3071.

Of asymptomatic volunteers who had had a previous limited discectomy for herniated disk, 40% had significant pain on experimental disk injection. Psychological features and pervious discectomy correlated with the risk of false-positive injection.

Carragee EJ, Paragioudakis SJ, Khurana S et al. (2000) Lumbar high-intensity zone and discography in subjects without low back problems (2000 Volvo Award winner in clinical studies). Spine 25(23): 2987-2992.

A HIZ lesion was found in approximately 25% of asymptomatic subjects, closely matched by age and risk of lumbar disk degeneration to chronic LBP illness patients. Disks with HIZ lesions were more likely than not painful on disk injection even in asymptomatic subjects.

Carragee EJ, Tanner CM, Khurana S et al. (2000) The rates of false-positive lumbar discography in select patients without low back symptoms. Spine 25(11): 1373-1380; discussion 1381.

This study of experimental discography in subjects asymptomatic for LBP found that psychological factors, chronic pain factors, and a history of disputed compensation claims predicted the degree of pain reported on injection of usually asymptomatic degenerative disks.

Carragee EJ, Tanner CM, Yang B et al.(1999) False-positive findings on lumbar discography: Reliability of subjective concordance assessment during provocative disc injection. Spine 24(23): 2542-2547.

This paper showed how subjects with iliac crest pain from bone graft harvesting were unable to reliably distinguish between the sensation from the bone graft site and the pain with disk injection. This study calls into question the reliability of the "concordancy" rating made during clinical discography.

Dreyfuss P, Halbrook B, Pauza K et al. (2000) Efficacy and validity of radiofrequency neurotomy for chronic lumbar zygapophyseal joint pain. Spine 25: 1270-1277.

This paper reported that approximately 60% of patients had 90% pain relief 12 months after a medial branch neurotomy for suspected facet joint pain. For diagnosis, this group used differential blocks with long- and short-acting agents. Interestingly, the duration of pain relief with long- and short-acting agents in the study was the same. This finding points out that the mechanisms of pain perception emanating from the lumbar spine are poorly understood.

Fukui S, Osheto K, Shiotani M et al. (1997) Distribution of referred pain from the lumbar zygapophyseal joints and dorsal rami. Clin J Pain 13: 303-307.

This study mapped the perceived location of pain with stimulation of the facet joints in the lumbar spine.

Gracely R, Dubner R, McGrath P et al. (1979) Narcotic analgesia: Fentanyl reduces the intensity but not the unpleasantness of painful tooth pulp stimulation. Science 203: 1261-1263.

This study demonstrated the effect of narcotics on both the pain intensity and the perceived unpleasantness of experimental pain stimulation.

Jensen M, Brant-Zawadzki M, Obuchowski N et al. (1994) Magnetic resonance imaging of the lumbar spine in people without back pain. N Engl J Med 331(2): 69-73.

This classic study of asymptomatic subjects graded MRI findings of the lumbar spine. The authors showed only 36% of subjects had normal disks at all levels. Although many degenerative changes were commonly found (including anular defects, disk degeneration, and arthrosis), extruded disk herniations were rare (1%).

Kaplan M, Dreyfuss P, Halbrook B et al. (1998) The ability of lumbar medial branch blocks to anesthetize the zygapophyseal joint: A physiologic challenge. Spine 23: 1847-1852.

This study demonstrated that lidocaine anesthetic applied to the medial branch effectively eliminated experimental facet joint pain in eight of nine volunteer asymptomatic subjects.

Kawakami M, Tamaki T, Hashizume H et al. (1997) The role of phospholipase A2 and nitric oxide in pain-related behavior produced by an allograft of intervertebral disc material to the sciatic nerve of the rat. Spine 22: 1074-1079.

This study showed the possible role of chemical mediators in the pathomechanism of radicular pain. Physical compression and chemical irritation may both cause radicular symptoms. Whether this finding is important in LBP symptoms (as opposed to radicular symptoms) was not tested.

Kibler R, Nathan P. (1960) Relief of pain and paraesthesiae by nerve block distal to a lesion. J Neurol Neurosurg Psychiatry 23: 91-98.

This classic paper from 1960 studied subjects with severe pain from a variety of lesions. The authors found that it was possible to obtain pain relief by the infiltration of anesthetic far from or in tissues unrelated to the lesion. Even central pain from a spinothalamic track lesion could be relieved with distal injections such as at the sacral roots. Furthermore, even skin or peripheral nerve injections in subjects with herniated disk pain appear to have their radicular pain from their central lesion relieved.

Marks R, Houston T, Thulbourne T. (1992) Facet joint injection and facet nerve block: A randomized comparison in 86 patients with chronic low back pain. Pain 49: 325-328.

   The facet joint and nerve injections were found to have approximately equal diagnostic potential. However, treatment with therapeutic injections appeared to be unsatisfactory.

McCall I, Park W, O'Brien J et al. (1979) Induced pain referral from posterior lumbar elements in normal subjects. Spine 4: 441-446.

   The facet joint discomfort in normal subjects was tested by stimulating the capsule and surrounding tissue. Maps were made, which suggest that gluteal pain is common with stimulation from the L4-L5 level; however, there is wide variation among subjects.

Nachemson A. (1989) Lumbar discography: Where are we today? Spine 14: 555-557.

   A theoretical critique of discography.

North R, Kidd D, Zahurak M et al. (1996) Specificity of diagnostic nerve blocks: A prospective, randomized study of sciatica due to lumbosacral spine disease. Pain 65: 77-85.

   These authors found that the radicular pain from root compression may be relieved with medial branch blocks, distal sciatic nerve blocks, or a selective block at or near the lesion. These findings point out the low specificity of this type of anesthetic blockade and the risk of false-positive results.

Ohnmeiss DD, Vanharanta H, Guyer RD. (1995) The association between pain drawings and computed tomographic/discographic pain responses. Spine 20(6): 729-733.

   These authors found a strong correlation between subjects with abnormal pain drawings (thought to be associated with increased emotional distress) and reports of pain on discography with anatomically normal disks. In those patients with abnormal pain drawing, 50% reported false-positive pain; 12% of those with normal pain drawings had false-positive injections.

Pincus T, Burton AK, Vogel S et al. (2002) A systematic review of psychological factors as predictors of chronicity/disability in prospective cohorts of low back pain. Spine 27(5): E109-E120.

   This is a comprehensive and thoughtful review of the psychological factors predicting chronicity of pain in patients with LBP. An extensive bibliography is provided.

Revel M, Poiraudeau S, Auleley G et al. (1998) Capacity of the clinical picture to characterize low back pain relieved by facet joint anesthesia: Proposed criteria to identify patients with painful facet joints. Spine 23: 1972-1976.

   This study demonstrates the poor correlation between clinical signs and symptoms of LBP and the response to anesthetic facet joint blockade in patients suspected of having facet joint pain. As in other studies, there is no gold standard to determine which patients in the study had facet joint pain and confirm either the clinical or the diagnostic injection diagnosis.

Saal JSM. (2002) General principles of diagnostic testing as related to painful lumbar spine disorders: A critical appraisal of current diagnostic techniques. Spine 27(22): 2538-2545.

   This paper gives a good general review of diagnostic injection techniques in patients with LBP.

Schwarzer A, Aprill C, Fortin J et al. (1994) The relative contribution of the zygapophyseal joint in chronic low back pain. Spine 19(7): 801-806.

   This study found that of eight patients with positive pain relief responses to facet joint blocks, three (32%) also had positive disk injection studies. Once again, whether these patients had discogenic pain, facet pain, both, or some other source for their pain is unknown.

Schwarzer A, Aprill C, Derby R et al. (1995) The prevalence and clinical features of internal disc disruption in patients with chronic LBP. Spine 20(17): 1878-1883.

   These authors found no correlation between the historical clinical findings in physical examination and the results of lumbar discography. This has been interpreted as demonstrating either that internal disk disruption has no clear clinical picture and can only be diagnosed on discography or that discography may be positive in patients with both discogenic and nondiscogenic causes of chronic LBP.

Schwarzer A, Bogduk N. (1996) The prevalence and clinical features of internal disk disruption in patients with low back pain (Letter to the editor). Spine 21: 776.

   This study found that sham injections of saline relieved greater than 50% of LBP in chronic LBP patients receiving placebo facet injections.

Schwarzer A, Wang S, Bog duk N et al. (1995) Prevalence and clinical features of lumbar zygapophyseal joint pain: A study in an Australian population with chronic low back pain. Ann Rheum Dis 54(2): 100-106.

   Here, 63 patients with chronic LBP illness were studied with facet joint injections of bupivacaine and paraspinal muscle injections of saline. Of all subjects 32% had more than 50% pain relief with saline injections. Of the subjects not showing the placebo response, 40% had relief with the anesthetic agent.

Siddall P, Cousins M. (1997) Spinal pain mechanisms. Spine 22(1): 98-104.

   This paper describes neuromodulators of chronic pain at multiple levels along the neuraxis. These authors make a compelling argument to shift the conceptualization of spinal pain from a simple "hard wired" system of stimulus–response.

Walsh T, Weinstein J, Spratt K et al. (1990) Lumbar discography in normal subjects: A controlled prospective study. JBJS 72-A(7): 1081-1088.

   In performing experimental discography on 10 asymptomatic young men with minimal lumbar disk degeneration, these authors found that 1 subject in 10 had pain rated as "bad" with disk injection and that 2 subjects had pain they rated as "moderate."

Low Back Pain
Nonoperative Treatment Strategies

Rebecca S. Ovsiowitz★, Priya Swamy★, Mitchell K. Freedman §, Guy W. Fried †, and Alexander R. Vaccaro ‡

★ M.D., Thomas Jefferson University, Philadelphia, PA
§D.O., Director of Physical Rehabilitation and Pain Management, The Rothman Institute; Clinical Instructor, Thomas Jefferson University Hospital, Philadelphia, PA
†M.D., Medical Director of Outpatient Services, Incontinence Program, and Respiratory Care Program, Magee Rehabilitation Hospital; Clinical Assistant Professor, Thomas Jefferson University Hospital, Philadelphia, PA
‡M.D., Professor of Orthopaedic Surgery, Thomas Jefferson University and the Rothman Institute, Philadelphia, PA

- The International Association for the Study of Pain defines pain as follows:
  - Pain is an unpleasant sensory and emotional experience associated with actual or potential tissue damage and described in terms of such damage.
  - Chronic pain lasts beyond three months and is associated with significant impairment of activities of daily living, work, or both.

Low Back Pain Epidemiology

- Lifetime incidence: 60%-90%
- Leading cause of disability in those 45 and younger
- Third leading cause of disability in those older than 45

Low Back Pain Generators

Disk

- The outer one third of the anulus fibrosus is innervated by afferent pain nerve fibers.
- Chondrocytes within the nucleus pulposus produce phospholipase A2, which regulates the arachidonic acid cascade and liberates arachidonic acid from cell membranes at the site of inflammation.
- Phospholipase A2 generates membrane-destabilizing products (unsaturated fatty acids), causing membrane injury and edema.

Bone

- Pain can result from a traumatic fracture in the setting of normal bone.
- A pathologic fracture can be caused by the following:
  - Osteoporosis
  - Multiple myeloma
  - Paget's disease
  - Primary spine tumor
  - Metastatic spine tumor
  - Osteomyeltis

Nerve Roots

- Secondary to disk compression and inflammation
- Lateral recess stenosis with nerve root compression
- Radiculitis
  - Radiculitis may manifest as peripheral nerve root motor and sensory abnormalities.

- A straight leg raise causes pain in a radicular pattern—the posterior aspect of the leg for lower lumbar root pathology.
- A reverse straight leg raise causes pain to radiate down the front of the thigh in the setting of lumbar root compression and inflammation (Fig. 5–1, Box 5–1).

Facet Joints

- Responsible for 15%-40% of chronic low back pain symptoms (i.e., facet syndrome).
- The anatomy consists of paired synovial joints lined with a synovial membrane, an articular surface covered with hyaline cartilage, a fibrous capsule, and mechanosensitive nociceptive fibers.
- Facet joints connect the inferior articular process of the vertebra above and the superior articular process of the vertebra below.
- They contain high-threshold mechanosensitive afferent nerve fibers serving as nociceptors and low-threshold afferent fibers that modulate proprioceptive feedback.
- They are innervated by the medial branches of the dorsal rami of the vertebrae above and at the same level.
- Facet joints are compressed with extension and lateral bending.
- Pain is often provoked with extension.
- Microfractures can result in post-traumatic lumbozygapophyseal pain.
- No unique physical exam findings were diagnostic of facet joint pathology (Fig. 5–2).

Spinal Muscles

- Pain can be induced by mechanical pressure or stretch and can be relieved by rest.
- Anaerobic exercise leads to the accumulation of potentially toxic metabolites.
- Ischemia results in intermittent claudication.

Sacroiliac Joint

- The sacroiliac joint represents the cause of low back pain in 5%-10% of patients.
- Pain in the sacroiliac joint can be elicited with palpation of the posterior inferior iliac spine, buttock, thigh, or groin region.
- No specific physical exam finding is considered sensitive or specific for the diagnosis of sacroiliac joint dysfunction.
- Sacroiliac joint dysfunction may result in axial and referred lower limb pain arising from the sacroiliac joint (Fig. 5–3).
- Examples of sacroiliac joint pathology include spondyloarthropathy, crystal and pyogen arthropathy, arthrosis secondary to sacral or pelvis fracture, and diastasis secondary to pregnancy or childbirth.

Spinal Ligaments

- Chronic lifting may stress the spinal ligamentous complex (supraspinous, interspinous, posterior longitudinal ligament, anterior longitudinal ligament, and ligamentum flavum).
- Ligamentum flavum contains nerve endings.
- The posterior longitudinal ligament has large numbers of free nerve endings and is innervated by the sinuvertebral nerves (a branch of the somatic ventral rami and autonomic grey ramus communicans).
- The anterior longitudinal ligament receives innervation from the grey ramus communicantes and ventral rami.

Visceral or Nonspinal Sources of Low Back Pain

- Retroperitoneal inflammation
- Gallbladder, pancreas, kidney, and stomach dysfunction
- Intrapelvic pathology

Nonoperative Treatment Strategies for Low Back Pain

Lifestyle Changes

Tobacco Cessation

- Smoking is a risk factor for low back pain in those with a 50 pack per year history, especially if younger than 45.
- Chronic coughing can lead to increased intradiscal pressure.
- Smoking impairs the spinal vertebral arterial supply through functional vasoconstriction, arterial atheromatous changes, or both.
- Cigarette smoke inhalation reduces solute exchange capacity and oxygenation, leading to impaired nutrition to the disk.
- Smoke inhalation reduces the cellular uptake rate of nutritional substances.
- Smoke inhalation has been shown to reduce metabolite production within the intervertebral disk in pigs.
- A greater rate of disk degeneration is noted in smokers.

Limited Alcohol Intake

- Abuse of alcohol is related to deterioration of muscle strength and histologic injury to muscle; falls may lead to further tissue damage.
- Patients have less ability to perceive tissue damage.

Weight Management

- Patients who are overweight place greater stress on the musculoskeletal system and spine.
- Patients with spinal injuries may gain weight because of less caloric expenditure from inactivity. Medications used for spinal pain may have the side effect of weight gain.

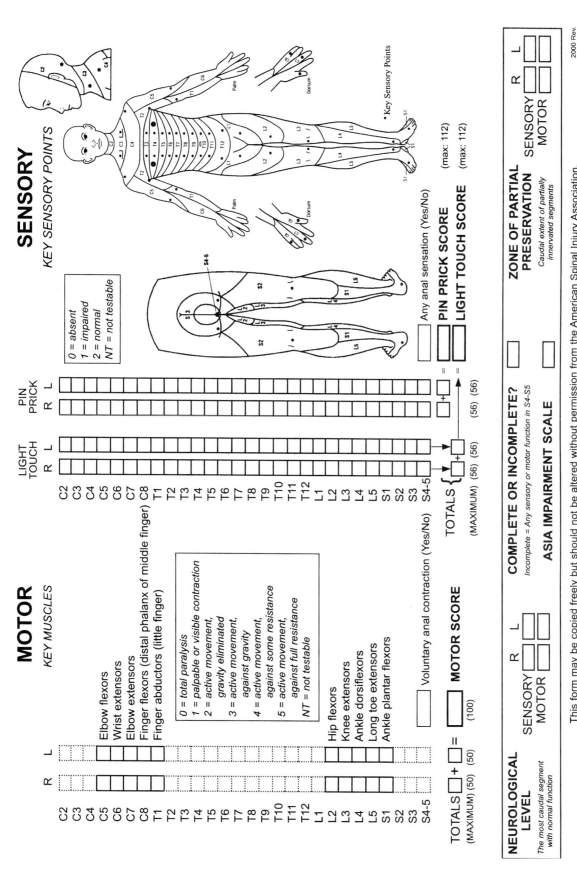

Figure 5–1: Dermatomal chart of lower extremities. Standard neurological classification of spinal cord injury. (American Spinal Injury Association 2002).

Box 5–1:	Test Key Muscles for Motor Strength

- L2, L3—Hip flexors
- L3, L4—Knee extensors
- L4, L5—Ankle dorsiflexors
- L5—Great toe dorsiflexor
- S1—Ankle plantar flexor

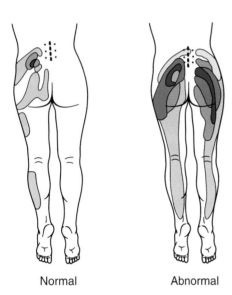

Normal   Abnormal

Figure 5–2: Pain referral patterns. Produced by intra-articular injections of hypertonic saline in asymptomatic (normal) and symptomatic (abnormal) patients. (Mooney V, Robertson J. (1976) Facet joint syndrome. Clin Orthop 115:149-156.)

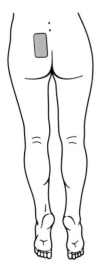

Figure 5–3: Primary referral pattern after provocative injection of the sacroiliac joint. (Fortin JD, Dwyer AP, West S, Pier J. (1994) Sacroiliac joint: pain referral maps upon applying a new injection/arthrography technique. Part I: asymptomatic volunteers. Spine 19:1475-1482.)

Exercise

- Exercise is the keystone to treatment of lower back pain.
- Adequate flexibility is believed to prevent excessive stress to the lower lumbar spine.
- Patients who are not physically fit may be more likely to have lower back pain.

Goals

- Attempt to centralize pain in the setting of radiculopathy.
- Strengthen lumbar extensors and abdominal flexor musculature.
- Strengthen weak muscles.
- Stretch tight muscles.
- Provide an aerobic program.
- Review and educate the patient on proper body mechanics.
- Evaluate ergonomics for home, work, and play.
- Address specific functional activities (e.g., ambulation, activities of daily living, homemaking).

Precautions

- Avoid the philosophy "no pain, no gain."
- Spinal stenosis and spondylolisthesis—Avoid excessive trunk extension.
- Osteoporosis—Avoid trunk flexion or rotation.

Pilates

- Developed by Joseph Pilates in the 1920s; incorporates Zen meditation and yoga
- Uses specialized resistive equipment to provide open and closed kinetic chain exercises
- Includes home-based program that uses a mat and gravity to strengthen and elongate muscles
- Increases joint proprioception, strengthens muscles, and increases flexibility
- Includes exercises for abdominal and trunk muscle strengthening, bridging, and spinal stabilization
- Reported to cause less muscle soreness than other forms of exercise

Transcutaneous Electric Nerve Stimulation (TENS)

- TENS is pulsed electric stimulation to the skin through electrodes attached to a small battery-powered device.
- The conventional mode uses 10-30 mA of current at a 50-100 Hz current. Amplitude can be varied.
- There are several theories of the mechanism of pain control.
  - The gate control theory states that the stimulation of large fibers (Aβ) activates the dorsal horn of the spinal cord to inhibit pain generated by small diameter, afferent nociceptive fibers (Aδ and C fibers).

- Electric stimulation may provoke the release of endogenous opiates.
- TENS is useful as an adjuvant method of pain control for back pain.

Acupuncture

- The technique of acupuncture was used for pain relief for centuries in Eastern cultures.
- The disruption of energy flow, or Qi, is thought to cause pain.
- Acupuncture involves the placement of solid needles at various points.
- The number of needle placements and treatments vary greatly among patients. Early responders have better success rates.
- The technique is effective in some patients.

Osteopathic Manipulation

- Osteopathic manipulation is performed by osteopathic physicians, specially trained physical therapists, and allopathic physicians.
- Manipulation is used as an adjuvant to conventional pain treatment.
- Nonthrusting manipulation techniques are presented in Table 5–1.
- High velocity, low amplitude techniques of spinal manipulation require experienced practioners and are contraindicated in certain conditions, including fracture and malignancy.
- Manipulation techniques may reduce the amount of medication required to treat back pain.
- Osteopathic manipulation has been shown to be effective in subacute injury.

Magnets

- There are two types of magnetic therapy—static and electromagnetic.
- Static magnets vary in strength from 300-5000 gauss.

Table 5–1:	Nonthrusting Manipulation Techniques	
TECHNIQUE	MECHANISM	METHOD
Soft tissue	Addresses soft tissue restrictions	Force is applied by kneading tissue, stretching, oscillating compression, and release.
Muscle energy	Approaches restrictive tissue directly; also known as contract-relax	The joint is held directly against the restrictive tissue and the patient moves from the barrier.
Myofascial release	Applies pressure to muscle, tendons, and fascia	The affected part is held in a position of ease; this is repeated until better range of motion or the restriction of motion is relieved.

- Electromagnetic therapy has been used to promote bone healing, wound healing, and sleep.
- Theories of action
  1. Magnets create an electromagnetic field that induces a mild current to stimulate nerve endings.
  2. Magnets decrease sensitivity of nociceptive fibers and increase localized blood flow.
- Magnets are available in unipolar and bipolar styles, arranged in various configurations, and made of different materials.
- Only one randomized, controlled study evaluating the effectiveness of magnets in the treatment of back pain has been done. It did not find magnets more effective than a placebo.

Intradiscal Electrothermal Anuloplasty (IDET)

- A flexible electrode is fluoroscopically guided percutaneously into the disk to coagulate the anulus fibrosus.
- IDET results in thermal destruction of nociceptive fibers.
- This procedure is not universally accepted. At least one study reports that patients have more than 50% pain reduction with this nonoperative technique.

Medications

Nonsteroidal Anti-Inflammatory Drugs (NSAIDs)

- NSAIDs block prostaglandin synthesis by reversible inhibition of cyclooxygenase.
- Prostaglandin E2 sensitizes nerve endings to bradykinin, histamine, and other inflammatory mediators.
- NSAIDs are effective in relieving mild to moderate pain.
- They can be used continuously short term to calm inflammation or on an as-needed basis for pain relief.
- NSAIDs are metabolized by the liver and excreted via the kidney.
- Patients who do not respond to one NSAID may respond to another.
- There is no additive effect with aspirin.
- Class side effects include gastrointestinal (GI) ulcers and renal failure (Table 5–2).

Tramadol

- Centrally acting synthetic opioid for moderate to severe pain
- Works through μ-receptor binding and weak inhibition of reuptake of serotonin and epinephrine
- Low risk of dependence
- Liver and renal excretion
- Dose: 50-400 mg daily
- Available as Ultracet with 37.5-mg tramadol and 325-mg acetaminophen

Table 5–2:	Examples of NSAIDS		
NAME	**DOSE**	**ADVANTAGES**	**SIDE EFFECTS**
Ibuprofen	400-3600 mg *per os* (PO) daily	Over the counter	GI side effects, renal insufficiency, liver toxicity
Diclofenac	Delayed or immediate release—50-150 mg PO daily Extended release—100 mg daily	Available in slow and immediate release formulations	Hepatotoxicity, GI side effects, renal insufficiency
Celecoxib cyclooxygenase-2 (COX-2) inhibitor	200-800 mg PO daily	COX-2 selective inhibitor; lower risk of GI complications, no antiplatelet activity	Fluid retention, renal toxicity, hepatic toxicity

Table 5–3:	Examples of Membrane Stabilizers		
NAME	**DOSE**	**ADVANTAGES**	**SIDE EFFECTS**
Carbamazepine	100-1200 mg PO daily	History of use with other pain disorders	Dizziness, nausea, drowsiness Rare—Aplastic anemia
Gabapentin	100-3600 mg PO daily	Minimal end-organ damage, can easily titrate	Dizziness, fatigue, peripheral edema, weight gain
Topiramate	12.5-400 mg PO daily		Fatigue, dizziness, somnolence, urinary calculi, weight loss Rare—Myopia, narrow angle glaucoma

- Use with caution with concurrent selective serotonin reuptake inhibitor (SSRI) or in patients with a history of seizures

Membrane Stabilizers

- Class of medications that are anticonvulsants
- Most useful for lancinating or burning pain associated with radiculopathy or neuropathy
- Unknown mechanism of action for pain relief
- Requires continuous use for effectiveness, and must be withdrawn slowly to prevent possible seizures (Table 5–3)

Antidepressants

- Tricyclic antidepressants are most effective for pain modulation (Table 5–4).
- Selective serotonin reuptake inhibitors have not been shown to be effective for back pain modulation.
  - They block the uptake of norepinephrine and serotonin into presynaptic nerve terminals.

- They are thought to act as sodium channel blockers of neuropathic pain.
- Doses for pain are lower and time of onset is faster than for depression.
- Side effects are anticholinergic symptoms and sedation.

Topical Medications

- Examples of topical medications are presented in Table 5–5.

Opiates (Table 5–6)

- Interact with receptors in the central nervous system and GI tract
- Most potent analgesic agents available
- Act at the μ receptors located in the substantia gelatinosa in the spinal cord
- Decrease the release of substance P, a potent modulator of pain perception
- Useful short-term relief to break the pain cycle and enable the patient to start physical therapy

Table 5–4:	Examples of Antidepressants	
NAME	**DOSE**	**SIDE EFFECTS**
Nortriptyline	10-375 PO mg daily	Sedation, hypotension, arrhythmias, confusion, anticholinergic side effects such as urinary retention and constipation
Amitriptyline[AU2]	25-250 mg daily	Sedation, nausea, arrhythmias, anticholinergic effects

Table 5–5:	Examples of Topical Medications		
NAME	**DOSE**	**ADVANTAGES**	**SIDE EFFECTS**
Lidoderm patch	Apply to affected area for a maximum of 12 hrs/day	Can be applied to desired area	Increased absorption with heat
Capsaicin cream	Apply cream to affected area	Available over the counter	Burning sensation

Table 5–6: Examples of Opiates

NAME	DOSE	ADVANTAGES	SIDE EFFECTS
Morphine sulfate	15-30 mg PO every 4 hours, titrate up as needed	Short- and long-acting formulations available respiratory depression	Sedation, dizziness, constipation, tolerance,
Oxycodone	5-10 mg PO every 12 hours, titrate up as needed	Short- and long-acting formulations available	
Fentanyl patch	25-150 mg every 72 hours	3-day dosing regimen, nonoral formulation, not for acute pain	

- Can be safely used in chronic conditions
- Available in short- and long-acting formulations such as pills, patches, and lollipops
- Can be titrated up slowly as necessary

Muscle Relaxants (Table 5–7)

- This nonhomogenous class of medications can be helpful for painful muscle spasms that may exist in the presence of muscle or nerve injury.
- All have sedative side effects and can be used to promote sleep.
- All have short half-lives and a dosage may need to be administered several times a day.

Injections

- Useful as diagnostic tool for facet or sacroiliac joint pain
  - Anesthetic agents may be injected into the joint cavity (intra-articular) on the affected side.
  - The patient performs pain provocative maneuvers after injection.
  - Relief of 50%-75% of pain is considered diagnostic.
  - The length of pain relief must correspond to the duration of anesthetic injected.
  - Injection is repeated a second time with a different duration anesthetic to decrease the false-positive rate.

Medial Branch Blocks

- These blocks include the medial branches of the L1-L4 dorsal rami and the L5 dorsal rami proper.
- The goal is to anesthetize the nociceptive fibers that innervate the facet joints.
- One must anesthetize two levels of the medial branch of the dorsal ramus for each facet joint evaluated; for example, the L3-L4 facet joint needs to have medial branch blocks at L3 and L4 (Fig. 5–4).

Facet Joint Injections

- This combination of steroids and anesthetic is injected at the most likely level based on pain patterns.
- The average time for relief is 3-4 months.
- Side effects of injections include hyperglycemia, dizziness, and localized hematoma.

Sacroiliac Injections (Fig. 5–5)

- Diagnostic injections are performed fluoroscopically with anesthetics of two different durations on separate occasions.
- A steroid and anesthetic combination may be therapeutic in some patients.

Epidural Injections

- Most effective in those with a radicular
- Must be performed under fluoroscopy for accurate placement
- Transforaminal approach (Fig. 5–6)
  - Advantage—Anesthetic and steroid are placed at the ventral aspect of the nerve root and can reach the ventral pain generators
  - Useful for disk herniations and foraminal stenosis with radiculopathy
  - Less risk of dural puncture
- Translaminar approach
  - Requires less injectate than the caudal approach
  - Injection site close to pathology
- Caudal approach
  - Reliable only up to the L5-S1 disk level
  - Requires large amounts of injectate

Table 5–7: Examples of Muscle Relaxants

NAME	DOSE	ACTION	SIDE EFFECTS
Cyclobenzaprine	10-60 mg PO daily	Chemically related to tricyclic antidepressants; primarily exerts effect centrally in the brain stem	Dizziness, drowsiness, central nervous system depression, anticholinergic effects, diarrhea
Diazepam	2-40 mg PO daily	True skeletal muscle relaxant	Sedation, fatigue, respiratory depression, hypotension
Tizanidine[AU3]	2-36 mg daily	Selective α blocker	Drowsiness, dizziness, dry mouth, hypotension

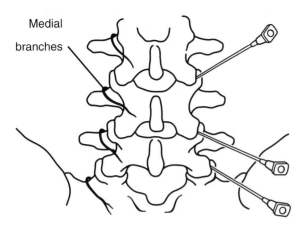

Figure 5–4: Posterior view of the lumbar spine, showing the location of the z-joints and their innervation by the medial branches of the dorsal rami.
On the left, needle positions for the L3 and L4 medial branch blocks used to anesthetize the L4/L5 z-joint are shown. On the right, needle positions for L3/L4, L4/L5, and L5/S1 intra-articular z-joint injections are shown. (Bogduk N. (1989) Back pain: zygaphysial blocks and epidural steroids. In: Neural Blockade in Clinical Anaesthesia and Management of Pain (Cousins MJ, Bridenbaugh PO, eds.), 2nd edition. Philadelphia: Lippincott, pp. 935-954.)

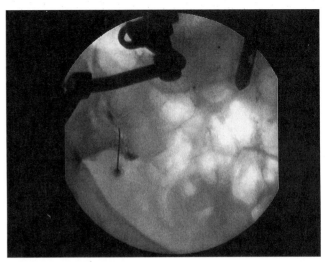

Figure 5–5: Left sacroiliac joint injection.

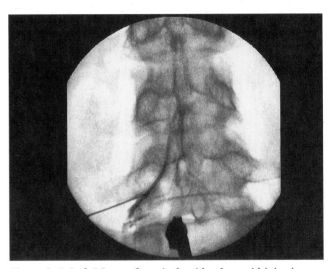

Figure 5–6: Left L5 transforaminal epidural steroid injection.

Trigger Points

- Trigger points are hyperirritable foci in muscles and fascia in areas of muscle tightness.
- Palpation produces referred pain.
- Trigger points can respond to a stretching program and the correction of dysfunctional postural mechanics.
- Injections with saline or a local anesthetic can be performed at the site of irritation.

References

Bogduk N, Karasek M. (2002) Two-year follow-up of a controlled trial of intradiscal electrothermal anuloplasty for chronic low back pain resulting from internal disc disruption. Spine J 2: 343-350.

This was a prospective cohort study that compared a conventional rehabilitation program with IDET for the treatment of low back pain. This study demonstrated approximately 50% pain reduction maintained over two years in more than half of the IDET treatment group.

Brosseau L, Milne S, Robinson V et al. (2002) Efficacy of the transcutaneous electrical nerve stimulation for the treatment of chronic low back pain: A meta-analysis. Spine. 27(6): 596-603.

Five studies with 419 patients enrolled found TENS did not statistically decrease low back pain. However, patients who used TENS reported that they felt better, had less pain, and were more satisfied with the care.

Dreyfuss P, Michaelson M, Pauza K et al. (1996) The value of medical history and physical examination in diagnosing sacroiliac joint pain. Spine 21: 2594-2602.

This prospective study evaluated 12 sacroiliac joint tests for their diagnostic usefulness. In the study, 85 patients were evaluated by 12 manual examinations and diagnostics blocks (68 unilateral blocks and 17 bilateral blocks). No exam or combination of tests increased the likelihood of a correct diagnosis with the exception of the diagnostic block.

Feldman DE, Rossignol M, Shrier I et al. (1999) Smoking: a risk factor for development of low back pain in adolescents. Spine 24: 2492-2496.

This was a prospective study that evaluated 810 high school students from Montreal, Canada. The association with low back pain increases with the amount of cigarettes smoked.

Leboeuf-Yde C. (2000) Body weight and low back pain. Spine 25: 226-237.

This was a systematic literature review of 56 journal articles reporting on 65 epidemiologic studies. Overall, this review reported a positive association between body weight and low back pain in 32% of the studies. Bias may be related to "the healthy worker effect," because obese people with low back pain are more likely to seek health care than nonobese people with similar pain.

Leboeuf-Yde C, Kyvik KO, Bruun NH. (1998) Low back pain and lifestyle; Part I: Smoking—Information from a population-based sample of 29,424 twins. Spine 23: 2207-2214.

Longworth W, McCarthy PW. (1997) A review of research on acupuncture for the treatment of lumbar disk protrusions and associated neurological symptomatology. J Alt Comp Med 3: 55-76.

Malanga GA, Nadler SF. (1999) Nonoperative treatment of low back pain. Mayo Clin Proc 74: 1135-1148.

McPartland J, Miller B. (1999) Bodywork therapy systems. Phys Med Rehab Clin N Am 10(3): 583-602.

Saal JA. (1996) Natural history and nonoperative treatment of lumbar disc herniation. Spine 21: 2S-9S.

Saal JS, Franson RC, Dobrow R et al. (1990) High levels of inflammatory phospholipase A2 activity in lumbar disc herniations. Spine 15: 674-678.

Vad VB, Bhat AL, Lutz GE et al. (2002) Transforaminal epidural steroid injections in lumbosacral radiculopathy: A prospective randomized study. Spine 27(1): 11-16.

Weinstein S, Herring S. (1993) Rehabilitation of the patient with low back pain. In: Rehabilitation Medicine: Principles and Practice (Delisa JA, ed.), 2nd edition. Philadelphia: JB Lippincott Co., pp. 996-1013.

This was a twin control method using a Danish register of 29,424 twins. The 3,751 monozygotic pairs demonstrated that the smoking monozygotic twin did not have more low back pain than the nonsmoking twin. This study did not show a causal link between low back pain and smoking.

A review article with information from many worldwide studies on the use of acupuncture. Acupuncture can be helpful for those who have had unsuccessful results with other conservative treatment. It is useful as an adjuvant therapy for sciatica and disk prolapse.

Summary article on conservative treatment of low back pain that covers patient history, physical, diagnostic studies, medications, modalities, therapeutic injections, and acupuncture.

A good review of various manual medicine techniques including osteopathic manipulation, movement therapies, and muscle energy.

This is a literature review article on lumbar disk herniation with an emphasis on nonoperative care. It highlights the prognostic factors of positive outcomes, describing favorable, unfavorable, and neutral factors in deciding which candidates are appropriate for nonoperative care.

This study demonstrated high levels of phospholipase A2 in human intervertebral disk material obtained from five patients. Phospholipase A2 is an enzyme responsible for liberating inflammatory mediators causing tissue and membrane injury. The histopathologic findings in this study focus on the biochemical basis of pain mediation in lumbar disk herniation.

Comparative study of transforaminal epidural steroid injections versus trigger point injections in 48 patients with radiculopathy because of a herniated disk. Of the patients in the steroid injection group, 84% had pain decreased by 50% and satisfaction for more than one year. Of the saline injection group, 48% had improvement.

This is a detailed chapter on low back pain rehabilitation presenting epidemiology, anatomy, biochemistry, diagnosis, and treatment options.

CHAPTER 6

Herniation of the Nucleus Pulposus in the Cervical, Thoracic, and Lumbar Spine

Matthew Rosen*, John M. Beiner §, Brian K. Kwon †, Jonathan N. Grauer ‡, and Alexander R. Vaccaro ‖

* B.A., Thomas Jefferson University College of Medicine, Philadelphia, PA

§M.D., B.S., Attending Surgeon, Connecticut Orthopaedic Specialists, Hospital of Saint Raphael; Clinical Instructor, Department of Orthopaedics, Yale University School of Medicine, New Haven, CT.

† M.D., Orthopaedic Spine Fellow, Department of Orthopaedic Surgery, Thomas Jefferson University and the Rothman Institute, Philadelphia, PA; Clinical Instructor, Combined Neurosurgical and Orthopaedic Spine Program, University of British Columbia; and Gowan and Michele Guest Neuroscience Canada Foundation/CIHR Research Fellow, International Collaboration on Repair Discoveries, University of British Columbia, Vancouver, Canada

‡ M.D., Assistant Professor, Co-Director Orthopaedic Spine Surgery, Yale-New Haven Hospital; Assistant Professor, Department of Orthopaedics, Yale University School of Medicine, New Haven, CT

‖ M.D., Professor of Orthopaedic Surgery, Thomas Jefferson University and the Rothman Institute, Philadelphia, PA

Anatomy and Physiology of the Intervertebral Disk (Fig. 6–1)

- Each disk consists of a nucleus pulposus and a surrounding anulus fibrosus (Table 6–1).
- The centrally located nucleus pulposus consists of collagenous and reticular fibers enmeshed in mucoid material.
- The anulus fibrosus, composed of concentric layers of fibrous connective tissue and fibrocartilage, retains the mucoid nucleus.
- The nucleus pulposus functions as a dynamic shock absorber, moving posterior with flexion of the vertebral column (either from sudden movement or chronic stress such as prolonged obesity).
- Structural deterioration begins in early adult life with dehydration, intradiscal fissuring, and fragmentation progressing to anular disruption and tearing with possible herniation.

Terminology

- The nomenclature of disk pathology has evolved over the last five decades from early reports because of newer imaging modalities (chiefly magnetic resonance imaging, or MRI) (Fig. 6–2).

Figure 6–1: Anatomy of the intervertebral disk.

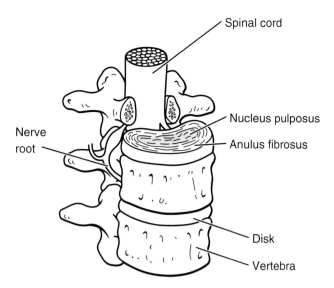

- Spinal cord
- Nucleus pulposus
- Anulus fibrosus
- Nerve root
- Disk
- Vertebra

- Terminology concerning herniation often differs across institutions (Table 6–2, Boxes 6–1 and 6–2).

Herniation of the Nucleus Pulposus in the Cervical Spine

Epidemiology

- Although all levels of the subaxial cervical spine (Box 6–3) may be affected, disk herniation (Fig. 6–3) most often involves the C5-C6 disk followed by the C6-C7 disk and the C4-C5 disk.
- People in the fourth decade of life are affected most often (Kelsey et al. 1984).
- Men outnumber women by a ratio of 1.4 to 1 (Kelsey et al. 1984).

- Proven factors associated with cervical disk herniation include the following (Kelsey et al. 1984):
  - Lifting heavy objects
  - Smoking cigarettes
  - Diving
- Possible, but unlikely, factors associated with cervical disk herniation include the following (Kelsey et al. 1984):
  - Operating or driving vibrating equipment (specific frequency is important)
  - Spending significant time driving automobiles

Clinical Presentation

- Acute—A history of trauma or specific episodes such as motor vehicle accidents, lifting, or pulling something (generally younger patients)
- Subacute or chronic—No such history (generally older patients)
- Symptoms (Table 6–3)
  - Neck pain
  - Stiffness
  - Shoulder, arm, or hand pain or paresthesia
  - Muscle weakness
- Symptoms can be generalized and diffuse in a mesodermal distribution or can be localized and specific with nerve root radiculopathy (sclerotomal distribution)(Figs. 6–3 and 6–4).
- Patients can also present the following with myelopathy and long tract findings:
  - Clumsiness
  - Clonus
  - Positive Hoffman's and Babinski's reflex
  - Hyperreflexia in lower and possibly upper extremities depending on the level of lesion
  - Gait or balance disturbance
- Other signs include the following:
  - Muscle atrophy
  - Weakness

Table 6–1:	Anatomy and Physiology of the Intervertebral Disk	
	NUCLEUS PULPOSUS	**ANULUS FIBROSIS**
Collagen content	Type II	Type I
Water content	High	Low
Proteoglycan content	High	Low
Pain fibers	No	Yes
Healing potential	No	Yes
Function	Load bearing	Structural containment of nucleus
	Load distribution to end plates and anulus	Transfer of load from compression to
	Shock absorption tension	
Comments	Inflammatogenic properties (when exposed to the extracellular environment)	Fibers perpendicular to each other to increase tensile strength
	Leukotactic	
	Increases vascular permeability	

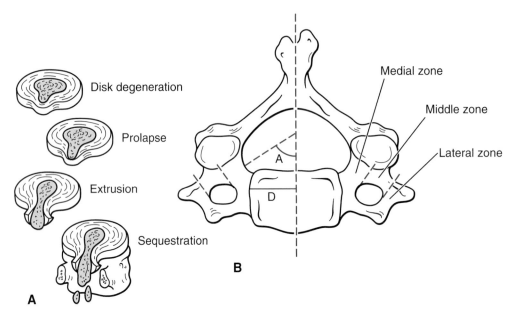

Figure 6–2: Herniated and cervical disks. **A,** Herniated disks may take the form of protrusion, extrusion, or sequestration. See the text for details. **B,** A cervical disk may impinge upon the nerve root at several zones.

Table 6–2:	Terminology of Disk Pathology*		
TERM	**DEFINITION**	**SYNONYMS**	**COMMENTS**
Normal	Disk does not protrude beyond vertebral end plates	Nonbulging	Incidence of abnormal findings in "normal" patients
Bulge	Circumferential, symmetric disk extension around the vertebral border	Prolapse	Usually <3 mm beyond end plates Can be a normal variant NOT a herniation
Protrusion	Focal or asymmetric extension of the disk beyond the vertebral border Disk origin broader than any dimension of the protrusion	Anulus involvement is generalized or broad based versus localized or focal based	
Extrusion	More extreme extension of the disk beyond the vertebral border Base of disk extrusion at the site of disk origin is narrower than the diameter of the extruding material Connection exists between the extruded material and the disk of origin	"Ruptured," though the term is ill-defined	
Sequestration	No connection between disk fragment and parent disk Intermediate signal on T1, increased signal on T2	Free fragment	May be difficult to determine presence or absence of connection between disk and fragment
Migration	Displacement of disk material from the site of extrusion	May or may not be sequestered	
Contained	Displaced disk is covered by outer anulus	"Subligamentous" refers to posterior longitudinal ligament (PLL) covering	Distinction may be hard even with modern MRI
Uncontained	Anulus covering is absent over displaced disk	May still be subligamentous, meaning under intact PLL	

* See Fig. 6–2, A.

<table>
<tr><td>

Box 6–1: **Definitions of Common Descriptive Terms***

- Internal disk derangement
  - Anular injury in an otherwise normal-appearing disk
- Anular tear
  - Anular disruption to the outer edge of the anulus
  - Thought to be related to low back pain that does not improve
  - After a "pop," a patient may feel relief of pain when the pressure in the disk is relieved
  - A.k.a. anular fissure; the term does not imply traumatic origin
- Anular rupture
  - Clearly defined traumatic origin (e.g., distraction injury)
- High intensity zone
  - High signal area on T2 MRI image usually involving the posteroinferior disk
  - Relation to anular tears and pain is controversial

_____

* (Fardon et al. 2001.)

</td></tr>
</table>

Box 6–2: **Nerve Root Terminology Associated with Disk Herniations**

- No contact
  - Normal fat signal surrounds the root on T1 images
- Contact without deviation
  - Nerve is not displaced but disk material abuts it
- Contact with deviation
  - Nerve root is displaced but not compressed
- Compression
  - Disk material compresses the nerve root against adjacent structures

Box 6–3: **Unique Anatomy of the Cervical Spine**

- The cervical spine can be distinguished from the rest of the vertebral column:
  - Cervical vertebrae contain foramina transversarium in each transverse process to allow passage of the vertebral arteries (except in C7, which 95% of the time contains smaller transversaria that only permit accessory vertebral veins) (Fig. 6-2, *B*).
- Each nerve root exits the spinal canal *above* the pedicle of its named vertebra.
- The nerve roots exit at an angle of approximately 90 degrees from the spinal cord.
- A herniated disk compresses the *exiting* nerve root in the cervical spine (e.g., a disk herniation at C5-C6 compresses the C6 nerve root) (Fig. 6–3)
- The first, second, and seventh thoracic vertebrae are atypical.

C1

- The atlas is a circular, ring-shaped bone.
- The superior facets articulate with the occipital condyles of the skull.
- The atlas has no spinous process or body, but it does have anterior and posterior arches (each with a tubercle and a lateral mass).

C2

- The second cervical vertebra, the axis, is the strongest cervical vertebra.
- The atlas rotates on two flat bearing surfaces of the axis, the superior articular facets.
- The dens is held in position by the transverse ligament of the atlas, thereby preventing horizontal displacement of C1.

C7

- The seventh cervical vertebra is called the vertebra prominens because of its long, nonbifid spinous process.
- C7 also has large transverse processes.

- Positive Lhermitte's sign—Cervical flexion–extension produces electric-like pain down the arm in a dermatomal pattern
- Positive Spurling's test—Rotation toward the side with the pain with extension of the neck, reproducing the radicular pain down the arm (Fig. 6–5)
- Often, a complete physical examination will allow relatively accurate diagnosis of the level affected (Fig. 6–4).

Imaging

- Radiography may show antero- or retrolisthesis, narrowed disk spaces, or osteophytes.
- Computed tomography (CT) gives the best detail of the bony overgrowth of joints of Luschka.
- MRI is the method of choice for diagnosing cervical disk herniations (Takhtani et al. 2002) (Fig. 6–6).
- Sagittal T2 weighted gradient-recalled echo imaging allows excellent visualization of an acute herniation (Takhtani et al. 2002, Scherping 2002)
- If the use of MRI is contraindicated (such as in pacemaker patients), myelography with postcontrast computed

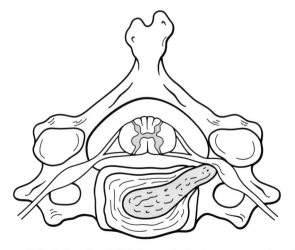

Figure 6–3: A herniated disk in cervical spine compressing the exiting nerve root.

Table 6–3: Cervical Disk Herniation Findings

LEVEL	NERVE ROOT COMPRESSED	SENSORY OR PAIN FINDINGS (FIG. 6–5)	MOTOR	REFLEX
C2-C3	C3	Mastoid process and dorsal surface of neck	None	None
C3-C4	C4	Dorsum of neck, levator scapulae, and along anterior chest	Diaphragm	None
C4-C5	C5	Lateral neck pain extending to the top of the shoulder Axial nerve involvement manifested as numbness in the medial deltoid	Deltoid, biceps	Biceps
C5-C6	C6	Pain along the side of the arm and forearm extending into thumb and index fingers Numbness over the tip of thumb and first interosseous muscle on the dorsum of the hand	Wrist extension	None
C6-C7	C7	Pain along the middle of the forearm extending into the middle, index, and ring fingers	Triceps	Triceps
C7-C8	C8	Pain radiating along the medial forearm extending to the ring and small fingers	Interossei	None

tomography scanning (Fig. 6–7) is recommended if cervical disk disease is suspected (Scherping 2002).
- Abnormality or herniation of a disk is not necessarily a symptomatic event (Table 6–4).

Treatment

Nonsurgical Methods

- Many patients with cervical disk herniations, with or without radiculopathy, can be treated without surgical intervention.
- Both traction and soft collars prevent extreme movement of the neck, thereby reducing nerve root compression.
- Nonsteroidal anti-inflammatory drugs and occasionally a short course of oral steroids (in older patients) may reduce the severity of symptoms.
- Physical therapy may alleviate patient discomfort, but it has not been shown to affect the long-term outcome.

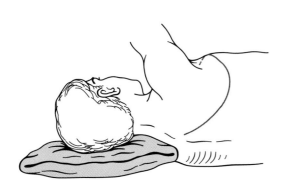

Figure 6–4: Anterior and posterior dermatomes corresponding to the cervical nerve root innervation. (Borenstein et al. 2004.)

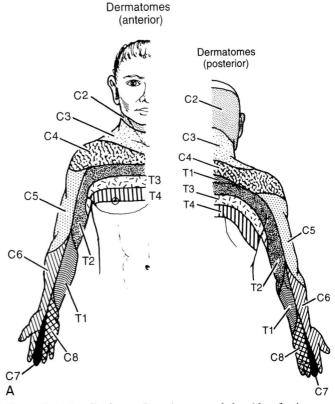

Figure 6–5: Spurling's test. Rotation toward the side of pain, with extension of the neck and sight downward pressure on the skull, reproduces the patient's radicular pain.

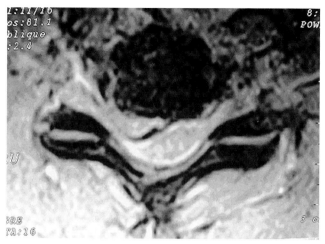

Figure 6–6: T2-weighted axial MRI. A right paracentral herniated cervical disk is impinging on the exiting nerve root and spinal cord.

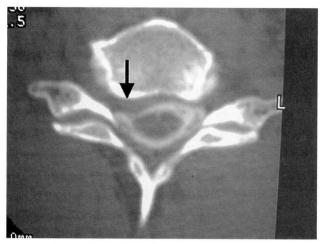

Figure 6–7: Myelography with postcontrast axial CT. Reveals a right paracentral herniated disk effacing the contrast in the cerebrospinal fluid but not compressing the spinal cord.

Surgical Methods

- If nonsurgical techniques fail, the patient with cervical disk herniation may be a candidate for surgical decompression of the affected nerve root.
- Historically, posterior foraminotomy or laminoforaminotomy was used to treat isolated radicular symptoms. These techniques allow indirect posterolateral decompression of the nerve root with little morbidity.
- Modern techniques of anterior discectomy have improved and are now the standard of care for herniated disks in the cervical spine (Table 6–5, Box 6–4).

Thoracic Spine (Box 6–5)

Epidemiology

- Symptomatic thoracic disk herniations are relatively rare—1 person in 1 million people per year (0.25%-0.75% of the total disk herniations).
- Thoracic disk herniations peak in the fourth through sixth decades.
- There is slight male predominance.

Table 6–4:	Abnormal Cervical Disk MRI Findings in Asymptomatic Subjects*			
AGE	ANY "MAJOR" ABNORMALITY	HERNIATED DISK	BULGING DISK	DEGENERATED DISK
<40	14%	10%	0%	25%
>40	28%	5%	3%	60%

* (Boden et al. 1990a.)

- Approximately 37% of patients report a history of trauma (Stillerman et al. 1998).
- Scheuermann's disease predisposes to thoracic disk herniations.
- Most common levels are T9-T12.
- Many thoracic disk herniations are asymptomatic (Box 6–6).

Clinical Presentation

- Patients with thoracic disk herniations present a variety of symptoms and signs, from pain, burning, numbness, and paresthesia to frank myelopathy and spinal cord dysfunction.
- The clinician must be aware that many potentially life-threatening medical causes of these symptoms exist (Table 6–6).
- Patients with symptomatic thoracic disk herniations seem to present three overlapping forms (Vanichkachorn et al. 2000).
  - **Predominantly axial pain**—Most (75%) patients will experience pain localized to the middle or lower thoracic region, which may radiate up or down in a nondermatomal pattern.
  - **Radicular pain**—Discomfort radiates to the front of the chest in a band-like dermatomal pattern (the T10 region is the most common) (Fig. 6–8).
  - **Myelopathy**—Motor impairment is found in 61% of patients, hyperreflexia and spasticity in 58%, sensory impairment in 61%, and bladder dysfunction in 24% (Stillerman et al. 1998).
- High thoracic disk herniations can produce symptoms or signs including the following:
  - Upper arm pain or radiculopathy
  - Horner's syndrome
- Often, the only truly objective finding is change in the pinwheel sensation along the back.

Table 6–5:	Surgical Approaches in the Treatment of Cervical Disk Disorders*			
APPROACH	**TECHNIQUE VARIATIONS**	**INDICATIONS**	**ADVANTAGES**	**DISADVANTAGES**
Anterior	Anterior cervical discectomy Anterior cervical discectomy, fusion	Disk herniation with symptomatic myelopathy or radiculopathy at one, two, or three levels	Avoids morbidity of posterior exposure Direct decompression of spinal nerve root Minimized intrusion into spinal canal	Risk of injury to esophagus, trachea, recurrent and superior laryngeal nerves Transient sore throat, difficulty swallowing are common Vertebral arteries are at risk, though uncommonly injured
Posterior	Posterior foraminotomy, laminoforaminotomy Laminaplasty Laminectomy, fusion Posterior cervical discectomy (abandoned)	Posterolateral disk herniation Failed anterior spinal surgery with radicular symptoms Multilevel cervical spondylosis **with lordotic sagittal alignment**	Causes less instability than anterior discectomy without fusion Allows multilevel decompression Avoids potential for injury to anterior structures (especially nerves to larynx)	Only indirectly decompresses nerve roots Postlaminectomy kyphosis is common with resection of >50% of facets without fusion Significant paraspinal muscle pain is common (because of extensive dissection of paraspinal muscles) Multilevel decompressions must be lordotic to allow the cord to float back

* (Rushton et al. 1998, Narayan 2001.)

Natural History

- Similar to the case in the cervical and lumbar spine, many patients will get better with nonoperative treatment.
- Stillerman et al. (1998) reported that 0.2%-1.8% of all symptomatic herniations are treated surgically each year.
- Younger patients presenting an acute soft disk herniation related to an acute traumatic event will often experience pain, myelopathic symptoms, or both, prompting surgical intervention.
- Older patients with a longer duration of symptoms representing degenerative disk bulges or herniations will more often than not get better without surgery.

Box 6–4: Anterior Cervical Discectomy: Is Fusion Necessary?

- Most surgeons now routinely include an interbody fusion with structural bone graft when doing an anterior cervical discectomy. Reasons for this include the following:
  - Restoring sagittal lordosis
  - Increasing height of intervertebral foramen by distraction
  - Stabilization of the motion segment to decrease inflammation and nerve irritation
  - Faster relief of radiculopathy
- Some neurosurgeons, however, advocate disk excision without arthrodesis (Sonntag et al. 1996, Dowd et al. 1999). Arguments include the following:
  - No graft-related and fewer overall complications
  - Faster operative times with less blood loss
  - Faster recovery time and return to work
  - No clinical or psychological issues with graft healing or pseudarthrosis

---

Box 6–5: Unique Anatomy of the Thoracic Spine

- The thoracic spine has several features that distinguish it from the cervical and lumbar regions:
  - Rigid zone secondary to the rib cage
  - Vertically oriented facets (permit lateral bending and rotation but little flexion or extension)
  - A spinal cord/canal ratio of only 40% (smaller than cervical and lumbar)
  - Dentate ligaments that connect spinal cord and nerve roots—tether cord to anterior structures, more sensitive to ventral compression
  - Kyphosis that drape cord over anterior elements
- The blood supply to the thoracic spinal cord is less redundant than in the cervical or lumbar regions (Dommisse 1974):
  - One anterior and two posterior longitudinal arteries
  - Segmental vessels
  - Artery of Adamkiewicz—usually T9-T11, left-sided
  - A particularly tenuous cervicothoracic junction blood supply; the spinal cord from T4-T9 is very sensitive to injury

Box 6–6:	**Abnormal Thoracic Disk MRI Findings in Asymptomatic Subjects***

- 90 asymptomatic subjects
- 73% had one or more abnormal disks on MRI scans
- 37% had disk herniations
- 20 patients followed for 26 months; no patient became symptomatic
  - Large herniations were resorbed
  - Small herniations were unchanged or increased in size

* (Wood et al. 1995.)

Location of Thoracic Disk Herniations

- Disk herniations in the thoracic spine may be central, centrolateral, and lateral (Stillerman et al. 1998).
  - 94% were centrolateral—more likely to produce myelopathy.
  - 6% were lateral—more commonly present with radicular symptoms.
  - 65% of patients showed evidence of calcification.
  - 7% intradural extension was noted at surgery.
  - 14% were found to have multiple herniations.

Diagnostic Imaging

- Plain radiographs—Intradiscal calcification (Fig. 6–9)
- MRI—A combination of T1- and T2-weighted images in the sagittal and axial planes revealing disk material bulging posteriorly or laterally into the spinal canal

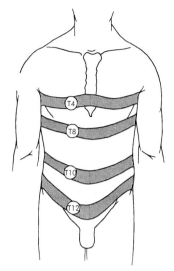

Figure 6–8: Sensory dermatomes thoracic spine. (Williams et al. 2003.)

- CT myelography—Used less in the thoracic spine but an important modality for determining the extent of canal compromise in those patients with equivocal MRI scans or those in whom MRI scanning is not possible (e.g., pacemakers) (Fig. 6–10)

Nonsurgical Treatment

- Initial management—Nonsteroidal anti-inflammatory medication, activity modification, and a short course of hyperextension bracing may be beneficial (severe cases in older patients may warrant a short taper of oral steroids).
- Once symptoms have partially subsided—Use physiotherapy with modalities; a range of motion, flexibility, and strengthening of erector spinae; then aerobic conditioning.
- Steroid injections—Epidurals not routinely used, but selective nerve root injections offer good symptomatic relief.

Surgical Indications

- Myelopathic symptoms or signs
- Persistent radicular pain unresponsive to conservative therapy (for at least 4-6 weeks) with imaging consistent with clinical findings
- Axial pain—Controversial; surgical treatment is less likely to relieve back pain than radicular symptoms or myelopathy

Surgical Treatment

- The sensitivity of the thoracic spinal cord to injury (see Box 6–5) limits the ability of the surgeon to gain access to the disk space from the traditional posterior approaches used in the lumbar spine.
- Anterior and lateral approaches have been developed that limit dissection of the cord from the herniated disk (Table 6–7, Box 6–7).

Table 6–6:	**Differential Diagnosis of Thoracic Pain***

NONSPINAL CAUSES	SPINAL CAUSES
Cardiovascular	Infection
Pulmonary	Neoplastic
Neoplastic	Primary
Hepatobiliary	Metastatic
Gastrointestinal	Degenerative
Retroperitoneal	Spondylosis
Polymyalgia rheumatica	Spinal stenosis
Fibromyalgia	Facet syndrome
Rib fractures	Disk disease
Intercostal neuralgia	Costochondritis
	Metabolic
	Osteoporosis
	Osteomalacia
	Deformity
	Kyphosis
	Scoliosis
	Trauma
	Neurogenic
	Herniation
	Spinal cord neoplasm
	Arteriovenous malformation
	Inflammatory (herpes zoster)

* (Adapted from Vanichkachorn et al. 2000.)

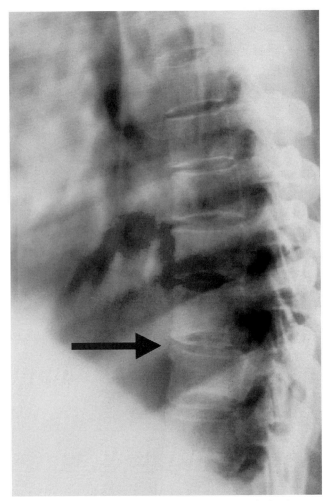

Figure 6–9: Radiograph showing thoracic disk calcification.

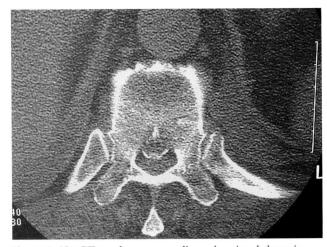

Figure 6–10: CT myelogram revealing a herniated thoracic disk.

- Results of thoracic discectomy are generally good, in terms of both pain relief and recovery of motor function in those patients with myelopathy (Bohlman et al. 1988, Simpson et al. 1993).
- The overall complication rate for thoracic discectomy is 15% (Stillerman et al. 1998).
  - Major—Death, permanent neurological deterioration, medical complications, need for reoperation
  - Minor—Neuralgia, pneumothorax, continued pain, wound infection

Lumbar Spine

- A symptomatic lumbar disk herniation occurs during the lifetime of 2% of the general population.
- Risk factors for sustaining a lumbar herniated disk include the following:
  - Male gender
  - Age 30-50
  - Heavy lifting, especially in a twisting motion
  - Poor job satisfaction or low income
  - Cigarette smoking
  - Prolonged vibration exposure
- Of lumbar disk protrusions, 90%-95% are observed at the L4-L5 or L5-S1 level.
- Not all disk pathology has clinical importance (Table 6–8).

Clinical Presentation

- Usually, in mild or moderate disk herniations, patients first notice lower back pain corresponding to anular pressure and fissuring.
- This can progress to frank tears in the anulus and herniation of inflammatogenic material; the severity of the lower back pain may lessen, but a radiculopathy in the form of pain, paresthesia, or weakness can appear because of pressure on the nerve root.
- With severe herniations, the patient may experience immediate lower extremity pain with little or no lower back involvement.
- Lower back pain will be intermittent and is often brought on by physical activity and made worse by prolonged sitting, moving from a seated to a standing position, or bending and twisting (each of these movements increases lumbar disk pressure).
- In patients experiencing herniation of lumbar disks with radiculopathy, Valsalva maneuvers may exacerbate pain in the lower extremity (Box 6–8).

Diagnosis–Clinical Exam

- Posture—Standing (sitting hurts); a possible spasm causes a pseudoscoliotic list to one side or a straightening of the lumbar lordosis.

Table 6–7: Surgical Approaches for Thoracic Disk Herniations

SURGICAL APPROACH	VARIATIONS	INDICATIONS	ADVANTAGES	DISADVANTAGES

Anterior	Transsternal
	Thoracotomy or
	  transthoracic
	Detachment of diaphragm
	  for access to lower levels
		Central or centrolateral disks
		Transsternal T1-T4
		T4-T12 rib resection or
		  rib-splitting
			Excellent midline exposure
			Multiple levels accessible
			Facilitates instrumentation
				Violates pleura
				Significant perioperations
				  Morbidity
				Diaphragm takedown
				  significantly slows recovery

Posterior	Laminectomy (abandoned)
	Pediculofacetectomy
	Transfacet pedicle-sparing
		Lateral, some centrolateral
		  disks
		Upper thoracic spine
			Avoids morbidity of
			  thoracotomy
				Limited visualization of disk
				Access not possible to
				  midline or intradural disks
				Higher incidence of segmental
				  instability, pain

Lateral	Extracavitary
	Costotransversectomy
		Lateral or centrolateral disks	Pleura is not violated—less
			  morbidity, etc.
			Diaphragm remains intact
				Technically difficult
				Relatively large posterior
				  dissection
				Complete anterior decompression
				  is difficult

Video-assisted
  thoracoscopic surgery
	Conversion to open
	  always possible
		Lateral or centrolateral disks	Avoids morbidity of
			  thoracotomy
			Avoids posterior muscle,
			  bone dissection
			Shorter ICU stays,
			  rapid recovery
				Increased operative time
				Steep learning curve
				Limited decompression, no
				  ability to instrument
				High incidence of intercostal
				  neuralgia or visceral injury

Box 6–7: Role of Arthrodesis in Thoracic Disk Herniations

- Anatomy
  - Rib cage stability may make fusion unnecessary
- Relative indications
  - Scheuermann's kyphosis patients (prone to further kyphosis)
  - Lower levels (rib cage stability not present)
  - Partial corpectomy performed to access disk
  - Multiple levels removed
- Advantages
  - Low morbidity, easy to perform
  - Increases stability to prevent collapse (controversial)
- Disadvantages
  - Requires bone graft (autograft or allograft) unless rib can be used
  - Slightly longer operative time
- Instrumentation (used almost exclusively for lower levels)
  - Increases cost and operative time
  - Provides stability at a high-stress junctional zone

Table 6–8: Abnormal Lumbar Disk MRI Findings in Asymptomatic Subjects*

AGE	HERNIATED DISK	BULGING DISK	DEGENERATED DISK
20-39	21%	56%	34%
40-59	22%	50%	59%
60-80	36%	79%	93%

* (Boden et al. 1990b.)

- Heel and toe gait should be observed to detect weakness of L5 or S1 (see Figs. 6–11 and 6–12).
- Tension signs are useful in diagnosing a lumbar disk herniation; a straight leg raise (SLR) in patients under 35 is specific and sensitive to a symptomatic disk herniation.
- Maximal tension is created in the sciatic nerve and transmitted to the nerve roots between 35 and 70 degrees of leg elevation.
- For a true, positive SLR, patients should experience radicular pain or paresthesia below the knee within the leg elevation range above (Fig. 6–11).

Box 6–8: Lumbar Disk Herniation and Cauda Equina Syndrome*

- Typically large midline herniations in older patients with spinal stenosis
- 1-2.4% of symptomatic lumbar disk herniations
- Symptoms or signs
  - Bowel or bladder difficulties
  - Saddle anesthesia
  - Diminished rectal tone
  - Lower extremity sensory and motor deficits
- Should be treated as a surgical emergency; decompression within 48 hours provides best outcome

* (Ahn et al. 2000.)

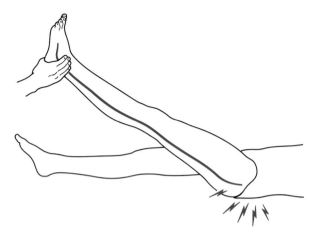

Figure 6–11: L5 nerve root functions.

- Femoral stretch testing (performed by extending the hip with a bent knee and with the patient prone) can reproduce radicular pain from compression of a higher lumbar root (L2-L4).
- The following Waddell signs should be noted:
  - Nonanatomic distribution of pain or tenderness to light touch
  - Low back pain when standing with a downward force on the head
  - Change in findings with posture, distraction, etc. (e.g., SLR)
  - Overreaction or symptom magnification

Figure 6–12: S1 nerve root functions.

Motor and Sensory Examination

- See Figs. 6–11, 6–13 and 6–14 for L4, L5, and S1 nerve functions.

Localization of Lumbar Disk Herniation

- A neurologic physical examination can help determine the likely location of a herniated lumbar disk.
- Several classification systems exist for describing where a disk herniation occurs.
- Wiltse et al. (1997) proposed an anatomic system familiar to most surgeons (Figs. 6–15 and 6–16).

Anatomic Features of the Lumbar Spine

- Lumbar roots exit the dural sac at an acute angle and travel inferiorly to exit under the pedicle of the vertebral body (Fig. 6–17).
- Depending on the location of the disk herniation, pressure may be exerted on the *exiting* or the *traversing* nerve root.
- Only far-lateral or extraforaminal disk herniations should exert pressure on the *exiting* nerve root

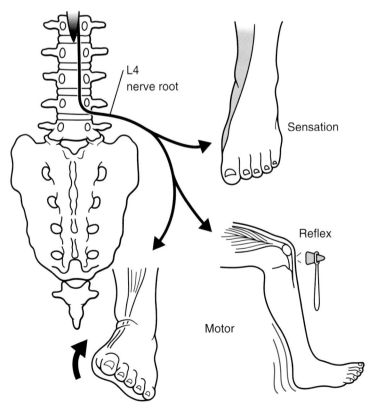

L4 nerve root

Sensation

Reflex

Motor

Tibialis anterior muscle

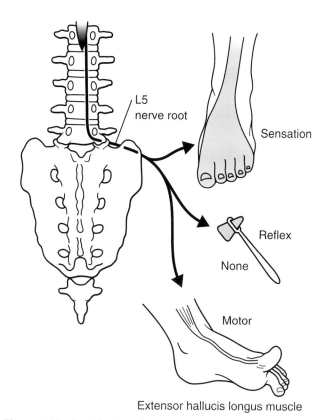

Figure 6–13: Straight leg raise to test nerve tension.

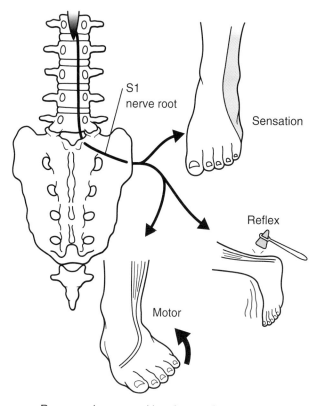

Figure 6–14: L4 nerve root functions.

- (e.g., an extraforaminal disk herniation at L4-L5 may compress the L4 nerve root) (Fig. 6–18).
- Central, posterolateral, subarticular, or foraminal lumbar disk herniations will compress the *traversing* nerve root (e.g., a foraminal disk herniation at L4-L5 will compress the L5 nerve root) (Fig. 6–19, Box 6–9).

Treatment

Nonsurgical Treatment

- Initial therapy consists of the following:
  - Bed rest for 1-3 days only
  - Nonsteroidal anti-inflammatory medications
  - Judicious and sparing use of stronger analgesics or muscle relaxants
  - Progressive return to normal activity; both extremes of continued bed rest and rapid strenuous physical activity or physiotherapy have been shown to worsen symptoms
- Oral steroids can provide symptomatic relief for leg pain more than for back pain because of acute inflammation of a nerve root.

- Steroid use in patients under 50 must be weighed against the potential for avascular necrosis of the hip and other side effects.
- Epidural steroids—Randomized clinical trials and meta-analysis indicate short-term improvement, but long-term relief is lacking (Watts et al. 1995).
- Manipulative therapy and physiotherapy have been found equivalent to medical management (medication or activity modification) of lumbar disk herniation in terms of significant short-term pain relief compared with a placebo, but there has been no proven long-term benefit.

Surgical Treatment

- See Table 6–9 and Box 6–10 for surgical treatment.
- The following are positive predictive factors (preoperatively) in lumbar disk surgery:
  - No worker's compensation claim
  - Nonsmoker
  - Absence of back pain
  - Pain extending to the foot (true radicular pain)
  - Positive SLR
  - Larger herniation
  - Good social support system

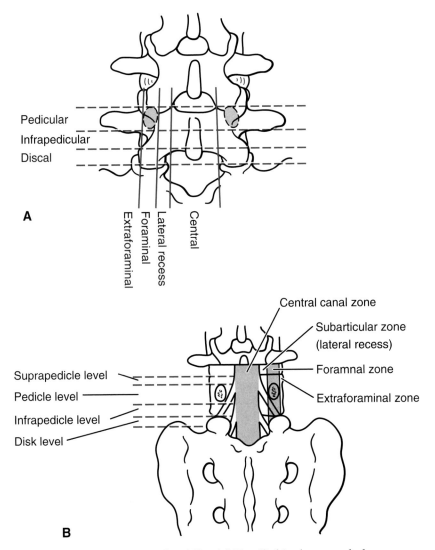

Pedicular

Infrapedicular

Discal

Extraforaminal
Foraminal
Lateral recess
Central

A

Central canal zone

Subarticular zone
(lateral recess)

Foramnal zone

Extraforaminal zone

Suprapedicle level

Pedicle level

Infrapedicle level

Disk level

B

Figure 6–15: Anatomic "zones" and "levels" identified in the coronal plane.

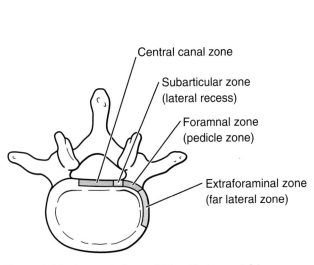

Central canal zone

Subarticular zone
(lateral recess)

Foramnal zone
(pedicle zone)

Extraforaminal zone
(far lateral zone)

Figure 6–16: Anatomic "zones" identified on axial images.

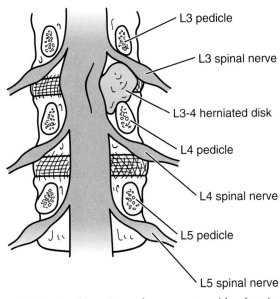

L3 pedicle

L3 spinal nerve

L3-4 herniated disk

L4 pedicle

L4 spinal nerve

L5 pedicle

L5 spinal nerve

Figure 6–17: Cauda equina and nerve roots with a herniated disk.

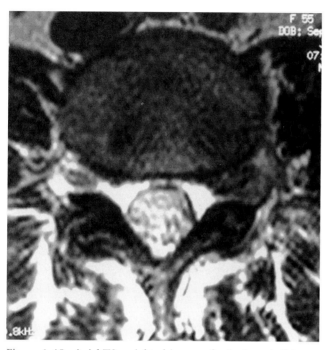

Figure 6–18: Axial T2-weighted image of a far-lateral disk herniation compressing the exiting nerve root.

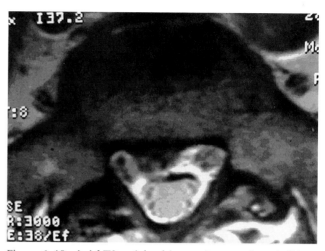

Figure 6–19: Axial T2-weighted image. A posterolateral disk herniation causing effacement of the surrounding fat and partial displacement the traversing nerve root.

Box 6–9: **Natural History of Lumbar Disk Herniations***

This was a prospective, randomized trial of nonoperative treatment versus surgical discectomy for isolated lumbar disk herniations. All patients that "beyond doubt required surgical therapy" and those with "no indication for operative intervention" were excluded from the randomized group and results.

- Nonsurgical
  - 25% were cured, 36% improved significantly.
  - Therefore, these 60% would have had unnecessary surgery if all went to operation.
  - On the flip side, the 40% of patients who needed surgery would suffer for months if all were required to wait for operative intervention.
  - Three months were sufficient to decide.
- Surgical
  - Significantly better outcomes occurred at a follow-up of one year.
  - Insignificantly better outcomes occurred at four years.
  - Only minor changes took place in patients during the last six years of observation.

* (Weber 1983.)

Table 6–9: **Comparison of Techniques for Lumbar Discectomy**

TECHNIQUE	PROS	CONS
Open discectomy	Standard of care Better visualization of nerve	More muscle dissection Longer hospital stay, increased pain Potential for iatrogenic instability
Open microdiscectomy	Becoming more standard Limits muscle damage Decreased pain Headlamps, loupe magnification commonly available	Limited visualization of nerve Potential for nerve injury because of smaller incision size
Microscope-assisted discectomy	Limited muscle dissection Better lighting, magnification Potentially shorter inpatient stays, less time off work, better results reported by some authors	Increased time, cost Equipment may not be available
Percutaneous discectomy	Muscle dissection limited to portals Theoretically less morbidity, blood loss, etc.	Increased cost Steep learning curve Longer operative time

Box 6–10:	Indications for Operative Disk Excision

- A general review of the literature can provide the following indications for surgical intervention:
  - Major or progressive muscle weakness
  - Symptoms or signs of cauda equina syndrome
  - Radiculopathy and severe pain unrelieved by conservative management and persisting at least 4-6 weeks
- Evidence exists that pain and radiculopathy that persist more than six months can develop into chronic nerve pain poorly treated even with surgical intervention at that point. Some authors believe, therefore, that a window of opportunity for surgical treatment is present in the face of persistent pain or radicular findings.

References

Ahn UM, Ahn NU, Buchowski JM et al. (2000) Cauda equina syndrome secondary to lumbar disk herniation: A meta-analysis of surgical outcomes. Spine 25: 1515-1522.

> Pooled outcomes were analyzed in 322 patients. There was a significant advantage to treating patients within 48 hours versus more than 48 hours after the onset of cauda equina syndrome. A significant improvement in sensory and motor deficits and in urinary and rectal function occurred in patients who underwent decompression within 48 hours versus after 48 hours. Older age and pre–existing bowel or bladder dysfunction were associated with worse outcomes.

Boden SD, McCowin PR, Davis DO et al. (1990a) Abnormal magnetic-resonance scans of the cervical spine in asymptomatic subjects. A prospective investigation. J Bone Joint Surg Am 72:1178-1184.

> MRI scans of 63 volunteers with no history of symptoms indicative of cervical disease and 37 patients with asymptomatic lesion of the cervical spine were mixed randomly and studied by 3 independent neurologists. The scans were interpreted as demonstrating an abnormality in 19% of the asymptomatic subjects; 14% of those less than 40 years old and 28% of those older than 40. Of the subjects less than 40, 10% had a HNP and 4% had foraminal stenosis. Of the subjects older than 40, 5% had a HNP, 3% bulging of the disk, and 20% foraminal stenosis. The disk was degenerated or narrowed at one level in more than 25% of the subjects less than 40 and in almost 60% of those who were older than 40. The prevalence of abnormal MRI's of the cervical spine as related in age to asymptomatic individuals emphasizes the dangers of predicting operative decisions on diagnostic tests without precisely matching those findings with clinical signs and symptoms.

Boden SD, Davis DO, Dina TS et al. (1990b) Abnormal magnetic-resonance scans of the lumbar spine in asymptomatic subjects. A prospective investigation. J Bone Joint Surg Am 72:403-408.

Bohlman HH, Zdeblick TA. (1988) Anterior excision of herniated thoracic discs. JBJS 70: 1038-1047.

> MRI scans of 63 volunteers with no history of symptoms indicative of cervical disease and 37 patients with asymptomatic lesion of the cervical spine were mixed randomly and studied by 3 independent neurologists. The scans were interpreted as demonstrating an abnormality in 19% of the asymptomatic subjects; 14% of those less than 40 years old and 28% of those older than 40. Of the subjects less than 40, 10% had a HNP and 4% had foraminal stenosis. Of the subjects older than 40, 5% had a HNP, 3% bulging of the disk, and 20% foraminal stenosis. The disk was degenerated or narrowed at one level in more than 25% of the subjects less than 40 and in almost 60% of those who were older than 40. The prevalence of abnormal MRI's of the cervical spine as related in age to asymptomatic individuals emphasizes the dangers of predicting operative decisions on diagnostic tests without precisely matching those findings with clinical signs and symptoms.

> The authors treated 22 thoracic disk herniations in 19 patients with excision using an anterior transthoracic decompression or a costotransversectomy, and they reported a 48-month follow-up. Of the patients, 16 had an excellent or a good result, 1 had a fair result, and 2 had a poor result. Of the 14 patients who had had motor weakness preoperatively, 12 had varying degrees of improvement in motor function postoperatively. Pain was relieved or reduced in 18 patients. The authors conclude that although the results were good, the procedure is associated with some risk of damage to the spinal cord. It therefore requires meticulous preoperative planning and careful surgical technique.

Borenstein DG, Wiesel SW, Boden SD, eds. (2004) Low Back and Neck Pain: Comprehensive Diagnosis and Management, 3rd edition. Philadelphia: Saunders.

Dommisse GF. (1974) The blood supply to the spinal cord: A critical vascular zone in spinal surgery. JBJS 56B: 225-235.

> The author studied cadavers and radiographs of patients to outline the normal variants of the blood supply to the spinal cord. Descriptions of three longitudinal vessels, the differential metabolic demands of grey and white matter, and the radicular arteries reinforcing the longitudinal arterial channels at various levels, including the artery of Adamkiewicz, are presented.

Dowd GC, Wirth FP. (1999) Anterior cervical discectomy: Is fusion necessary? J Neurosurg (Spine 1) 90: 8-12.

> A prospective, randomized trial of anterior cervical discectomy with and without fusion found no difference in patient satisfaction and return to preoperative activity levels. Though the fusion rate was higher in the fusion group, this did not correlate with the outcome. The authors suggest that the addition of fusion to the procedure may be unnecessary.

Fardon DF, Milette PC. (2001) Nomenclature and classification of lumbar disk pathology: Recommendations of the combined task forces of the North American Spine Society, American Society of Spine Radiology, and American Society of Neuroradiology. Spine 26: E93-E113.

> This work represents the collaborative efforts of the three societies, offering recommendations for standardized nomenclature involving disk pathology in the lumbar spine.

Kelsey J, Githens PB, Walter SD et al. (1984) An epidemiology study of acute prolapsed cervical intervertebral discs. J Bone Joint Surg Am 66(6): 907-914.

> The authors conducted an epidemiological study in a patient population of acute prolapsed cervical disks. It was concluded

that individuals in the fifth decade were more likely to experience cervical disk herniation, and men were more likely to be affected than women. Factors that may contribute to the development of the condition were also described.

Narayan P, Haid RW. (2001) Treatment of degenerative cervical disk disease. Neurol Clin 19: 217-229.

The article explains both the surgical and the nonoperative approaches to the treatment of various types of cervical disk disease. Information regarding the radiologic evaluation of each abnormality is also given. The article focuses on the treatment of cervical disk disease to relieve any associated radiculopathy or myelopathy.

Rushton SA, Albert TJ. (1998) Cervical degenerative disease: Rationale for selecting the appropriate fusion technique (anterior, posterior, and 360 degrees). Ortho Clin N Am 29: 755-777.

This article reviews the rationale and indications for various spinal surgery techniques. Success rates for various procedures, as well as the results and complications associated with each, are described.

Scherping SC. (2002) Cervical disk disease in the athlete. Clin Sports Med 21: 37-47.

This article reviews cervical disk disease and presents information on clinical presentation, imaging and diagnosis, and management. Although the article concludes with information regarding the management of cervical disk disease in the athlete, much of the article is concerned with general cervical spine abnormalities.

Simpson JM, Silveri CP, Simeone FA et al. (1993) Thoracic disk herniation: Reevaluation of the posterior approach using a modified costotransversectomy. Spine 18: 1872-1877.

Using a posterolateral approach (costotransversectomy or transpedicular), 23 thoracic disk herniations were decompressed with a follow-up averaging 58 months. An excellent or good result was achieved in 16 patients; 3 patients had a fair result. There were no poor results. All 6 patients with significant preoperative lower extremity weakness improved. Pain was relieved in 16 patients and reduced in 3. There were no significant neurologic complications associated with the procedure. The authors conclude that posterolateral decompression for thoracic disk herniation remains a viable alternative without the inherent risk and morbidity of a transthoracic approach.

Sonntag VKH, Klara P (1996) Is fusion necessary after anterior cervical discectomy? Spine 21: 1111-1113.

Sonntag and Klara express opposing views on the need for fusion after discectomy and support their perspectives with clinical experience and a review of the pathoanatomy of disk disease. Sonntag believes that most patients are well served with discectomy alone, avoiding the complications of graft harvest and potential nonunion. Klara thinks that the interposed graft restores foraminal height and maintains cervical lordosis, both of which are important to a good outcome.

Stillerman CB, Chen TC, Couldwell WT et al. (1998) Experience in the surgical management of 82 symptomatic herniated thoracic discs and review of the literature. J Neurosurg 88: 623-33.

The authors surgically treated 71 patients with 82 herniated thoracic disks. The most common sites of disk herniation

requiring surgery were from T8 to T11. Evidence of antecedent trauma was present in 37% of the patients; 94% were centrolateral and 6% were lateral. Evidence of calcification was present in 65% of patients, and in 7% intradural extension was noted at surgery. The authors found that 10 patients (14%) had multiple herniations. Four surgical approaches were used for the removal of these 82 disk herniations: transthoracic in 49 (60%), transfacet pedicle-sparing in 23 (28%), lateral extracavitary in 8 (10%), and transpedicular in 2 (2%). Postoperative evaluation revealed improvement or resolution of pain in 47 (87%) of 54, hyperreflexia and spasticity in 39 (95%) of 41, sensory changes in 36 (84%) of 43, bowel or bladder dysfunction in 13 (76%) of 17, and motor impairment in 25 (58%) of 43. Complications occurred in 12 (14.6%) of the 82 disks treated surgically. Major complications were seen in 3 patients and included perioperative death from cardiopulmonary compromise, instability requiring further surgery, and an increase in the severity of a preoperative paraparesis.

Takhtani D, Melhem ER. (2002) MR imaging in cervical spine trauma. Clin Sports Med 21: 49-75.

A review of the continuous improvements in MRI as it applies to spine surgery. The specific types of MRI sequence appropriate for various spinal conditions are described.

Vanichkachorn JS, Vaccaro AR. (2000) Thoracic disk disease: Diagnosis and treatment. JAAOS 8: 59-169.

This is a review of the anatomy, epidemiology, clinical presentation, imaging, natural history, and treatment of thoracic disk disease. The authors emphasize the natural tendency of these patients to improve with nonsurgical care, give indications for operative intervention, and explain the relative merits of the various surgical approaches in terms of outcome and complications.

Watts RW, Silagy CA. (1995) A meta-analysis on the efficacy of epidural corticosteroids in the treatment of sciatica. Anesth Intensive Care 23: 564-569.

This meta-analysis included 907 pooled patients. Significant pain relief (75% on average) occurred in patients treated with epidural steroid injections for the treatment of sciatica. Short-term results were significantly different than controls.

Weber H. (1983) Lumbar disk herniation: A controlled, prospective study with ten years of observation. Spine 8: 131-140.

In this study, 126 patients with uncertain indications for surgical treatment had treatment chosen by randomization in surgical or nonsurgical management. Statistically better outcomes were reported in the surgical group at one year, less difference was seen at four years, and no real changes in the last six years were observed. A high crossover rate, imprecise definitions of nonsurgical care, and author-evaluated outcomes are criticisms of this article. The author concludes that it is safe to wait on uncomplicated lumbar disk herniations because many patients get better without surgery.

Williams KD, Park AL. (2003) Lower back pain and disorders of intervertebral disks. In: Campbell's Operative Orthopaedics (Canale ST, ed.), 10th edition. Philadelphia: Mosby.

Wiltse LL, Berger PE, McCulloch JA. (1997) A system for reporting the size and location of lesions of the spine. Spine 22: 1534-1537.

Anatomic zones and levels are defined, using a system intuitive to most surgeons, and recommendations are made for reporting pathology in the spine, particularly in relation to lumbar disk herniations.

Wood KB, Garvey TA, Gundry C et al. (1995) Magnetic resonance imaging of the thoracic spine: Evaluation of asymptomatic individuals. JBJS 77: 1631-1638.

Two studies examine a group of 90 asymptomatic patients with MRI scans of their thoracic spines. The authors describe the incidence and epidemiology of thoracic disk herniations and follow a subgroup of these patients for an average of 26 months.

Wood KB, Blair JM, Aepple DM et al. (1997) The natural history of asymptomatic thoracic disk herniations. Spine 22: 525-529.

This study examines a group of 90 asymptomatic patients with MRI scans of their thoracic spines. Based on the results of this study, the authors believe that asymptomatic disk herniations may exist in a state of relative flux yet exhibit little change in size and remain asymptomatic. There was a trend, however, for small disk herniations either to remain unchanged or to increase in size and for large disk herniations often to decrease in size.

CHAPTER 7

Cervical, Thoracic, and Lumbar Degenerative Disk Disease
Spinal Stenosis

Brady T. Vibert★ and Jeffrey S. Fischgrund §

★ M.D., Resident, Orthopaedic Surgery, William Beaumont Hospital, Royal Oak, MI
§ M.D., Spine Surgeon, William Beaumont Hospital, Royal Oak, MI

Introduction

- Degenerative disk disease is manifested as loss of fluid, height, and integrity of the intervertebral disk. It may result in osteophyte formation, ligament hypertrophy, and synovial cyst formation.
- Spinal stenosis, the narrowing of the spinal canal or neural foramina, may occur because of degenerative disk disease and resulting hypertrophic changes. Spinal stenosis may result in radiculopathy, myelopathy, or both in the cervical and thoracic spine. Spinal stenosis in the lumbar spine may result in radiculopathy, neurogenic claudication, or cauda equina syndrome—that is, saddle anesthesia (perineal) and loss of bowel and bladder function in severe cases.
- Radiculopathy is a nerve root dysfunction that results in a lower motor nerve lesion only in the affected nerve's distribution.
- Myelopathy is a condition affecting the spinal cord and resulting in upper motor neuron dysfunction.
- Spinal stenosis in the cervical and thoracic spine may result in myelopathy
- Thoracic spinal stenosis caused by degenerative changes is rare because the rib cage, which provides rigid structural support, minimizes motion at the thoracic intervertebral motion segments.

Pathophysiology

- Spinal stenosis can come from advanced degenerative disk disease.
- All disks age, but pathologic disk degeneration is an accelerated and exaggerated course of normal aging (Fig. 7–1).

Classification
Arnoldi Classification of Spinal Canal Stenosis

I.   Congenital or developmental
     a. Idiopathic
     b. Achondroplastic
     c. Osteopetrosis
II. Acquired
     a. Degenerative
         i.   Central
         ii. Lateral recess and foraminal
     b. Iatrogenic
         i.   Postlaminectomy
         ii. Postfusion
         iii. Postdiscectomy
     c. Miscellaneous disorders
         i.   Acromegaly
         ii. Paget's

Disk Degeneration Flow Chart

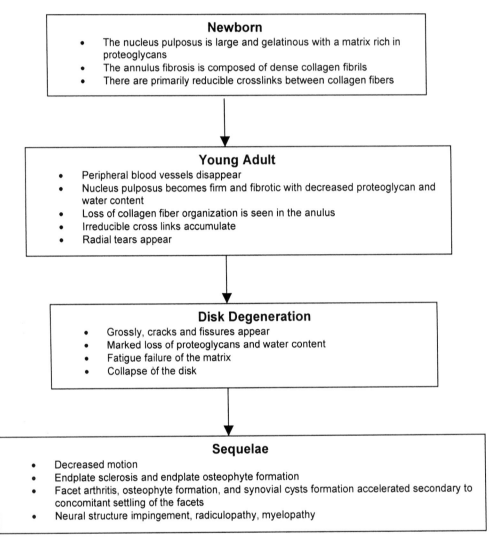

Newborn
- The nucleus pulposus is large and gelatinous with a matrix rich in proteoglycans
- The annulus fibrosis is composed of dense collagen fibrils
- There are primarily reducible crosslinks between collagen fibers

Young Adult
- Peripheral blood vessels disappear
- Nucleus pulposus becomes firm and fibrotic with decreased proteoglycan and water content
- Loss of collagen fiber organization is seen in the anulus
- Irreducible cross links accumulate
- Radial tears appear

Disk Degeneration
- Grossly, cracks and fissures appear
- Marked loss of proteoglycans and water content
- Fatigue failure of the matrix
- Collapse of the disk

Sequelae
- Decreased motion
- Endplate sclerosis and endplate osteophyte formation
- Facet arthritis, osteophyte formation, and synovial cysts formation accelerated secondary to concomitant settling of the facets
- Neural structure impingement, radiculopathy, myelopathy

Figure 7–1: Disk degeneration flow chart.

  iii. Fluorosis
  iv. Ankylosing spondylitis
 d. Traumatic
III. Combined—Any combination of congenital, developmental, or acquired stenosis

Lumbar Stenosis

Anatomy

- The spinal cord usually ends at the L1 level with the nerves of the cauda equina remaining in the dural sac until they exit their respective foramina.
- Osteophyte formation from the vertebral body endplates and facet joints, synovial cysts from the facet joints, ligamentum flavum hypertrophy, and disk bulging may all impinge the dural sac and exiting nerve roots.

- Fig. 7–2 is a schematic that illustrates normal anatomic relationships in the lumbar spine.
- Fig. 7–3 is an artist's illustration revealing advanced lumbar spine degeneration with central and foraminal stenosis.

Diagnostic Tools

History

- Age—Usually over 50

Symptoms

- Low back pain
- Low back stiffness
- Mechanical symptoms
- Radiculopathic pain
- Lower extremity weakness
- Neurogenic claudication

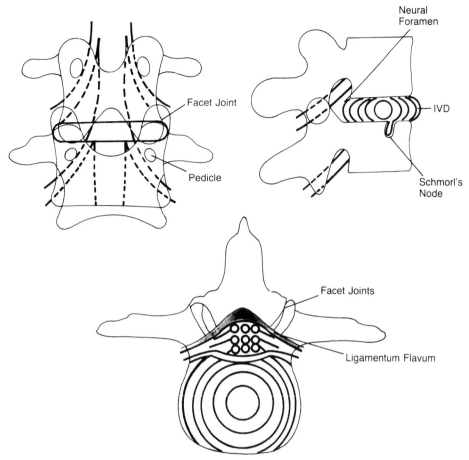

Figure 7–2: Anatomic relations in the lumbar spine. (Reproduced from Wiesel et al. 1982.)

- Symptoms of neurogenic claudication must be differentiated from vascular claudication and degenerative disk disease, as described in Table 7–1.
- Table 7–2 differentiates spinal stenosis from disk herniation.

Physical Examination and Signs (Table 7–3)

- A complete physical examination, focusing on the neurologic examination, is critical in diagnosing lumbar stenosis and differentiating it from other disease processes.
- Decreased lumbar extension
- Rarely, muscle atrophy (especially calf)
- Difficulty with toe or heel walking
- Usually no muscle weakness
- Negative long tract signs
- Sensory examination is usually normal but may be abnormal in advanced cases.
- Patients walk with lumbar flexion and do not like to lie flat or stand straight.

Imaging
Plain Films

- An anteroposterior (AP) and lateral lumbar spine, as well as an AP pelvis, should be acquired for all patients with neurologic signs or symptoms and those with more than six weeks of back pain.
- Plain films frequently reveal the following:
  - Disk space narrowing or degenerative disk disease
  - Endplate osteophytes and sclerosis
  - Facet enlargement or osteophyte formation
  - Narrowed neuroforaminal canals
  - Loss of lumbar lordosis
- Plain films occasionally reveal the following:
  - Degenerative scoliosis
  - Spondylolisthesis, usually at L4-L5
- Figs. 7–4 and 7–5 reveal these changes.
- Although plain films may help rule out unusual causes of stenosis, such as ankylosing spondylitis and possibly tumors, they are limited in their ability to evaluate the encroachment of neural structures and other bony pathology.

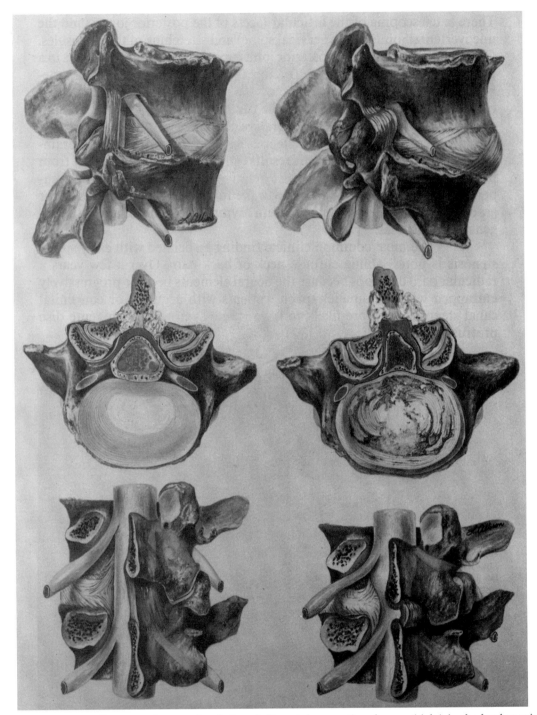

Figure 7–3: Illustrations revealing normal anatomic relations (left) and degenerative changes (right) in the lumbar spine. (Reproduced from Rothman et al. 1982.)

Magnetic Resonance Imaging

- Magnetic resonance imaging (MRI) is the best modality for evaluating lumbar spinal stenosis (Schnebel et al. 1989).
- Both axial cuts and sagittal cuts should be obtained.
- Gadolinium is only necessary in postsurgical patients or when differentiating from infection, tumor, or other pathologic processes.

- MRI is excellent for viewing the following:
  - Spinal stenosis
  - Lateral recess stenosis
  - Disk bulges and herniations
  - Nerve root impingement
  - Facet degeneration, hypertrophy, and cyst formation
  - Maintenance or loss of epidural fat (lost in stenosis)

Table 7–1: Differential Diagnosis of Symptoms*			
FINDINGS PAIN	**NEUROGENIC CLAUDICATION**	**VASCULAR CLAUDICATION**	**DEGENERATIVE DISK DISEASE**
Type	Vague cramping, aches, sharp burning in legs	Tightness, cramping (usually calf)	Dull low back pain
Location	Back, buttocks, legs	Leg muscles	Back
Radiation	Common, proximal to distal	Localized in legs, distal to proximal	Localized to back, anterior thighs
Exacerbation	Standing, walking (less so); none with bicycling unless the trunk is extended	Walking, bicycling	General activities—Bending, standing twisting, lifting
Improvement	Sitting, flexing, squatting	Standing, cessation of activity	Decreased activity, rest
Time to relief	Slow	Rapid	Slow
Walking uphill	No pain (trunk flexed)	Pain	Pain possible
Back pain	Common	Uncommon	Common

*(Adapted from Herkowitz et al. 1999.)

Table 7–2: Lumbar Stenosis versus Disk Herniation*		
CONDITION	**STENOSIS**	**DISK HERNIATION**
Age	>50	<50
Sex	Mostly female	Mostly male
Onset	Insidious	Acute
Pain location	Diffuse	Dermatomal
Weakness	Uncommon	Common
Straight leg raise	Negative	Positive

*(Adapted from Herkowitz et al. 1999.)

- Ligamentum flavum hypertrophy (contributes to stenosis)
- Tumors
- Infections
- Figs. 7–6 and 7–7 are MRI studies of a patient with extensive degenerative changes.

Computed Tomography and Computed Tomography Myelogram

- Computed tomography (CT) myelogram is still useful in patients unable to obtain MRI (brain aneurysm clips, metal shavings in the eye, large body habitus, occasionally severe claustrophobia, and some postfusion patients with instrumentation).
- CT and CT myelogram are both sensitive for spinal stenosis, lateral recess stenosis, and disk herniations.

- The primary weaknesses of CT are decreased resolution compared with MRI, the inability of CT to demonstrate intrathecal pathology (tumors), and radiation exposure to the patient.
- CT myelogram has the added disadvantage of being an invasive procedure.

Electromyogram

- Limited use for diagnosing lumbar stenosis
- May be helpful when diagnosing or excluding other disease processes, such as diabetic neuropathy, polyradiculopathies, and amyotrophic lateral sclerosis

Nonoperative Treatment of Lumbar Spinal Stenosis

- Although studies reveal that patients with symptomatic spinal stenosis have improved outcome with surgical intervention, patients with mild symptoms and those who refuse surgery may benefit from conservative treatment (Johnsson et al. 1991).
- Pharmacologic therapy—Attempts to decrease pain and nerve irritation or inflammation
  - Anti-inflammatories (nonsteroidal anti-inflammatory drugs or salicylates)
  - Steroid dose packs (controversial but may decrease symptoms)
  - Antidepressants (occasionally)

Table 7–3: Differential Diagnosis of Physical Findings*			
TEST	**NEUROGENIC CLAUDICATION**	**VASCULAR CLAUDICATION**	**LUMBAR SPONDYLOSIS**
Neurologic examination	Occasionally abnormal, usually asymmetric	Rarely abnormal; symmetric finding if present	Normal
Straight leg raise	Rarely positive	Negative	Negative
Femoral stretch	Rarely positive	Negative	Negative
Pulses	Present or symmetrically diminished	Diminished or absent; often asymmetric	Symmetric
Skin	Normal appearance	Hair loss	Normal appearance

*(Adapted from Herkowitz et al. 1999.)

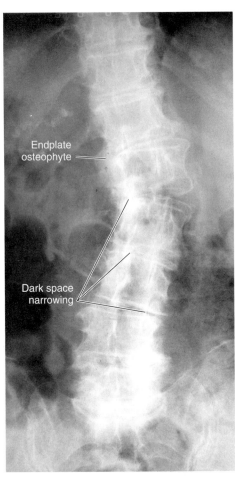

Figure 7–4: AP x-ray film. A lumbar spine with degenerative scoliosis, degenerative disk disease, and endplate osteophytes.

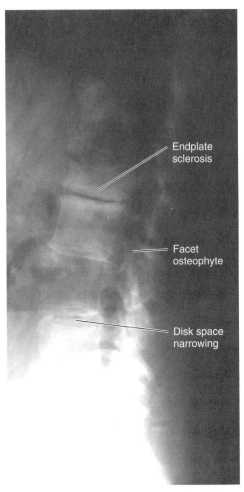

Figure 7–5: Lateral lumbar spine plain film. **Reveals disk space narrowing, facet hypertrophy, facet degeneration with osteophytes, and neuroforaminal encroachment.**

- Narcotics (avoid if possible because of the risk of dependence)
- Muscle relaxants
- Injection therapy
  - Steroid (Depo-Medrol) injections into the epidural space may benefit those with radicular components to their stenosis.
  - This therapy is given in a series of three injections.
  - It is relatively easy and safe.
- Physical therapy
  - Focus on flexion exercises, strengthening, and flexibility of the abdominal muscles and hamstrings.
  - Cardiovascular training may help the patient's overall health.
  - Physical therapy may decrease recovery time if the patient comes to surgery.
  - Modalities, such as heat, cold, massage, and transcutaneous electrical nerve stimulation units, may provide a short-term benefit.
- Traction, lumbosacral braces, and chiropractic manipulation have no proven long-term benefit.

Surgical Treatment

- Indications for surgical intervention include radicular pain or neurogenic claudication with MRI or CT myelogram revealing stenosis in the same distribution as the patient's symptoms in a patient who fails to improve with nonoperative treatment.
- The goals of surgery are pain relief, increased mobility, prevention of further neurological deficit, and improvement in the patient's quality of life.
- Appropriate medical clearance should be obtained for all patients over 50 or in younger patients with medical comorbidities.
- In decompressions requiring less than 2 operative hours, a spinal anesthetic may be used. A general anesthetic is required for longer cases.

Surgical Technique

- Surgical options are dependent upon the following:
  - Level of the stenosis
  - Number of involved segments

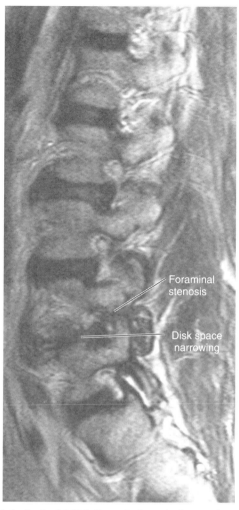

Figure 7–6: Sagittal MRI. **Reveals foraminal stenosis caused by facet hypertrophy and disk herniation.**

- Location of the stenosis (central, lateral, or foraminal)
- Associated deformities (degenerative spondylolisthesis or degenerative scoliosis)
- Presence of instability
- In general, stable spines require only decompression. Unstable spines may also require fusion.

Surgical Options for Decompression (see Fig. 7–8)

- Central stenosis—This requires decompressive lumbar laminectomy for adequate decompression.
- Lateral recess and foraminal stenosis—If there is no central stenosis, the surgeon may perform decompression through one or several laminotomies, decompressing individual roots; some prefer this procedure for bilateral single-level and ipsilateral two- or three-level radicular symptoms to preserve the midline structures.

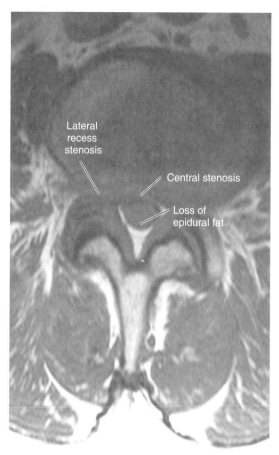

Figure 7–7: Axial MRI revealing central and lateral recess stenosis.

- Most authors show more than 85% of good to excellent results following decompressive lumbar laminectomy. Hansraj et al. reported 95% patient satisfaction in 103 cases (Hansraj et al. 2001).
- Katz et al. revealed progressive return of symptoms in many patients, with 23% requiring revision surgery from 7 to 10 years later (Katz et al. 1996).

Decompression with Fusion

- The goal is to decompress neural elements and to decrease mechanical back pain.
- Fusion is recommended when there is stenosis in conjunction with the following conditions.

Unstable Degenerative Scoliosis or Kyphosis

- Only curves of a certain magnitude, or unstable curves or progressive curves, require fusion.
- If proceeding with fusion, the need for realignment is not established.
- Relative indications for fusion are as follows:
  - Progressive curves
  - Curves greater than 20 degrees
  - Painful curve with back pain

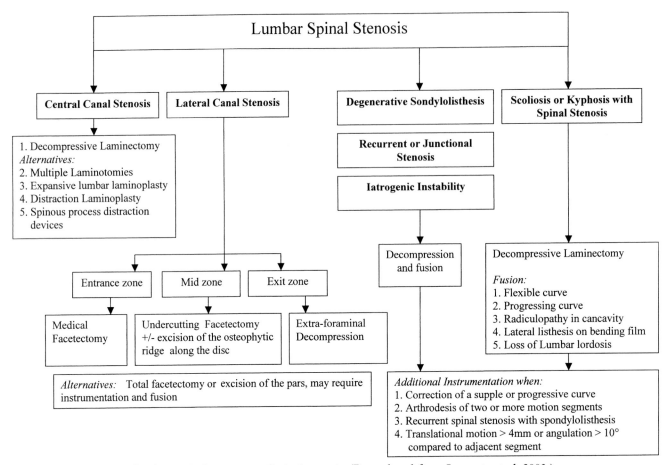

Figure 7–8: Flow chart for the surgical treatment of spinal stenosis. (Reproduced from Sengupta et al. 2003.)

- Loss of sagittal balance and lumbar lordosis
- Lateral listhesis in the side bending film
- Flexible curves
- Patients with radicular symptoms on the concave side of the curve

Degenerative Spondylolisthesis

- Herkowitz and Kurz, in a prospective randomized trial, reported in 1991 better outcomes in patients who had concomitant degenerative spondylolisthesis and underwent a fusion than in those who had decompressions alone (Herkowitz et al. 1991).
- In 1997, Fischgrund et al. performed a randomized prospective trial. They showed that instrumenting lumbar fusions increased fusion rates (45% to 83%) but that there was no significant difference in the clinical outcome of the patients (Fischgrund et al. 1997).
- Bridwell et al. studied 44 patients with stenosis and degenerative spondylolisthesis. They found better fusion rates and better functional outcomes in those who underwent instrumentation compared with those who did not (Bridwell et al. 1993).

Iatrogenic Instability Following Decompression

- Abumi et al. revealed that the removal of greater than 50% of both facets at one level led to instability (Abumi et al. 1990).
- Most believe that the removal of either one complete facet or up to 50% of both facets at a given level is acceptable.
- If these limits are exceeded, fusion of the affected levels is recommended.

Recurrent Same Level or Adjacent Level Stenosis (Revision Decompressions)

- Herno et al. recommended fusion with instrumentation after decompression at previously decompressed levels because further decompression of the facets may lead to increased instability of the motion segment (Herno et al. 1995).
- Sengupta and Herkowitz recommended, in the absence of instability and when no significant facet excision is

necessary, that adjacent level stenosis may be treated with decompression alone; otherwise, fusion is indicated (Sengupta et al. 2003).
- Fig. 7–8 is a flow chart for patients with degenerative lumbar spine stenosis.

Postoperative Care

- Patients remain in the hospital for 1-3 days after an operation.
- All patients should have sequential compression devices and thigh-high thromboembolic deterrent stockings to prevent deep venous thrombosis and pulmonary embolus; Anticoagulants are avoided by some surgeons because of the increased risk of epidural hematoma.
- Patients ambulate on the day of surgery.
- Physical therapy may be initiated for education and gait training.
- Patients should be discouraged from bending, twisting, squatting, and lifting for six weeks.
- After six weeks, outpatient therapy may be instituted for abdominal and low back strengthening, cardiovascular conditioning, and stretching.
- Also at six weeks, patients may begin a slow progression to full activities.

Cervical Spondylosis

- Cervical spondylosis refers to the degeneration of the cervical spine intervertebral disks and may result in radiculopathy or myelopathy.

Anatomy

- Cervical spine anatomy
  - Each motion segment in the subaxial cervical spine consists of five "joints:" the intervertebral disk space, two facets, and two false uncovertebral joints (joints of Luschka).
  - Impinging osteophytes may form at each of these "joints," and synovial cysts may form at the facets, all of which may impinge upon the surrounding neurologic structures.
- Fig. 7–9 shows a typical cervical vertebra. Note the relationship between the facet joint and the uncovertebral "joint." The cervical nerves exit between these two joints and may be impinged by osteophytes from either structure.

Diagnostic Tools

History

- Age—Degeneration in the cervical spine usually becomes radiographically apparent in the fourth or fifth decade and becomes more prevalent with increasing age.

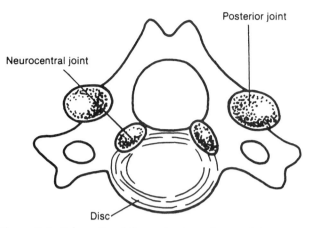

Figure 7–9: Schematic of the anatomic positions of the uncovertebral and facet joints. (**Reproduced from Brower RS 1999.**)

- Men have a slightly higher incidence of cervical disk degeneration, and they tend to have more severe degeneration than women.

Symptoms

- Symptoms of cervical spondylosis are usually chronic or subacute in nature in contrast to herniations, which are usually acute in nature.
- Patients will often have axial neck pain and stiffness.
- Radiating arm pain, weakness, and numbness occurs most often in the C5, C6, and C7 distributions.

Differential Diagnosis

- Cervical spondylosis (Table 7–4 differentiates cervical spondylosis from cervical disk herniation)
- Disk herniation
- Cervical strain or mechanical pain
- Tumor
- Multiple sclerosis
- Amyotrophic lateral sclerosis
- Guillain-Barré syndrome
- Nerve entrapment syndromes
  - Thoracic outlet syndrome

Table 7–4:	Cervical Spondylosis versus Disk Herniation	
CONDITION	**CERVICAL SPONDYLOSIS**	**DISK HERNIATION**
Age	>50	<50
Sex	Male > female	Male = female
Onset	Insidious	Acute
Pain location	Neck and arm	Arm
Neck stiffness	Yes	No
Weakness	Yes	Yes or no
Myelopathy	More common	Less common
Dermatomes	One or multiple	One

- Brachial plexopathy or neuritis
- Pronator syndrome
- Anterior interosseous nerve syndrome
- Carpal tunnel syndrome
- Ulnar nerve compression (cubital tunnel or Guyon's canal)
- Radial nerve compression
- Long thoracic nerve compression
- Suprascapular nerve compression

Physical Examination and Signs (Table 7–5)

- Decreased range of motion for the neck
- Dermatomal numbness and weakness (most commonly C6-C7)
- Diminished reflex
- Myelopathy
- Wide, ataxic gait pattern
  - Poor hand dexterity
  - Weakness
- Lhermitte's phenomena—A sensation of electric shocks radiating down the arms when axial pressure is applied to the head
  - Dysdiadochokinesia—Loss of coordination and dexterity of the hands, especially during rapid movements
  - Bowel or bladder dysfunction
  - Hyperreflexia
  - Positive Babinski's sign—Extension of great toe when plantar foot is stimulated
  - Positive Hoffman's sign—"Flicking" the distal phalanx of the middle finger causes the thumb to adduct
  - Diminished proprioception

Imaging

Plain Films

- This cervical spine series includes an AP view, a lateral view (neutral, flexion, and extension views), obliques, and an open mouth view.

- Use swimmer's view if the initial films do not show the C7-T1 junction.
- Evaluate overall alignment; those with spondylosis will often have loss of lordosis or spondylolisthesis.
- Evaluate for degenerative disk disease and disk space narrowing on the laterals.
- The obliques reveal the foramen, and they should be evaluated for stenosis.
- Figs. 7–10 and 7–11 are plain films illustrating degenerative changes in the cervical spine.

Magnetic Resonance Imaging

- MRI is the best modality for imaging the cervical spine.
- Axial and sagittal sections should be obtained.
- Evaluate the space available for the cord; less than 13 mm is relative stenosis and less than 10 mm is critical stenosis.
- MRI is excellent for viewing the following:
  - Herniated disks
  - Degenerative disk disease and spur formation
  - Facet arthritis and spur formation
  - Uncovertebral joint degeneration and spur formation
  - Nerve root impingement
  - Cord compression or impingement
  - Myelomalacia
  - Tumor
- Infection
  - Syrinx and other cord pathology
- Figs. 7–12 and 7–13 are sagittal and axial MRI photos showing degenerative disk disease, spur formation, nerve root impingement, and cord compression.

Myelography and CT Myelography

- Modality of choice for those who cannot undergo an MRI
- Good for postoperative imaging if hardware was placed
- Advantages—Good patient tolerance, excellent imaging of the cervical spine, and may be performed in many situations in which an MRI is contraindicated
- Disadvantages—Invasive, requires a dye load, requires radiation, difficult for those with a large body habitus, and difficult for patients with claustrophobia

Table 7–5: Physical Examination Findings by Level				
ROOT LEVEL	**PAIN LOCATION**	**MUSCLE WEAKNESS**	**REFLEX**	**NOTES**
C2	Occipital region	None	None	Very rare
C3	Posterior neck, ear	None	None	Uncommon
C4	Base of neck, medial shoulder	None	None	Uncommon
C5	Base of neck, top of shoulder, lateral upper arm	Deltoid, some biceps weakness	None or biceps	Difficult to distinguish from cuff tear
C6	Base of neck, anterior arm, lateral forearm, radial hand	Wrist extensors, biceps	Biceps	Most common
C7	Middle finger, posterior arm, posterolateral forearm	Triceps	Triceps	Common
C8	Ulnar hand	Finger flexors, intrinsics	None	Uncommon

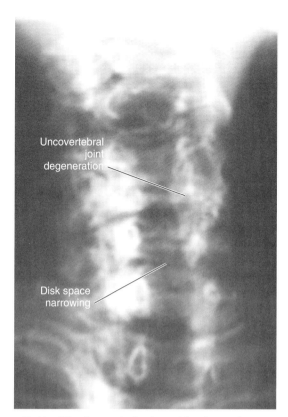

Figure 7–10: AP of a cervical spine with advanced degenerative changes.

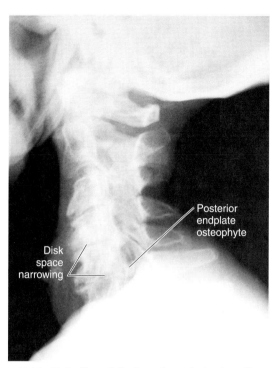

Figure 7–11: Plain film of the lateral cervical spine. Illustrates extensive degenerative disk disease and loss of lordosis.

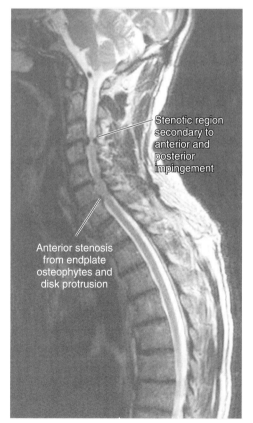

Figure 7–12: Sagittal MRI of the cervical spine revealing multilevel stenosis.

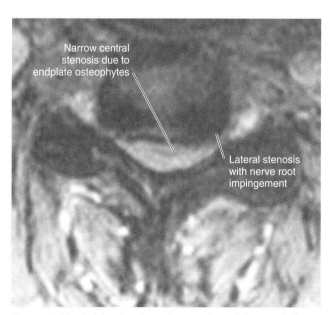

Figure 7–13: Axial MRI through a portion of the cervical spine. Reveals central and foraminal stenosis.

Electromyogram

- Unlike lumbar spinal stenosis, the electromyogram (EMG) plays a role when evaluating cervical stenosis or radiculopathy.
- EMG is useful for including or excluding peripheral neuropathies and central causes of weakness when the diagnosis is not clear.

Nonoperative Treatment

- Nonoperative treatment of cervical spondylosis without myelopathy will frequently improve or completely resolve neck pain and radiculopathy.
- In general, patients with myelopathy are surgical candidates; nonoperative treatment is of limited value.
- Goals—Decrease pain and improve function
- Physical therapy—the mainstay of nonoperative treatment, it should be performed 2-3 times per week for 4-6 weeks
  - Range of motion exercises
  - Progressive resistance training
  - Modalities (heat, ultrasound, and massage)
  - Home exercise education
- Medical treatment
  - Anti-inflammatories—Nonsteroidal anti-inflammatory drugs and celecoxib cyclooxygenase-2 inhibitors are useful for decreasing the inflammation around the entrapped nerve root or roots; a regular dosing protocol should be instituted.
  - Narcotics should be avoided except for limited use in acute flare-ups.
  - Antidepressants may be necessary for emotionally depressed patients with chronic cervical spine conditions.
  - Muscle relaxants have been shown to have some benefit when there is a component of cervical muscle spasm; however, sedatives should be avoided because of their high risk for the development of dependency.
- Chiropractic care may be contraindicated; it has not been proved to be of any long-term benefit.

Surgical Treatment of Cervical Spondylosis

- Indications for surgical intervention include the following:
  - Failed nonoperative treatment of radiculopathy (minimum 3 months)
  - Progressive neurologic deficit
  - Presence of myelopathy
  - Unrelenting pain
- Goals include pain relief, improved function, and prevention of further neurologic deficit.

- Note that for cervical spondylotic myelopathy, surgery may not improve neurologic function but is aimed at preventing a progressive deficit.
- Appropriate medical clearance should be obtained.
- A general anesthetic is required.

Surgical Options for Cervical Decompression

- Anterior cervical discectomy and fusion with or without instrumentation
- Anterior cervical corpectomy and fusion with instrumentation
- Laminaplasty
- Laminectomy
- Laminectomy and fusion with or without instrumentation
- A combination of the preceding options
- The surgical technique of choice depends upon the level or levels involved, the number of levels involved, the presence of central canal stenosis, the presence of foraminal stenosis, and other associated factors such as spondylolisthesis, kyphosis, instability, and ossification of the posterior longitudinal ligament (OPLL). Table 7-6 analyzes the various techniques.

Anterior Cervical Discectomy and Fusion

- Cloward (1958) and Smith and Robinson (1958) independently described techniques of anterior cervical discectomy and fusion in 1958.
  - The Smith-Robinson technique entails using a tricortical iliac crest bone graft to lever open the disk space and, thereby, indirectly decompressing the neural foramina; the osteophytes then resorb over time.
  - Cloward recommended manually removing impinging osteophytes, removing a central core of bone from adjacent vertebral bodies, and replacing it with a similar sized and shaped iliac crest bone graft.
  - Today, many surgeons perform a direct decompression and fuse with a Smith-Robinson–type bone graft.
- There has been no definitive study showing an autograft to be superior to an allograft; in single-level surgery, the allograft is becoming more popular based upon favorable fusion rates and the lack of donor site morbidity.
- Allografts may be fibular wedge, tricortical iliac wedge, or patellar wedge.
- Some studies have shown that discectomy alone, without fusion, is adequate for single-level disease in the treatment of cervical radiculopathy but that it leads to long-term neck pain (Maurice-Williams et al. 1996).
- Use of instrumentation is also controversial; no study has shown a definitive long-term benefit for instrumenting single-level fusion; two-level or more fusions should usually be instrumented.

Table 7–6:	Techniques for Cervical Spondylosis Decompression				
SURGERY*	**INDICATIONS**	**CONTRA-INDICATIONS**	**ADVANTAGES**	**DISADVANTAGES**	**INSTRUMENTATION**
ACDF	Single- or two-level radiculopathy Instability (single level)	Three-level or more stenosis	Safe, well-tolerated Good long-term results	Risk of pseudarthrosis	+/– for single level
ACCF	Broad areas of stenosis (multilevel OK) Instability Deformity (including swan neck) Kyphosis	Isolated foraminal stenosis	Common procedure Excellent anterior and foraminal decompression	Risk of vertebral artery injury Risk of iatrogenic instability Risk of graft extrusion Pseudarthrosis	Yes
Laminaplasty	Long area of canal stenosis OPLL Buckled ligamentum flavum	Instability Kyphosis	Maintains stability Long decompressions	C5 palsy	No
Laminectomy	Long area of canal stenosis Degenerative anterior ankylosis	Kyphosis Instability	Long decompressions Best surgery for those with anterior ankylosis	C5 palsy May create instability	Yes or no

*ACDF, anterior cervical discectomy and fusion; ACCF, anterior cervical corpectomy and fusion.

Anterior Cervical Corpectomy and Fusion (ACCF)

- Areas of spondylotic change may result in cervical myelopathy.
- If the canal is congenitally narrow, there is a broad area of cervical stenosis; if there is OPLL, ACCF is indicated because it allows wider decompression.
- Anterior stabilization of the cervical spine following anterior corpectomy requires the placement of a strut graft (an iliac crest autograft or allograft or a fibular autograft or allograft) (Bernard et al. 1987).

Complications of the Anterior Approaches

- Pseudarthrosis
- Graft dislodgement, resumption, or collapse
- Dysphasia
- Hoarseness
- Vertebral or carotid artery injury
- Neurologic injury, including injury to the recurrent laryngeal nerve
- Iliac crest donor site morbidity (infection, hematoma, pain, lateral femoral cutaneous nerve palsy, bowel herniation, or iliac wing fracture)
- Hardware complications (pull out or screw breakage)
- Dural tears
- Inadequate decompression
- Esophageal or tracheal injury
- Respiratory embarrassment caused by hematoma formation

Laminaplasty

- Laminaplasty has become more popular because of the lower incidence of postoperative kyphosis when compared with laminectomy.
- Goals—Decompress the spine while maintaining cervical spine stability
- Indications—Myelopathy caused by degenerative stenosis, OPLL, or multilevel spondylotic myelopathy
- Contraindications—Presence of kyphosis
- Types of laminaplasty include the Z-plasty and the open door laminaplasty, which has many modifications.
- A long-term follow-up study found that postsurgical improvement was relatively maintained after almost 13 years (Miyazaki et al. 1996). Subsequent studies have questioned the maintenance of improvement for those with OPLL (Kawai et al. 1998).

Laminectomy

- Goal—Decompress the spine
- Indications—Similar to those for laminaplasty, especially in the presence of anterior ankylosis
- Contraindications—Kyphosis
- Biomechanical alterations may result in cervical spine instability following laminectomy and concomitant fusion.

Complications of the Posterior Approaches

- Neurologic deficit
- Redevelopment of stenosis
- Instability after laminectomy because of kyphosis
- C5 nerve root palsy can occur; when the spinal cord migrates posteriorly, the C5 root can be stretched,

resulting in shoulder pain and possibly deltoid or biceps weakness. The palsy usually has a decent recovery within 1 year.

Postoperative Care

- Patients generally remain hospitalized for at least one evening and longer for more extensive procedures.
- A rigid cervical collar is often used for all anterior fusions greater than one level and is often replaced with a soft collar for single-level cases with instrumentation. However, if no instrumentation is used for a single-level fusion, a rigid collar should be prescribed.
- For anterior approaches, the head of the hospital bed should be elevated at least 30 degrees for the first 24 hours to help prevent hematoma formation.
- Regular neurologic examinations should be performed.
- Patients should be advised against bending or twisting their head, heavy lifting, strenuous activity, and overhead activity.
- Rigid collars should be discontinued by 6 weeks after the operation, and outpatient physical therapy for range of motion and strengthening should be started.
- Patients may begin to slowly advance to regular activities at the 6-week mark.

References

Abumi K, Panjabi M, Kramer K et al. (1990) Biomechanical evaluation of lumbar spinal stability after graded facetectomies. Spine 15: 1142-1147.

Fresh human lumbar spines were biomechanically evaluated following unilateral facetectomy, bilateral facetectomy, unilateral medial facetectomy, or bilateral medial facetectomy. Testing revealed that medial facetectomy (unilateral or bilateral) did not affect lumbar spinal stability. Conversely, either unilateral or bilateral complete facetectomy rendered the lumbar spine unstable.

Bernard T, Whitecloud T. (1987) Cervical spondylitic myelopathy and myeloradiculopathy: Anterior decompression and stabilization with autogenous fibula strut graft. Clin Orthop 221: 149-160.

Twenty-one patients were followed for an average of 32 months after having anterior decompression and fusion with autogenous fibular strut graft. Of the 21 patients, 16 showed functional improvement. The authors recommend fibular strut autograft over iliac crest autograft because of the excellent structural stability afforded by the fibular strut and high union rates.

Bridwell K, Sedgewick T, O'Brien M et al. (1993) The role of fusion and instrumentation in the treatment of degenerative spondylolisthesis with spinal stenosis. J Spinal Disorders 6(6): 461-472.

Forty-four patients with degenerative spondylolisthesis underwent decompressive lumbar laminectomy. Of those patients, 9 did not have a fusion performed, 11 underwent concomitant posterolateral fusion, and 18 had fusions with instrumentation. The group with fusion and instrumentation had a significantly better fusion rates than those without instrumentation.

Brower RS. (1999) Cervical disk disease. In: The Spine (Herkowitz HN et al. eds.), 4th edition. Philadelphia: W.B. Saunders. Fischgrund

J, Mackay M, Herkowitz H et al. (1997) Degenerative lumbar spondylolisthesis with spinal stenosis: A prospective, randomized study comparing decompressive laminectomy and arthrodesis with and without spinal instrumentation (1997 Volvo Award winner in clinical studies). Spine 22: 2807-2812.

This was a prospective, randomized study of 66 patients with degenerative lumbar spondylolisthesis and spinal stenosis who underwent decompressive lumbar laminectomy with fusion either with or without instrumentation. At a follow-up after 2 years, the fusion rate was much higher in instrumented patients, 82% versus 45%, but successful fusion did not significantly improve back or leg pain.

Cloward RB. (1958) The anterior approach for removal of ruptured cervical disks. J Neurosurg 15:602–617.

Hansraj K, Cammisa F, O'Leary P et al. (2001) Decompressive surgery for typical lumbar spinal stenosis. Clin Orthop 10-17.

The authors evaluated 103 consecutive patients who underwent decompressive laminectomy for typical lumbar spinal stenosis. Patients younger than 65 had greater improvement in function and severity scores, but overall satisfaction was similar in both groups. Only 5% required revision surgery.

Herkowitz HN, Garfin SR, Balderston RA et al. (eds.) (1999) In: Rothman-Simeone: The Spine, 4th edition. Philadelphia: Saunders.

Herkowitz H, Kurz L. (1991) Degenerative lumbar spondylolisthesis with spinal stenosis: A prospective study comparing decompression with decompression and intertransverse process arthrodesis. J Bone Joint Surg (Am) 73: 802-808.

This prospective, randomized study looked at 50 patients who underwent either decompression alone or decompression with posterolateral fusion without instrumentation. The patients were followed for approximated 3 years, and results showed improved back and leg pain relief in the group that had concomitant arthrodesis.

Herno A, Airaksinen O, Saari T et al. (1995) Surgical results of lumbar spinal stenosis: A comparison of patients with or without previous back surgery. Spine 20(8): 964-969.

This retrospective study revealed that patients undergoing revision surgery for recurrent spinal stenosis had a significantly worse outcome than those undergoing a primary procedure. Of those undergoing a primary procedure, 67% stated excellent to good results versus 46% of those undergoing revision surgery.

Johnsson KE, Uden A, Rosen I. (1991) The effect of decompression on the natural course of spinal stenosis: A comparison of surgically treated and untreated patients. Spine 16: 615.

Nineteen patients with spinal stenosis were treated without surgery and were compared with a cohort of 44 patients treated surgically with decompression at follow-up times of 31 and 53 months. Of the patients who elected surgery, 60% felt better based on a visual analog scale versus only 33% of those treated without surgery. No proof of deterioration was found in the untreated patients.

Katz J, Lipson S, Chang L et al. (1996) Seven- to ten-year outcome of decompressive surgery for degenerative lumbar spinal stenosis. Spine 21: 92-98.

This study was a retrospective review of 88 patients who had decompressive laminectomies with or without fusion. A 7- to

10-year follow-up revealed that 23% required reoperation and 33% complained of severe back pain but that 75% were satisfied with the results of surgery.

Kawai S, Sunago K, Doi K et al. (1988) Cervical laminaplasty (Hattori's method): Procedure and follow-up results. Spine 13: 1245.

> This paper describes the Z-shaped laminaplasty developed by Hattori in 1971 and provides a follow-up for 78 patients who received the procedure. Satisfactory results were maintained for long periods.

Maurice-Williams R, Dorward N. (1996) Extended anterior cervical discectomy without fusion: A simple and sufficient operation for most cases of cervical degenerative disease. Br J Neurosurg 10: 261-266.

> This retrospective review evaluated 187 patients who had been treated by extended anterior discectomy without fusion for cervical radiculopathy or myelopathy. Of the patients, 94.5% showed clear neurologic improvement and only 1% complained of persistent neck pain.

Miyazaki K, Hirohuji E, Ono S et al. (1986) Extensive simultaneous multisegment laminectomy for myelopathy due to the ossification of the posterior longitudinal ligament of the cervical region. Spine 11(6): 531-542.

> The study followed 155 patients who underwent multilevel laminectomies for the treatment of OPLL. In all, 81.9% showed some improvement and almost 65% had good or excellent results.

Rothman RH, Simeone FA. (1982) The Spine, 2nd edition. Philadelphia: Saunders.

Schnebel B, Kingston S, Watkins R et al. (1989) Comparison of MRI to contrast CT in diagnosis of spinal stenosis. Spine 14: 332-337.

> A retrospective review of MRI and CT scans from 41 patients. The studies were reviewed by a single, blinded examiner and were evaluated for stenosis (central and lateral) and disk disease. Results showed a 96.6% correlation between CT and MRI for evaluating stenosis, but MRI revealed disk disease almost three times more often than CT.

Sengupta D, Herkowitz H. (2003) Lumbar spinal stenosis: Treatment strategies and indications for surgery. Orthop Clin N Am 34: 281-295.

> This is a review article evaluating the diagnosis and treatment from lumbar spinal stenosis.

Smith G, Robinson R. (1958). The treatment of certain cervical spine disorders by anterior removal of the intervertebral disc and interbody fusion. J Bone Joint Surg 40A: 607-624.

Wiesel SW, Bernini P, Rothman RH. (1982) The Aging Spine. Philadelphia: Saunders.

Surgical Management of Low Back Pain

Brian K. Kwon*, Eric Levicoff §, and Alexander R. Vaccaro †

* M.D., FRCSC; Orthopaedic Spine Fellow, Department of Orthopaedic Surgery, Thomas
Jefferson University and the Rothman Institute, Philadelphia, Pa.; Clinical Instructor,
Combined Neurosurgical and Orthopaedic Spine Program, University of British Columbia;
and Gowan and Michele Guest Neuroscience Canada Foundation/CIHR Research Fellow,
International Collaboration on Repair Discoveries, University of British Columbia,
Vancouver, Canada
§ M.D., Orthopaedic Surgery Resident, University of Pittsburgh Medical Center, Pittsburgh, PA
† M.D., Professor of Orthopaedic Surgery, Thomas Jefferson University and the Rothman
Institute, Philadelphia, PA

"The decision is more important than the incision."

Introduction

- Low back pain is an extremely common source of disability worldwide, with an enormous societal and health care effect (Frymoyer 1996) (Box 8–1).
- More than 14% of all new-patient visits to physicians are for problems related to the lower back, and the lifetime incidence of low back pain in the general population has been estimated at nearly 70%.
- Low back pain ranks only behind upper respiratory infections as the most common cause of work absence.
- Low back pain is the fifth most common cause of hospitalization and the third most common reason for surgical procedures in the United States, with an estimated economic effect of between $25 and $85 billion annually.
- As the natural history of low back pain is generally favorable, surgery is seldom offered as an initial treatment option.
- Despite this, approximately 165 lumbar spine operations per 100,000 individuals occur each year in the United States, a rate that has been estimated to be more than 5 times that of England and Scotland (Cherkin et al. 1994).

- Lumbar fusion for discogenic pain or lumbar laminectomies for radicular symptoms are the most common spine surgeries performed; both have had estimated failure rates of between 15% and 40% (Turner et al. 1992).

Clinical Etiologies of Low Back Pain

- The etiologies of low back pain are extremely diverse.
  - **Idiopathic or Nonspecific**—Up to 85%, with no specific diagnosis, although the validity of this categorization has been recently questioned (Abraham et al. 2002)
  - **Degenerative disk disease**—A large category that includes discogenic pain, disk herniation, and degenerative scoliosis
  - **Developmental**—For example, isthmic spondylolisthesis and idiopathic scoliosis
  - **Congenital**—For example, scoliosis secondary to failures of formation and segmentation
  - **Traumatic**

- Previous history of low back pain
- Increasing age
- Smoking
- Medical comorbidities
- Lower socioeconomic status
- Psychological distress
- Heavy occupational demands

Box 8–2: **Red Flags in the Clinical Presentation That Require Further Investigation**

- History of significant trauma
- History of previous malignancy
- Age—older than 50 years
- Systemic symptoms—fever, chills, anorexia, and recent weight loss
- Severe or progressive neurologic deficit, particularly saddle anesthesia, bowel or bladder dysfunction, and multiroot deficits
- Ongoing infection
- History of immunosuppression (corticosteroids, immunosuppressant use, and HIV)

- **Infectious**—For example, osteomyelitis and discitis
- **Inflammatory**—For example, ankylosing spondylitis and other spondyloarthropathies
- **Neoplastic**—Benign, primary malignant, and metastatic
- **Metabolic**—Osteoporosis
- **Referred**—Dissecting aortic aneurysm, renal vein thrombosis, acute myocardial infarction, pancreatitis, and duodenal ulcer
- In general, the outcomes of operative intervention for the idiopathic or nonspecific category of patients are unsatisfactory because patients within this category inherently lack a firm diagnosis. The remaining spinal etiologies can, under certain circumstances, mandate surgical intervention.
- Although most patients have "mechanical low back pain" that requires little investigation, there are certain "red flags" in the clinical presentation that mandate further careful evaluation (Box 8–2).

Diagnostic Tools

- The key to successful outcomes after surgery for low back pain is to first establish a pathoanatomic diagnosis with an understanding of the components of the low back that can cause pain (Box 8–3).

Box 8–3: **What Structures Are Sources of Pain in the Lumbar Spine?**

- As surgery is largely an exercise in anatomic modification, it is useful to at least conceptually understand the anatomic components of the lumbar spine thought to contribute to the generation of pain signals.

Intervertebral Disks

- This is thought to be the primary pain generator in the setting of degenerative disk disease.
- Pain fibers have been demonstrated in the outer third of the anulus fibrosus but not in the deeper anulus or nucleus pulposus.
- A variety of biochemical factors are found in the disk that can mediate painful stimuli, including prostaglandins, lactic acid, and substance P.
- During the process of disk degeneration, nerve ingrowth has been observed to occur into the deeper aspects of the anulus fibrosus and even into the nucleus. It is thought that this expansion of sensory innervation within degenerative disks may significantly contribute to low back pain.

Facet Joints

- The facet joint capsule is extensively innervated with pain fibers that can be activated by pressure and stretch and sensitized by inflammatory mediators.
- The synovial folds of the joint lining also possess pain fibers.
- Also present are several types of proprioceptive nerve endings thought to mediate protective muscular reflexes.

Musculoligamentous Structures

- Both the anterior and posterior longitudinal ligaments possess sensory innervation; in particular, the PLL has been found to have substance P containing fibers.
- Unencapsulated nerve fibers are found in the paraspinal musculature; these may respond to metabolites accumulated during prolonged muscle contraction or spasm.

Neural Structures

- Pain from mechanical nerve root compression is thought to require the presence of inflammation.
- The dorsal root ganglion itself has been shown to be extremely responsive to both direct pressure and vibratory forces. An increase in the genetic expression of neuropeptides such as substance P or other inflammatory mediators in response to mechanical nerve root compression may be an important element of increased pain signaling.

- Many diagnostic tools are available, but to use them effectively you must recognize both the advantages and limitations of each.
- Unfortunately, because of our incomplete understanding of the pathophysiology of low back pain (Box 8–4), arriving at a conclusive diagnosis is not possible in as many as 85% of patients who are categorized as having "idiopathic low back pain" (Deyo 2002). You must resist the temptation to offer such individuals an operation.
- Not unlike the rest of clinical medicine, a thorough history and detailed physical examination are the most important diagnostic tools.

Plain X-ray Film

- At a low cost, plain x-ray films provide a tremendous amount of information about the general anatomy of the vertebral bodies, spinal alignment, bone quality, and disk height.
- Flexion–extension films are used frequently to demonstrate dynamic instability, particularly among degenerative motion segments (Fig. 8–1). Their role in the routine evaluation of low back pain is limited. Lateral bending films are useful in the preoperative planning of adult scoliosis patients undergoing corrective surgery.
- Oblique x-ray films may be helpful in evaluating integrity of the pars intra-articularis in the setting of spondylolisthesis.

Box 8–4: Neurophysiology of Low Back Pain

- Though much research has been done recently on the neurophysiology of pain in the lumbar spine, it is still relatively poorly understood (Cavanaugh 1996).
- Painful stimuli are mediated by one of two nerve types, both with unencapsulated endings:
  1. Small, myelinated (A-delta) fibers
  2. Unmyelinated C fibers
- It is assumed that structures containing either of these nerve types have the capacity to cause pain. Many elements of the lumbar spine contain such pain fibers.
- The recurrent sinuvertebral nerve is thought to be an important sensory nerve for transmitting painful stimuli from pain fibers within the anulus and the posterior longitudinal ligament.
- The threshold at which these pain fibers are stimulated is normally quite high.
- Inflammatory biochemical factors such as bradykinin, histamine, substance P, prostaglandins E1 and E2, and leukotrienes lower this threshold, thus promoting pain transmission.
- This biochemical "sensitization" of pain fibers is likely a key component of back pain. Also, the increased ingrowth of pain fibers into structures of the lower back may contribute to low back pain.
- Individual differences in this phenomenon of nerve ingrowth and sensitization might explain why some people with degenerative disk disease in their lower back have severe pain but others do not.

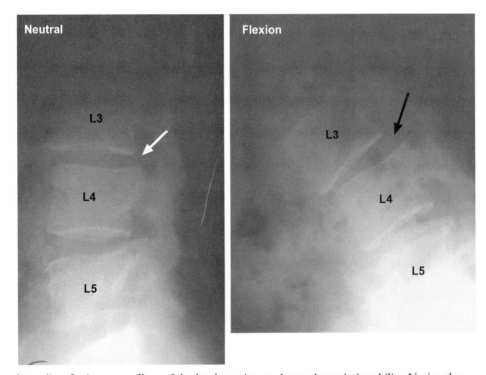

Figure 8–1: Lateral standing flexion x-ray films of the lumbar spine to detect dynamic instability. Notice that the patient has a subtle anterolisthesis of L3 on L4 when standing in the neutral position (shown by the white arrow), suggestive of a mild degree of instability at this level. The extent of the dynamic instability, however, is more clearly delineated on the flexion view (note the increase in anterolisthesis, indicated by the black arrow).

- For the patient who has new onset low back pain but does not have any of the red flags, lumbar spine films have been viewed as unnecessary for at least 4 weeks (Andersson 1998).

Computed Tomography

- Computed tomography (CT) provides excellent visualization of the bony anatomy of the vertebral column.
- Soft tissue windows and the use of intravenous contrast can help with the delineation of disk material, but soft tissues are generally better visualized with magnetic resonance imaging (MRI).
- CT myelography is an excellent investigation for spinal stenosis, rivaling MRI for visualization (although the invasiveness of myelography is a substantial drawback).

Magnetic Resonance Imaging

- MRI provides excellent axial, coronal, and sagittal visualization of soft tissues and neural structures both surrounding and within the vertebral column.
- It provides excellent study for evaluating neural compression within the canal and foramen.
- MRI is noninvasive but relatively expensive. Patient factors such as claustrophobia and ferromagnetic bodies (e.g., cardiac pacemakers, cochlear implants, and intracranial aneurysm clips) may make it unsuitable.
- The loss of water content within intervertebral disks during the natural process of disk degeneration produces a low signal on T2-weighted MRI, a finding described as the "dark disk" (Fig. 8–2). It is important to interpret the MRI findings of dark disks or disk herniations or bulges because they are found in a high percentage of individuals with no previous history of low-back pain, sciatica, or neurogenic claudication (Boden et al. 1990).
- Similarly, the presence of these MRI findings in asymptomatic patients does not reliably predict the subsequent development of back pain or root compression (Borenstein et al. 2001).

Facet Injections

- Facet injections or facet nerve blocks have been rationalized by the hypothesis that facet arthrosis contributes to low back pain; hence joint provoking with saline injections or anesthetizing with local anesthetic, steroids, or both might be diagnostic and therapeutic.
- Well-designed studies to evaluate the efficacy of facet injections are rare; only one well-controlled prospective, randomized trial of methylprednisolone versus saline injection has been performed with no demonstrable efficacy for methylprednisolone (Carette et al. 1991).

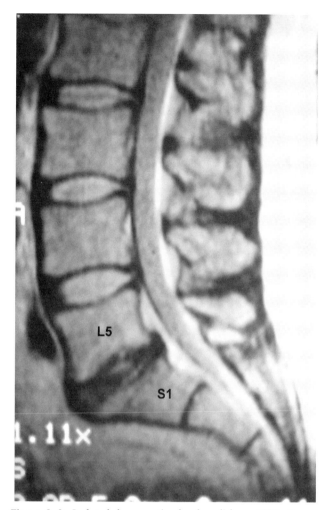

Figure 8–2: Isolated degenerative lumbar disk on MRI. On T2-weighted MRI images, water appears bright (hence the bright signal in the thecal sac within the spinal canal). During the process of degeneration, the disks lose their water content and thus appear darker on T2-weighted images. Notice the dark appearance of the L5-S1 disk in this patient compared with the appearance of the adjacent levels.

- The use of facet injections to predict surgical outcomes for patients with low back pain is not supported.

Discography

- The role of provocative discography as a method of identifying surgically amenable disk pathology in the setting of low back pain is highly controversial.
- Discography is performed by introducing a needle into the nucleus pulposus (Fig. 8–3). An injection of contrast medium confirms the accurate placement of the needle and visualizes internal fissures or tears in the disk that might not be shown with other imaging modalities. The significance of these morphologic findings is questionable.
- An injection of saline to distend the disk and stretch the anular fibers is performed to provoke the patient's pain. The

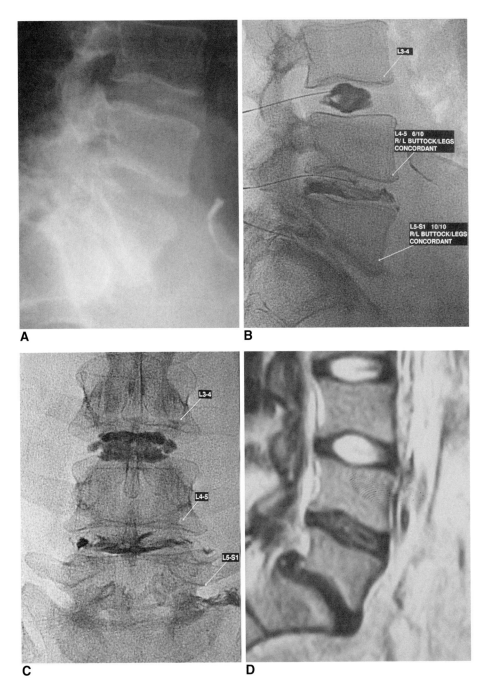

Figure 8–3: X-ray film, discogram, and MRI images of degenerative lumbar disks. Notice the radiographic loss of disk space height, most marked at L5-S1 but also evident at L4-L5 (A). The discogram (B and C) demonstrates the dye being inserted into the nucleus pulposus with normal containment at L3-L4 but extravasation at L4-L5 and L5-S1, suggestive of disk disruption at these levels. Upon injection of the dye, the patient reported concordant pain, which is recorded at the time of the procedure. The MRI findings (D) correlate with the discogram results, with the L3-L4 disk appearing normal but with dehydration and collapse at the L4-L5 and L5-S1 levels. Such correlation between MRI and discogram findings strongly suggests an etiologic role of that particular disk as a source of pain.

saline injection's reproduction of pain concordant with that typically experienced by the patient is thought to be useful for identifying disks that might benefit from fusion.

- The combination of concordant pain on discography with MRI findings of disk degeneration is not confirmatory, but it does strengthen the argument that a particular disk is a significant component of a patient's back pain.
- It has been suggested that the combination of concordant discographic pain with MRI findings predicts an increased likelihood for a good surgical outcome after fusion (Gill et al. 1992). This predictive value, however, is refuted by others who did not observe the predictive effect of positive discography on the surgical outcome (Parker et al. 1996).
- Furthermore, a retrospective review of 25 patients with single-level degenerative disk disease and positive discograms who were not operated on demonstrated that 68% improved with nonsurgical treatment at an average follow-up of 4.9 years, suggesting that the natural history of such "discogenic pain" is relatively favorable (Smith et al. 1995). Surgical interventions are compelled to improve upon this natural history.

General Surgical Indications

- In general, when faced with spinal pathology and trying to decide if surgical intervention is warranted, adhere to basic principles and ask yourself the following:
  1. Does this patient warrant an operation for **mechanical stability?**
  2. Does this patient warrant an operation for **neurologic reasons?**
  3. Are there **specific patient considerations** that influence the decision to operate or which operation to perform (e.g., psychological factors, nicotine exposure, and expectation of high physical demands)?
- The most difficult treatment decisions are in patients with degenerative disk disease and low back pain but without radicular symptoms. Whether surgery has a role in the management of such individuals, and what surgical technique to perform, are extremely contentious questions.
- Surgical indications proposed for patients with low back pain without radicular symptoms include the following:
  1. Unremitting pain and disability for more than 1 year
  2. Failure of a lengthy, aggressive trial of physical therapy and nonoperative treatment modalities (nonsteroidal anti-inflammatory drugs, nonnarcotic analgesics, local heat or ice, activity modification, and weight loss)
  3. Absence of psychiatric disorders and compensation or litigation issues
  4. Isolated single-level disk degeneration on MRI with concordant pain response on discography, demonstra-

ble single-level static or dynamic instability, or both (e.g., isthmic or degenerative spondylolisthesis)

Surgical Procedures

- The surgical management of low back pain largely focuses on **spinal fusion**.
- **Decompression** is indicated in the setting of leg pain and nerve root compression (e.g., disk herniations and spinal stenosis).
- **Nucleus pulposus or intervertebral disk replacement** are emerging options for low back pain secondary to single-level degenerative disk disease but are still being investigated.

Spinal Fusion Principles

- The basic goal of spinal fusion is **to prevent further segmental motion**; hence the objectives of spinal fusion are most appropriate for patients with evidence of spinal instability (e.g., spondylolisthesis of either an isthmic or a degenerative nature).
- The application of spinal fusion to patients with degenerative disk disease but without gross instability is based on the perception that low back pain is mediated by motion among spinal segments. As indicated previously, the disk itself is thought to be a major source of this pain (the "anterior pain generator"), so preventing motion across the disk or removing the disk altogether is postulated to relieve such discogenic pain.
- The keys to attaining a solid arthrodesis include the following:
  1. The meticulous preparation of the graft bed (i.e., decortication to maximize the surface area of cancellous bone)
  2. Supplementation with an appropriate type and amount of bone graft material—autograft, allograft, bone morphogenetic proteins, or bone substitutes (Table 8–1)
  3. Careful consideration of lumbar spine biomechanics—maintaining correct sagittal alignment and optimally placing the graft in compression rather than tension (Box 8–5)
  4. Optimizing systemic conditions that influence bone healing—nicotine, corticosteroids, nonsteroidal anti-inflammatory drugs, nutrition, and infection
- Problems with subsequent degeneration of levels adjacent to fused segments mandate that a minimum number of spinal levels fused, particularly in younger individuals.
- It is worth noting that despite the current obsession with technologies to promote lumbar spine fusion, it has been difficult to definitively prove that the clinical outcomes of patients undergoing lumbar spine procedures are significantly improved by the achievement of bony fusion. Although this suggests that patient outcome has little to do with whether bony ankylosis occurs or not,

Table 8–1: Choices for Bone Graft in Lumbar Spinal Fusion

TYPE	ADVANTAGES	DISADVANTAGES
Autograft	Osteogenic, osteoinductive, *and* osteoconductive properties Large trabecular surface provides optimal scaffold for bone remodeling No immune response or chance for blood-borne infection	Significant donor site morbidity (pain, infection, fracture, nerve damage during acquisition) Increased blood loss Increased operating room time Limited amount of available graft material; also, structural autograft is available only from iliac crest, fibula, tibia
Allograft	Historically the most successful and currently the gold standard against which all bone graft substitutes must be compared Eliminates the need for autogenous bone graft harvesting Potentially unlimited graft material Structural graft can be acquired from any bone (e.g., femur, humerus) Long shelf life	Provides osteoconductive scaffold without osteoinductivity and osteogenicity Small risk of disease transmission Lack of osteogenicity and decreased strength Potentially lower fusion rates than with autograft in the lumbar spine Prolonged incorporation time
Bone graft substitutes (both osteoinductive and osteoconductive)	Eliminates the need for autogenous bone graft harvesting Osteoinductive substances such as the bone morphogenetic proteins may equal autograft in their ability to facilitate fusion Potentially unlimited availability	Expensive Clinical efficacy has only been recently established in specific conditions Possible inflammatory or immune reaction

Box 8–5: Biomechanics of the Lumbar Spine

- The spinal column is made up of functional motion segments composed of adjacent vertebral bodies articulating with an intervertebral disk anteriorly and facet joints posteriorly (the "triple-joint complex").
- Most of the axial load (approximately 80%) is transmitted through the anterior column of the spine, consisting of the vertebral bodies, intervertebral disks, and longitudinal ligaments.
- The posterior elements, including pedicles, lamina, facets, transverse and spinous processes, and intervening ligaments resist tensile, shear, and rotational forces.
- The sagittal alignment of the lumbar spine normally demonstrates some degree of lordosis—maintaining or restoring this lordosis during spinal fusion is thought to be an important element of promoting normal spinal mechanics and function.

the spectrum of disorders subjected to spinal fusion and the difficulties in determining whether fusion has occurred make the literature hard to interpret.

Techniques for Achieving Fusion in the Lumbar Spine

- Several techniques have been developed and advocated for achieving fusion in the lumbar spine. Each has its own potential advantages and disadvantages (Table 8–2). In general, the more circumferential the fusion, the higher both the fusion and the complication rate.
- Fusion techniques include the following:
  1. Posterolateral intertransverse process fusion with or without adjunctive pedicle screw instrumentation
  2. Posterior lumbar interbody fusion (PLIF) with or without adjunctive pedicle screw instrumentation
  3. Transforaminal lumbar interbody fusion (TLIF) with or without adjunctive pedicle screw instrumentation
  4. Anterior lumbar interbody fusion (ALIF)
  5. Circumferential (combined anterior and posterior) fusion
- Interbody fusions in which bone graft material is placed into the intervertebral space enjoy higher fusion rates than posterolateral intertransverse process fusions because the interbody grafts are placed under compression and the posteriorly placed grafts are subject to more tension. Interbody fusion devices, however, incur the risk of extruding, settling into the endplate, or both with loss of disk space height.
- Successful fusion rates from 75% to 95% have been reported for each technique, but it is difficult to determine the superiority of one technique over another in terms of promoting fusion for several reasons:
  1. Most reports are retrospective reviews of a single institution's experience with one particular fusion technique. Few studies have performed comparisons of different techniques in a prospective randomized fashion.
  2. Reported fusion techniques have employed wide variations in surgical technique, particularly in choices of autograft, allograft, pedicle screw instrumentation systems, and interbody devices.
  3. Study subjects with low back pain represent a heterogeneous population, making it difficult to control across studies for variables such as age, symptomatology, radiographic diagnosis, psychological disturbances, and compensation or litigation status.

Table 8–2: Summary of Fusion Techniques

TECHNIQUE	ADVANTAGES	DISADVANTAGES	ADDITIONAL COMMENTS
Posterolateral intertransverse process fusion ± instrumentation	Technically straightforward with reasonable fusion rates marginally enhanced by the addition of instrumentation	Leaves the intervertebral disk intact, allowing it to potentially remain a source of pain Posterior approach inflicts damage to the dorsal paraspinal soft tissues	Most common method of lumbar fusion
Posterior lumbar interbody fusion (PLIF) ± instrumentation	Excises much of the disk, thus removing one potential pain generator Places bone graft in compression Increases disk height	Access to disk requires significant retraction of neural elements, with resultant radiculopathy secondary to epineural or perineural fibrosis Wide posterior exposure and anterior discectomy potentially destabilizes the motion segment, warranting additional pedicle screw fixation Technically demanding Incomplete disk excision (compared with ALIF)	Current versions commonly employ pedicle screw fixation to enhance the stability of the motion segment and "lock" the interbody device or graft in place to prevent extrusion
Transforaminal lumbar interbody fusion (TLIF) ± instrumentation	Similar to those of PLIF but approaches the disk more laterally, thus requiring less retraction of neural elements	Technically demanding Removes only part of the disk (compared with ALIF)	In comparative studies, fewer neurologic complications than with PLIF
Anterior lumbar interbody fusion (ALIF)	Near-total disk removal maximizes the surface area for bony fusion and allows maximal restoration of disk height Generally well-tolerated anterior approach compared with the posterior exposure May be accomplished with minimally invasive technology Circumferential stabilization increases fusion rates	Risk of catastrophic vascular injury or intra-abdominal injury during approach Risk of damaging autonomic fibers in presacral plexus, leading to retrograde ejaculation Relative lack of stability because it depends solely on compressive fit of interbody device or graft Does not reliably decompress neural elements posteriorly, although an increase in disk space height may provide some indirect decompression	Classically a low back pain operation because it is not designed to address leg symptomatology
Circumferential (anterior and posterior)	Combines the benefits of the wide surface area for interbody fusion (ALIF) with the ability to decompress and fuse with instrumentation posteriorly	Theoretically increased complications and morbidity than a single-stage procedure	Difficult to determine if the increased morbidity is sufficiently offset by the increased fusion rates to improve patient function

4. All reports of fusion rates are subject to uncertainty regarding the reliability of assessing bony fusion radiographically.

- In general, whether the fusion rate significantly influences the patient outcome after surgery for low back pain is highly debatable. As a good example of this, a recent prospective, randomized comparison was performed using 222 patients with chronic low back pain that underwent one of the following:
  1. Uninstrumented posterolateral fusion
  2. Instrumented posterolateral fusion (with pedicle screws)
  3. Instrumented posterolateral fusion (with pedicle screws) and an interbody fusion placed either posteriorly (PLIF) or anteriorly (ALIF)
- The authors found that although fusion rates increased with the more technically demanding procedures (72 %, 87 %, and 91%, respectively), there was no difference in clinical outcome in terms of pain, disability, depressive symptoms, and overall satisfaction 2 years after the operations (Fritzell et al. 2002).

Posterolateral Intertransverse Process Fusion

- Such a process is a time-honored, straight-forward method of promoting fusion among motion segments; it is likely the most common technique for fusion in the lumbar spine.
- This fusion, a posterior or a posterolateral muscle-splitting approach, involves decortication of the transverse processes, then the laying down of an autogenous bone graft along the transverse processes (Figs. 8–4 and 8–5).
- The pseudarthrosis rate for single-level uninstrumented fusions is estimated to be between 5% and 25%, although pseudarthrosis rates as high as 57% have been described (Lorenz et al. 1991).

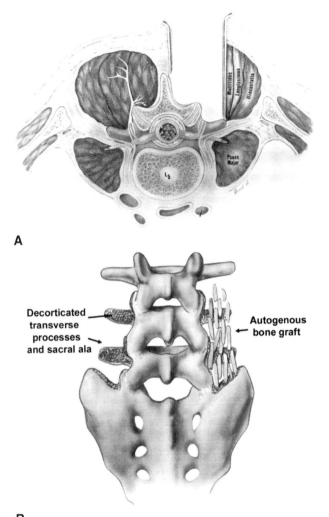

A

B

Figure 8–4: Schematic of posterior lumbar spine approach and uninstrumented posterolateral fusion. The posterior approach (A) requires dissection of the paraspinal musculature off the posterior elements of the spine out enough far enough to expose the transverse processes. It is important to visualize the transverse processes laterally because these need to be decorticated to promote the fusion posterolaterally (B).

- The addition of pedicle screw fixation (Figs. 8–6 and 8–7) has been popularized with the expectation that the increase in immediate stability would enhance the likelihood of bony fusion, lower the pseudarthrosis rate, and improve patient outcomes.
- Although it appears that the addition of instrumentation increases fusion rates for posterolateral intertransverse process fusion to some degree (pseudarthrosis rates from 5% to 10%), there is little evidence to suggest that this is accompanied by an improvement in clinical outcomes (Fritzell et al. 2002, Thomsen et al. 1997).
- Again, when interpreting results of fusion in the lumbar spine, remember the difficulties in radiographically evaluating bony fusion in the lumbar spine.

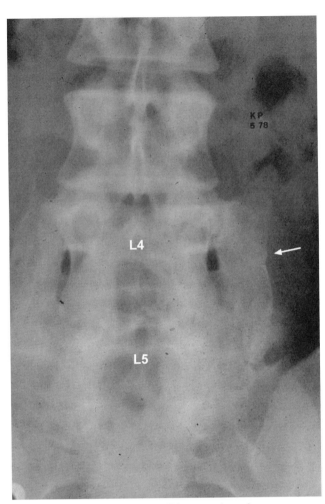

Figure 8–5: Radiograph of a solid posterolateral uninstrumented fusion. This AP x-ray film of a posterolateral uninstrumented L4-L5 fusion demonstrates full incorporation of the bone graft between the transverse processes (white arrow). Unfortunately, this degree of incorporation is not always present, often making it difficult to determine whether fusion has successfully occurred.

- The theoretical drawback to posterolateral intertransverse process fusion in the setting of low back pain is that although it reduces motion at the particular segment, some residual motion still occurs anteriorly in the otherwise intact intervertebral disk. If motion at the disk is indeed an element of pain generation, the posterolateral intertransverse process fusion—with or without instrumentation—does not completely address it.

Posterior Lumbar Interbody Fusion

- This approach was described by Cloward (1958) more than 50 years ago as a fusion technique that involved the extraction of much of the disk through a posterior approach and wide laminectomy, then the insertion of bone graft into the intervertebral space to achieve fusion of the anterior column. The approach can be widened by

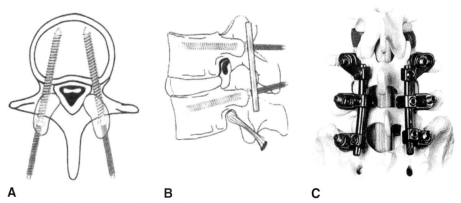

A **B** **C**

Figure 8–6: Schematic of posterolateral fusion with pedicle screws. Pedicle screws need to be inserted with great caution because they pass just lateral to the spinal canal (A) and just superior to the exiting nerve root (B). Rigid segmental fixation is achieved by connecting the screws to rods. Fusion is still performed by decorticating the transverse processes and laying bone in the posterolateral gutters.

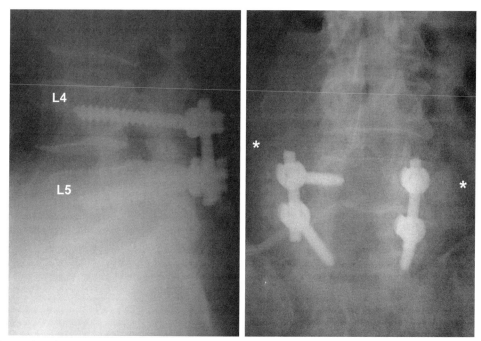

Figure 8–7: Radiographs of a L4-L5 posterolateral fusion instrumented with pedicle screws. This patient underwent a laminectomy and instrumented fusion at L4-L5. Note the slight degenerative spondylolisthesis at L4-L5, with 3-4 mm of forward translation of the body of L4. Notice the autogenous bone graft (asterisks) placed along the transverse processes. In the acute state, these cancellous and corticocancellous pieces of autogenous bone have a "fluffy" appearance, but over time, as the fusion mass matures, this consolidates to look more like that in Fig. 8–5.

removing the lower one third of the inferior facet and medial two thirds of the superior facet, although this increases the risk of iatrogenic instability.

• Current iterations of this technique involve the placement of a structural interbody device in addition to bone graft into the intervertebral space and the pedicle screw instrumentation posteriorly to provide immediate stability, offsetting to some extent the instability induced

by the wide decompression, which may involve some of the facet joint (Figs. 8–8 and 8–9).

• Many different interbody spacers have been used, including tricortical iliac crest graft, bone dowels, loose cancellous bone, and an increasing variety of interbody cage devices thought to provide structural support for the anterior column support and to maintain disk space height when the bone graft consolidates.

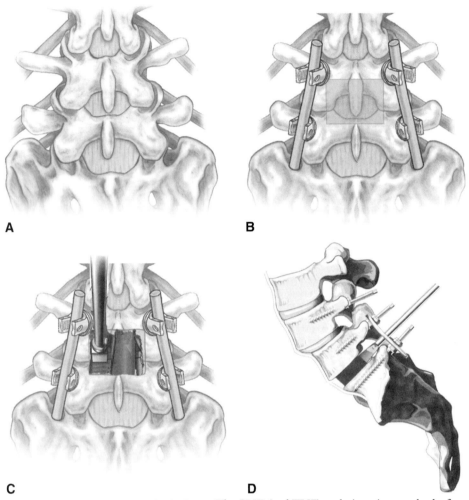

A

B

C

D

Figure 8–8: Schematic of posterior lumbar interbody fusion. The PLIF (and TLIF) technique is a method of performing both posterolateral and anterior interbody fusion all from the posterior approach. The posterior elements of the spine are exposed (A) and a wide laminectomy (shaded area in B) is performed. Currently, it is common to apply pedicle screw fixation, provide more rigid posterior fixation, prevent posterior graft migration, and allow some temporary distraction during the insertion of the graft. The disk is excised and removed through the laminectomy, and the graft is inserted (C and D). Great care must be exercised to limit the amount of medial dural retraction when putting in the cage device.

- Pedicle screw instrumentation allows one to distract across the disk space for improved access then compress after the insertion of the interbody graft to resist its extrusion and to restore lumbar lordosis.
- The advantages of the PLIF procedure include the following:
  1. Removal of much of the disk as a source of pain
  2. Increased disk space height that helps to restore sagittal alignment and increases the vertical height of the neural foramen (thus indirectly decompressing the exiting nerve root)
  3. Placement of the intervertebral bone graft in a setting of compression
  4. Increased fusion rates compared with the rates of posterolateral intertransverse process fusion

- The disadvantages of the PLIF procedure include the following:
  1. The need to extensively retract the neural elements to access the intervertebral disk and insert the interbody device and bone graft; this has resulted in a relatively high incidence of root injury and radiculopathy from forcible manipulation and epidural or perineural fibrosis, particularly of the traversing root descending around the pedicle of the distal vertebral body
  2. Destabilization created by the need to perform a wide laminectomy or decompression posteriorly and a complete discectomy anteriorly
  3. The potential for graft or interbody device extrusion; this and the destabilization are less of a concern with the use of pedicle screw instrumentation posteriorly

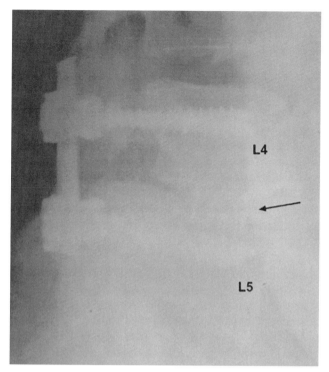

Figure 8–9: Radiograph of a posterior lumbar interbody fusion. This patient underwent a PLIF for discogenic back pain and L4 radicular symptoms. A titanium cylindrical mesh cage (black arrow) was used as the interbody device. Autogenous bone is packed into the anterior aspect of the disk space and into the cylindrical cage.

4. Although much of the disk is removed, the discectomy is incomplete; hence the surface area for bony fusion anteriorly is not maximized
5. Technically demanding

Transforaminal Interbody Fusion

- This modification of PLIF was developed by Harms to lessen the manipulation of neural elements during interbody fusion and thus reduce the rate of radiculopathy from the epineural and perineural scarring that had been observed with PLIF.
- Rather than a wide laminectomy, in TLIF, the pars inter-articularis and half of the facet are removed unilaterally, and the disk is then accessed along a path that lies beside the lateral aspect of the vertebral foramen (hence "transforaminal" interbody fusion). Because the access to the disk is more lateral than that of the PLIF technique, there is less need to retract the thecal sac and descending roots medially (Fig. 8–10).
- The approach can be done bilaterally to improve the completeness of disk excision and directly decompress the exiting and traversing nerve roots on both sides.
- Otherwise, TLIF differs little from PLIF. Both are typically performed with interbody devices to provide anterior column support when bony consolidation occurs. Both are often supplemented with pedicle screw instrumentation to provide distraction intraoperatively for interbody access then compression to restore lumbar lordosis and enhanced immediate stability.

Figure 8–10: Differences between PLIF and TLIF. With PLIF, a wide laminectomy is performed. Note on the left side that the exposure of the disk is limited even with the medial part of the facet resected. This requires fairly significant retraction of the neural elements medially to gain access to the disk (on the right side) for both the resection and the insertion of the interbody device. Alternatively, with TLIF, the facet is excised and the exposure to the disk is more lateral, requiring much less medial retraction of the dura to access the disk.

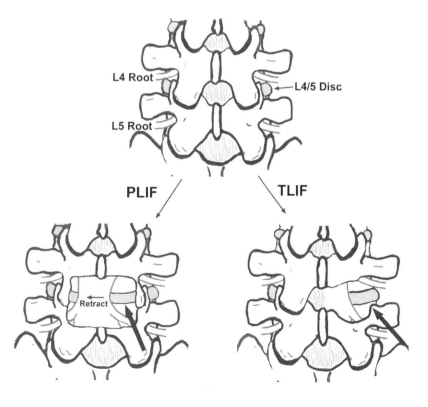

- In a relatively recent comparison of PLIF versus TLIF in 74 patients with degenerative disk disease, central disk herniations, or low grade spondylolisthesis, the PLIF group suffered far more complications, including four radiculopathies (compared with none in the TLIF patients) (Humphreys et al. 2001).
- The advantages of the TLIF procedure include the following:
  1. Less retraction on the neural elements than PLIF with lower incidence of iatrogenic nerve injury or damage
  2. Less destruction of posterior elements than PLIF
  3. Removal of part of the disk as a source of pain
  4. Increased disk space height, which helps to restore sagittal alignment and increases the vertical height of the neural foramen (thus indirectly decompressing the exiting nerve root)
  5. Placement of the intervertebral bone graft in a setting of compression
  6. Increased fusion rates compared with posterolateral intertransverse process fusion.
- The disadvantages of this TLIF procedure include the following:
  1. More lateral visualization of the disk space, making it difficult to excise much of it on the contralateral side—this can be resolved by performing bilateral TLIF
  2. Achieves an incomplete removal of the disk, potentially even less than with PLIF (although the TLIF approach to the disk can be performed bilaterally)
  3. Technically demanding

Anterior Lumbar Interbody Fusion

- The ALIF procedure is fundamentally a low back pain operation that focuses on eliminating the disk as a generator of pain and promoting fusion with an anterior graft placed under compression. It is not a procedure designed to address radicular symptoms secondary to root compression because the posteriorly located neural elements are not visualized. The restoration of disk space and foraminal height achieved with the ALIF procedure may indirectly reduce the exiting roots, but such a decompression is more reliably performed with a posterior procedure such as a PLIF or TLIF.
- Approaching the intervertebral disk anteriorly rather than posteriorly provides wider exposure to the disk and allows a more complete excision, thus providing a much larger surface area for fusion than the area that can be obtained with posterior procedures.
- An optimally sized interbody device can then be precisely placed to restore disk height and sagittal alignment.
- The intervertebral disks can be approached anteriorly through an open left-sided retroperitoneal approach, an open transperitoneal approach, or a laparoscopic approach. Transperitoneal approaches incur far more immediate postoperative morbidity than retroperitoneal approaches.
- After adequate exposure, the disk is excised as completely as possible and the disk space is distracted to restore height and lordosis. Morcellized autogenous bone graft and some form of structural interbody device are inserted to promote fusion (Fig. 8–11).
- Many of the same bone grafts and interbody devices used in PLIF and TLIF are used in ALIF—autogenous tricortical iliac crest bone, structural allograft (e.g., Femoral ring), and cages. The purpose of each is to provide structural support of the disk space while bony fusion occurs.

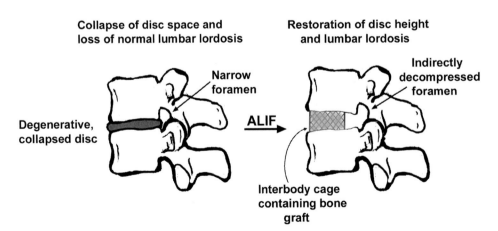

Collapse of disc space and loss of normal lumbar lordosis

Restoration of disc height and lumbar lordosis

Narrow foramen

Indirectly decompressed foramen

Degenerative, collapsed disc

ALIF

Interbody cage containing bone graft

Figure 8–11: Restoration of disk height and sagittal alignment with anterior lumbar interbody fusion. To some extent, all interbody fusions (ALIF, PLIF, and TLIF) can increase disk height and restore sagittal alignment. However, during ALIF, the most complete discectomy can be performed; hence the largest correction in height and alignment can be achieved. The restoration of disk height anteriorly increases the height of the foramen posteriorly and thus indirectly decompresses the exiting nerve root, although a nerve root decompression is more reliably done from a posterior approach. The interbody cage is one of many devices that can be inserted into the interbody space to provide structural support until fusion occurs.

- Strictly speaking, supplementary instrumentation is not added to the ALIF procedure. The stability rests on the compressive fit of the interbody device within the intervertebral space; hence a slightly oversized device is recommended after distraction of the disk space. An external orthosis may be used postoperatively to help to stabilize the motion segment.
- Bony fusion occurs readily with ALIF procedures, likely because of the biomechanical advantage of having the graft under compression.
- Significant complications may arise from the surgical approach. At L5-S1, the disk is shown between the iliac vessels, but autonomic nerves in the prevertebral space may be damaged, leading to retrograde ejaculation (Fig. 8–12). At L4-L5, the left common iliac vessels obscure access to the disk and must be moved out of the way. The left-sided iliolumbar vein is a major hazard in this area and must be identified and ligated prior to moving the common iliac vein. Peritoneal violation can lead to internal hernias and bowel obstruction.
- The advantages of the ALIF procedure include the following:
  1. Maximal removal of the disk as a source of pain, thus providing a larger surface area for interbody fusion than in PLIF or TLIF
  2. Optimal disk space distraction and hence optimal restoration of disk height and sagittal alignment
  3. Placement of the intervertebral bone graft in the biomechanically favorable setting of compression
  4. The avoidance of a posterior dissection to the spine, which inevitably damages the lumbar musculature and other soft tissues; in general, the anterior procedure has less blood loss and is better tolerated than posterior procedures and minimally invasive techniques further diminish operative morbidity
  5. Can be performed as a salvage procedure in the setting of previous posterior surgery; if a posterior laminectomy has been performed, an ALIF gains access to the disk without having to dissect the posterior scar that encases the dura
- The disadvantages of the ALIF procedure include the following:
  1. The potential for catastrophic vascular or intra-abdominal injury during the surgical approach
  2. The inability to reliably decompress neural elements
  3. The risk of retrograde ejaculation from injury to autonomic fibers
  4. Possibly a higher pseudarthrosis rate than instrumented fusions performed posteriorly because no additional instrumentation is placed to stabilize the interbody

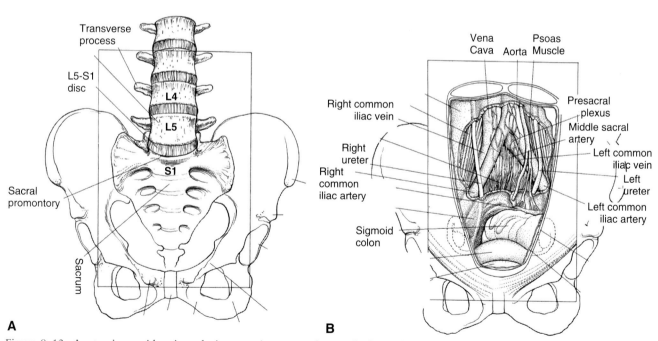

Figure 8–12: Anatomic considerations during anterior approaches to the lower lumbar spine. The anterior approach allows the most complete disk excision and restoration of disk height and avoids the muscle-damaging posterior approach. However, important neurologic, urologic, and vascular structures lay within the retroperitoneum in front of the lower lumbar spine. Damage to the presacral plexus of autonomic fibers can lead to retrograde ejaculation. Inadvertent damage to the large vessels, particularly the left common iliac vein that must be moved laterally, can lead to profuse, uncontrollable hemorrhage.

graft, which depends solely on compressive fit within the disk space

Circumferential (Anterior and Posterior) Fusion

- The supplementation of the ALIF procedure with pedicle screws and posterolateral intertransverse process fusion is considered to be a 360 degree fusion (Fig. 8–13); an ALIF plus pedicle screw stabilization without the intertransverse process fusion is described as a 270 degree fusion.
- The addition of posterior pedicle screws is thought to mitigate the relative lack of stability characteristic of otherwise uninstrumented ALIF, thus improving fusion rates.
- Because of the fairly extensive nature of the surgery, it has been applied to patients with previously failed lumbar surgery with the rationale that every measure should be taken to achieve fusion in what could be considered a last-effort salvage procedure for these patients (Leufven et al. 1999). In this rather challenging population of patients, circumferential

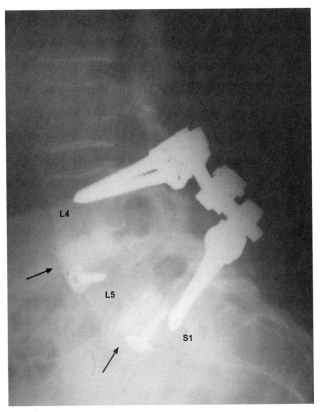

Figure 8–13: Circumferential fusion of L4-S1. Note the maintenance of disk height at L4-L5 and L5-S1 with the ALIF performed with structural allograft spacers (black arrows). The addition of pedicle screws at the back and posterolateral intertransverse bone grafting makes this a circumferential, 360 degree fusion.

fusion has had relatively high fusion rates and good clinical outcomes.

- The advantages of circumferential fusion include the following:
  1. Enhanced immediate stability and thus increased fusion rates and less graft extrusion
  2. Possibly a role as a salvage procedure to achieve fusion after previously failed surgery
- The disadvantages of circumferential fusion include the following:
  1. Increased operative time, blood loss, infection (two incisions), and acute postoperative morbidity
  2. Strong evidence that such an extensive effort to achieve bony fusion translates into better clinical outcome is lacking

Pedicle Screw Instrumentation

- The use of pedicle screws to provide segmental fixation in the lumbar spine is widespread in North America.
- The pedicle is the strongest point of screw fixation within the vertebral body; that is, the pedicle screw gains its rigidity primarily from its fixation within the pedicle, not from its length within the vertebral body.
- The increased construct stiffness is associated with slightly higher union rates for posterolateral intertransverse process fusion and helps to stabilize interbody devices or grafts in PLIF, TLIF, and ALIF.
- Pedicle screw strength and stability is related to several factors, including the inner and outer diameter of the threaded shaft and the quality of the host bone. Although wider screws are less prone to breakage, they are at a higher risk of plastically deforming or fracturing the pedicle.
- In the setting of osteoporosis, the interface between the pedicle screw threads and the host bone is weakened and may warrant supplementation with wires, hooks, or cement.
- Complications of pedicle screw instrumentation include late-onset discomfort requiring removal, neurologic injury, vascular injury, pedicle fracture, and screw fracture. Also, their use is associated with increased operative time, blood loss, infection, and cost. In experienced hands, the complication rate was reported as 2.4% in 4790 pedicle screws (Lonstein et al. 1999). Careful preoperative planning and attention to anatomic landmarks intraoperatively can reduce the risk of improper pedicle screw placement (Box 8–6 and Fig. 8–14).
- Circumstances in which the use of pedicle screws may have greater justification include the following:
  1. Revision surgery, particularly in patients with painful pseudarthrosis from previous attempts at lumbar fusion
  2. Correction of significant sagittal or coronal deformity
  3. Multilevel fusions—The rate of pseudarthrosis in non-instrumented fusions increases significantly as more levels are incorporated into the fusion mass

Box 8–6: Tips for Pedicle Screw Insertion in the Lumbar Spine

- Careful preoperative evaluation of axial imaging (CT or MRI) is helpful in determining the starting point, trajectory, and size of pedicles. Look at the where the widest part of the pedicle meets the transverse process.
- For the insertion of a screw in line with the axis of the pedicle, the starting point is located where the transverse process meets the base of the superior articular process; in the proximal–distal direction, this point is usually in line with the vertical midpoint of the transverse process (confirm this on the axial imaging). As an additional visual cue, in the medial–lateral direction, the insertion point is just adjacent to the lateral border of the pars. Expending the effort to clearly visualize the juncture of the transverse process, superior articular process, and pars is well worth the time!
- In degenerative spines, the facet joint are often osteophytic and will require some resection to identify the correct landmarks. The lateral aspect of the superior facet may need to be burred down to find the true juncture between the facet and the transverse process, or it may deceive you into starting too far to the side.
- The cortical bone at the starting point for screw insertion is removed with a burr or rongeur, and the channel or path for the screw is made initially with a solid, blunt-tipped probe with great care and control to prevent "plunging."
- From the preoperative images, you can estimate how medial the screw must be directed from the starting point at the lateral border of the superior articular process. Typically, the axis of the pedicles is aimed medially in the lower lumbar spine but becomes nearly perpendicular to the vertebral body at the thoracolumbar junction.
- In the lower lumbar spine in particular, where the pedicles are directed most medially, your hands must swing out laterally to sufficiently "toe in" the probe or screw. Do not let the soft tissue walls of the dorsal exposure push your hand medially, or you will fail to toe in and risk putting the screw out laterally. Alternatively, you can start the screw hole slightly more medially (in line with the actual joint surface of the facet) and direct the screw in a straighter trajectory.

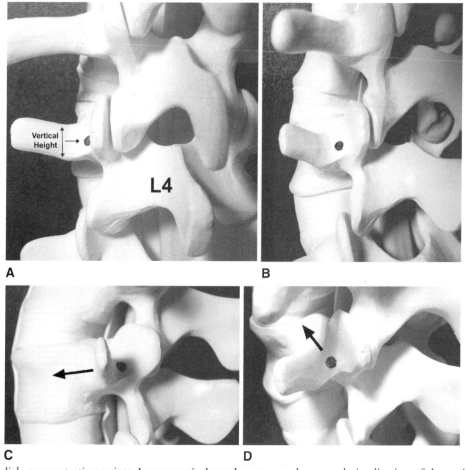

Figure 8–14: Pedicle screw starting points. Intraoperatively, make sure you have good visualization of the entire transverse process (it needs to be exposed anyway so that it can be decorticated and bone graft can be laid on top of it). For the superior–inferior position of the starting point, look at the vertical height of the transverse process and pick its midpoint when it arrives at the pedicle (A). The medial–lateral position is where the transverse process meets the superior articular process (B). Notice how this is just to the side of the lateral border of the pars (A and B). This point can be obscured in the degenerative spine if the articular processes are severely osteophytic. Note that from this starting point, the screw trajectory can be directed down the middle of the pedicle on both the lateral (C) and the axial (D) view.

4. Degenerative or isthmic spondylolisthesis or degenerative scoliosis requiring posterior decompression
5. Interbody fusions (PLIF, TLIF, and ALIF) to stabilize the segment and prevent extrusion of the interbody device or graft

Conclusions

- Low back pain is an extremely complex, multifactor problem that presents many diagnostic and therapeutic challenges.
- The role of surgical management is controversial and is constantly being redefined as surgeons attempt to intervene in a clinical entity whose natural history is not completely understood.
- It is felt that the key to successful surgical outcomes is a thorough diagnostic evaluation leading to the identification of anatomic pathology that may be amenable to surgical treatment. Operating without establishing such a diagnosis is unlikely to succeed.
- Numerous techniques for fusing the lumbar spine have been described. Each has its particular limitations and advantages. Interbody fusions that address the anterior pain generator are thought to be superior to posterior fusions alone.
- In general, large differences in fusion rates and clinical patient outcomes have not been demonstrated among the various types of lumbar fusions. In this regard, the decision about who to operate on is likely to be far more important than the particular fusion operation performed.

References

Abraham I, Killackey-Jones B. (2002) Lack of evidence-based research for idiopathic low back pain: The importance of a specific diagnosis. Arch Intern Med 162: 1442-1444.

This perspective provides an argument against the validity of the concept of idiopathic low back pain accepted as a diagnosis for a large percentage of patients for whom a more specific diagnosis has not been made. (See Deyo 2002 for the opposing argument). The authors contend that significant methodological flaws exist in the studies performed in the 1960s upon which the concept of idiopathic low back pain was based and that more refined research is needed now to rethink the pathogenesis and specific diagnoses of low back pain.

Andersson GB. (1998) Diagnostic considerations in patients with back pain. Phys Med Rehabil Clin N Am 9: 309-322.

This review emphasizes the importance of a careful history and physical examination in the diagnosis of low back pain and the need for a sensible, evidence-based approach to the use of diagnostic modalities (such as x-ray films, CT scan, and MRI). The author summarizes some of the guidelines for a thorough, diagnostic approach to low back pain established by a multidisciplinary panel commissioned through the Agency for Health Care Policy and Research.

Boden SD, Davis DO, Dina TS et al. (1990) Abnormal magnetic resonance scans of the lumbar spine in asymptomatic subjects: A prospective investigation. J Bone Joint Surg Am 72: 403-408.

This important and extensively quoted study demonstrates that a significant percentage of individuals with no previous history of low back pain, sciatica, or neurogenic claudication had disk abnormalities identified on MRI. This study highlights the importance of interpreting MRI findings with great caution and that they must be correlated to clinical signs and symptoms.

Borenstein DG, O'Mara JW Jr, Boden SD et al. (2001) The value of magnetic resonance imaging of the lumbar spine to predict low back pain in asymptomatic subjects: A 7-year follow-up study. J Bone Joint Surg Am 83-A: 1306-1311.

This is an important follow-up to the previous study of Boden et al. 1990 in which the asymptomatic individuals who had the MRI scans of their lumbar spines were followed for the next 7 years to determine whether their MRI findings predicted the later development of low back pain. Interestingly, the authors found that the MRI findings were not predictive for the subsequent development of low back pain, again emphasizing the need to carefully interpret the results of this imaging study.

Carette S, Marcoux S, Truchon R et al. (1991) A controlled trial of corticosteroid injections into facet joints for chronic low back pain. N Engl J Med 325: 1002-1007.

This was a randomized, placebo-controlled trial to evaluate the efficacy of fluoroscopically guided facet injections of either methylprednisolone or saline in patients with chronic low back pain. The authors conclude that there was no significant benefit from the methylprednisolone injection.

Cavanaugh JM. (1996) Neural mechanisms of idiopathic low back pain. In: Low Back Pain—A Scientific and Clinical Overview (Weinstein JN et al., eds.). Rosemont: American Academy of Orthopaedic Surgeons, pp 583-606.

This is an excellent review of the neurophysiology of low back pain in an outstanding textbook that comprehensively covers many clinical and basic science aspects of low back pain. The author describes the phenomenon of sensitization, which promotes an exaggerated pain response, and summarizes the neuroanatomy of potential pain generators in the lumbar spine.

Cherkin DC, Deyo RA, Loeser JD et al. (1994) An international comparison of back surgery rates. Spine 19: 1201-1206.

This interesting study reviewed lumbar spine surgery rates in 11 developed nations and found that the rate of such surgery was at least 40% higher in the United States than in any other country. Interestingly, the rates of back surgery also increased with the numbers of orthopedic and neurosurgical surgeons per capita.

Cloward RB. (1958) The anterior approach for removal of ruptured cervical disks. J Neurosurg 15:602-617.

Deyo RA (2002) Diagnostic evaluation of LBP: Reaching a specific diagnosis is often impossible. Arch Intern Med 162: 1444-1447.

This is the counterargument to the position statement of Abraham et al. 2002 in which Deyo contends that because anatomic abnormalities are readily identified by imaging studies in asymptomatic patients, assigning an exact pathoanatomic diagnosis to patients with low back pain is often impossible. The author emphasizes the need for a rationale, evidence-based approach to patients with low back pain.

Fritzell P, Hagg O, Wessberg P et al. (2002) Chronic low back pain and fusion: A comparison of three surgical techniques—A prospective, multicenter, randomized study from the Swedish Lumbar Spine Study Group. Spine 27: 1131-1141.

In the mid-1990s, the Swedish Lumbar Spine Study Group performed a large, prospective randomized study of patients with chronic low back pain, comparing nonoperative treatment to three forms of operative treatment. This study reports a comparison among the operatively treated groups. The comparison found no significant differences in 2-year outcomes among the three surgical treatments despite higher fusion rates in the more extensive procedures.

Frymoyer JW. (1996) Epidemiology—Magnitude of the Problem. In: The Lumbar Spine (Weisel SW et al., eds.). Philadelphia: W.B. Saunders Company, pp 8-16.

This is an excellent review of the epidemiology and societal effect of low back pain.

Gill K, Blumenthal SL. (1992) Functional results after anterior lumbar fusion at L5-S1 in patients with normal and abnormal MRI scans. Spine 17: 940-942.

This study attempted to determine the predictive value of preoperative discography and MRI findings for outcomes after ALIF in patients with chronic low back pain. These authors found that patients with abnormal MRI and discography had better surgical outcomes than those who underwent the same operation but with normal MRI findings.

Humphreys SC, Hodges SD, Patwardhan AG et al. (2001) Comparison of posterior and transforaminal approaches to lumbar interbody fusion. Spine 26: 567-571.

This study compared a consecutive series of patients who underwent either a TLIF or a PLIF. The authors found that the complication rate was higher in patients who underwent the PLIF. In particular, the incidence of radiculopathy postoperatively was higher with the PLIF group, in keeping with the smaller retraction of neural elements required for the TLIF.

Leufven C, Nordwall A. (1999) Management of chronic disabling low back pain with 360 degrees fusion: Results from pain provocation test and concurrent posterior lumbar interbody fusion, posterolateral fusion, and pedicle screw instrumentation in patients with chronic disabling low back pain. Spine 24: 2042-2045.

The authors present a 2-year follow-up using a consecutive series of patients in which a circumferential fusion was performed for chronic low back pain. High fusion rates were achieved, and approximately half of the patients had a good or excellent result.

Lonstein JE, Denis F, Perra JH et al. (1999) Complications associated with pedicle screws. J Bone Joint Surg Am 81: 1519-1528.

This is a retrospective review of the accuracy and associated complications from 4790 pedicle screws inserted over a 10-year period at the authors' institution. They describe a complication rate of 2.4%, with painful hardware being the most common complaint.

Lorenz M, Zindrick M, Schwaegler P et al. (1991) A comparison of single-level fusions with and without hardware. Spine 16: S455-S458.

This was one of many studies to evaluate fusion rates in lumbar spine surgery. Accepting the difficulties in determining fusion radiographically, these authors noted a 58.6% pseudarthrosis rate in patients undergoing an uninstrumented fusion; no instrumented fusions had a pseudarthrosis.

Parker LM, Murrell SE, Boden SD et al. (1996) The outcome of posterolateral fusion in highly selected patients with discogenic low back pain. Spine 21: 1909-1916.

This was a prospective analysis of a consecutive series of 23 patients undergoing posterior lumbar fusion for discogenic low back pain. All patients had MRI and discography. Of the patients, 48% had a poor result. Discography was not predictive of a good surgical outcome.

Smith SE, Darden BV, Rhyne AL et al. (1995) Outcome of unoperated, discogram-positive low back pain. Spine 20: 1997-2000.

This study retrospectively evaluated the outcomes of 25 patients who had discogram-positive disks and were considered surgical candidates but did not undergo operative treatment. After a mean follow-up of 4.9 years, the authors found that 68% of patients improved, suggesting that natural history is favorable and that operative treatment must surpass such results to be justifiable.

Thomsen K, Christensen FB, Eiskjaer SP et al. (1997) The effect of pedicle screw instrumentation on functional outcome and fusion rates in posterolateral lumbar spinal fusion: A prospective, randomized clinical study (1997 Volvo Award winner in clinical studies). Spine 22: 2813-2822.

This prospective randomized study compared uninstrumented and instrumented posterolateral lumbar spine fusions in 130 patients with grade 1 or 2 spondylolisthesis. Fusion rates were not significantly different, and the authors did not observe any significant improvement in patient outcomes with the addition of pedicle screws (the rate of significant complications from their insertion was 4.8%). The authors concluded that the use of pedicle screws was not justified to supplement posterolateral lumbar fusion.

Turner JA, Ersek M, Herron L et al. (1992) Patient outcomes after lumbar spinal fusions. JAMA 268: 907-911.

This was an extensive review of success and complication rates after lumbar spine surgery. The authors were unable to find literature to support that the achievement of or attempt at fusion conferred any advantage over surgery without fusion. Unfortunately, the literature at this time contained no sound prospective randomized studies.

CHAPTER 9

Management of the Failed Back Surgery Patient

David H. Kim★, Robert J. Banco §, Louis G. Jenis §, Frank F. Rand §, Kevin P. Sullivan †, and Scott G. Tromanhauser §

★M.D., Orthopaedic Spine Surgeon, The Boston Spine Group, Boston, MA
§M.D., The Boston Spine Group, New England Baptist Hospital, Boston, MA
†M.D., Metro West Medical Center, Framingham, MA; Nashoba Valley Medical Center, Ayer, MA; The Boston Spine Group, Southboro, MA

Introduction

- Patients with persistent, recurrent, or worsened symptoms following spinal surgery represent the most challenging diagnostic and therapeutic group in any adult spinal surgical practice. These patients are often severely frustrated, angry, and depressed. There is a high rate of narcotic dependence, and clinical evaluation is frequently confounded by the presence of secondary gain issues.

Definition

- Failed back syndrome (also failed back surgery syndrome)—Chronic and persistent unrelieved, worsened, or recurrent pain in the low back, lower extremity, or both of a patient following lumbar spinal surgery
- Persistent lower extremity weakness, sensory changes, or reflex abnormalities are **not** elements of failed back syndrome

Classification

Causes of Failed Back Syndrome (Table 9–1)

- Inappropriate patient selection
  - Presence of secondary gain issues (e.g., active litigation or workers' compensation)
  - Functional as opposed to clinical illness—Clues include positive Waddell's signs (Table 9–2), bizarre pain diagrams (Fig. 9–1), nonanatomic pain distribution, inconsistent history and examination, and a history of psychiatric diagnosis
  - Narcotic addiction and, for fusion surgery, nicotine addiction
  - Noncompliant behavior
- Incorrect diagnosis—Commonly missed causes of lower extremity pain, weakness, and sensory changes
  - Hip arthritis
  - Knee arthritis
  - Peripheral vascular disease (i.e., vascular claudication)
  - Diabetic peripheral neuropathy
  - Multiple sclerosis
  - Amyotrophic lateral sclerosis
  - Ankylosing spondylitis
- Incorrect surgical level—Check postoperative radiographic studies to correlate surgical level with preoperative symptoms
- Incorrect surgical procedure
  - Compressive radiculopathy or spinal stenosis requires appropriate decompression.
  - Preoperative spondylolisthesis may represent segmental instability that can be worsened by decompressive laminectomy alone, and many surgeons advocate including an instrumented or noninstrumented fusion in the surgical procedure for such patients; if fusion was not performed, flexion–extension radiographs should be checked for segmental instability.
- Inadequate surgery or poor surgical technique

Table 9–1:   Classification of Failed Back Syndrome

TYPE	CAUSE
Type I	Improper patient selection
Type II	Incorrect diagnosis
Type III	Incorrect indication
Type IV	Incorrect level
Type V	Incorrect surgery
Type VI	Iatrogenic
Type VII	Idiosyncratic

Table 9–2:   Waddell's Nonorganic Physical Signs

SIGN	FINDING
Tenderness	Broad lumbar tenderness to light touch
	Widespread tenderness to deep palpation in nonanatomic distribution
Simulation	Low back pain produced with axial loading of skull or shoulders
	Low back pain with passive rotation of shoulders and pelvis in plane through hips
Distraction	Negative seated straight leg raise test in a setting of a positive supine straight leg raise
Regional	Regional sensory and motor abnormalities in a nonneuroanatomic distribution (e.g., "give way" weakness and "stocking" sensory loss)
Overreaction	Overreaction during examination; excessive verbalization, facial expressions, tremors, collapse

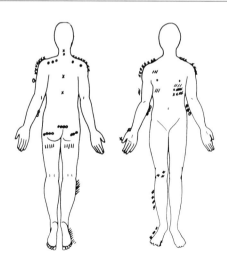

Figure 9–1: Characteristic "bizarre" pain drawing suggesting that the patient may be a poor candidate for surgical treatment. (Williams et al. 2003.)

- Inadequate decompression of foraminal or extraforaminal nerve root compression, especially with far lateral disk herniations
- Inadequate decompression of lateral recess in patients with disk herniation or central stenosis
- Iatrogenic nerve root injury (i.e., "battered root")

- Overly aggressive laminectomy
- Idiosyncratic
- Epidural fibrosis
  - Junctional degeneration
  - "Fusion disease"
- Three out of five positive Waddell's signs suggest that the patient may be a poor candidate for surgery (Waddell et al. 1980)
- Overreaction is the most significant Waddell's sign.

Additional Considerations for Specific Diagnoses

Lumbar Disk Herniation

History and Physical

- Timing of any period of symptomatic improvement and nature of recurrent symptoms are the most important diagnostic elements (Table 9–3).

Type I

- May be most common
- Consider the presence of secondary gain issues (e.g., active litigation or workers' compensation)

Type II

- High prevalence of disk protrusions and herniations in asymptomatic population
- Preoperative symptoms may be wrongly attributed to incidental herniation; consider alternative diagnoses

Type III

- Candidates for lumbar discectomy should have dominant lower extremity pain preoperatively, ideally pain radiating below the level of the knee (L4, L5, and S1 radiculopathy) and in a radicular pattern correlating with the side and location of herniation on preoperative magnetic resonance imaging (MRI).
- Dominant back pain is a relatively poor indication for decompression alone (Herron et al. 1985).
- Timing of surgery—Optimal results for discectomy occur when surgery is performed within 3 months of symptom onset; surgery delayed 1 year or longer is associated with inferior rates of symptomatic relief, possibly because of

Table 9–3:   Timing of Recurrent Symptoms

PERIOD OF POSTOPERATIVE IMPROVEMENT	POSSIBLE NONINFECTIOUS DIAGNOSES
None	Incorrect patient selection, diagnosis, level of surgery
Days to weeks	Postoperative scar tissue formation
Weeks to months	Recurrent disk herniation

permanent root injury, the formation of adhesions, and the development of chronic pain syndrome.
- Dysesthetic pain (hyperalgesia, or painful sensation provoked by light touch) may reflect permanent nerve root injury.

Type IV

- Compare preoperative and postoperative radiographic studies to confirm correct level or side of surgery.

Type V

- Review preoperative imaging studies for lateral and foraminal stenosis and for far lateral disk herniation (extraforaminal root compression). Review the operative report to determine whether all potential sites of root compression were appropriately addressed.

Type VI

- Dysesthetic pain may represent iatrogenic nerve root injury.

Type VII

- Epidural fibrosis—Symptomatic improvement for weeks to months followed by recurrent pain, often distributed across multiple roots and often described as "burning" pain with occasional lancinating pain and dysesthesia

Radiographic Studies

- Plain films—Check the site of laminotomy on the anteroposterior view and correlate with the patient's preoperative symptoms and location of herniation on preoperative MRI; check for subtle spondylolisthesis on the lateral view, indicating possible instability from aggressive facetectomy.
- Segmental instability can result in mechanical low back pain and may cause radicular pain from mechanical nerve root irritation (Kramer 1987).
- MRI—Such imaging is minimally informative within 3 months of surgery; the appearance typically is unchanged even in patients who are completely asymptomatic. Request a gadolinium contrast to differentiate residual or recurrent disk herniation from postoperative scar tissue and epidural fibrosis. Recurrent disk herniations or retained disk fragments will demonstrate minimal border enhancement and causes positive mass effect with the thecal sac and nerve root displaced from the herniation. Epidural fibrosis demonstrates diffuse enhancement and causes negative mass effect, with the thecal sac and nerve root displaced toward the scar tissue mass (Ross 2000) (Fig. 9–2).
- EMG or NCS—Utility is controversial. Studies are often normal in the setting of radiculopathic pain; appropriate changes following successful decompression are unknown.

Treatment

- Revisit the trial of conservative management for several months; symptoms may continue to improve up to 6 months following surgery.

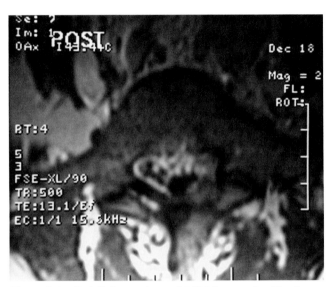

Figure 9–2: Gadolinium-enhanced MRI image of epidural fibrosis following lumbar microdiscectomy. **Note the enhancing scar tissue filling the left-sided laminotomy defect. Adhesion to the thecal canal contents is suggested by the displacement of the thecal sac and the nerve root** *toward* **the tissue.**

- Physical therapy, including aerobic conditioning and abdominal and back strengthening exercises—Consider specific gait assessment and retraining, especially with a chronic limp.
- Nonsteroidal anti-inflammatory drugs (e.g., ibuprofen, naproxen, or selective celecoxib cyclooxygenase-2 inhibitors)—If used continuously longer than 6 weeks, consider laboratory tests to evaluate renal and hepatic function.
- Avoid narcotic pain medication.
- Injection therapy (i.e., epidural steroids or selective nerve root block) may provide both therapeutic and diagnostic value; with extension-dominant back and buttock pain, consider facet block.
- Consider a trial of orthotic stabilization for segmental instability (Fritsch et al. 1996).
- Revision surgery
  - Microdiscectomy—The ideal candidate has a period of symptomatic relief lasting several months prior to recurrent lower extremity pain. MRI with gadolinium shows recurrent, nonenhancing disk herniation correlating with patient symptoms (may be the same or a different side or level). Surgery is often effective. With clear root impingement because of recurrent herniation, surgery has a 70%-80% success rate (Fager et al. 1980, Cauchoix et al. 1978) (Box 9–1).
  - In a setting of brief postoperative pain relief lasting days to weeks and with an MRI showing enhancing tissue compression of the nerve root, the patient may have postoperative epidural fibrosis. Surgery results in no change or worsening symptoms in 50%-80% of

Box 9–1:	**Factors Associated with Improved Results Following Revision Discectomy**

- Symptomatic relief for >6 months following initial surgery
- Radicular lower extremity pain greater than back pain
- MRI with gadolinium clearly showing recurrent disk herniation and nerve root impingement

patients (Fager et al. 1980, Spengler et al. 1980, Waddell et al. 1979, Benoist et al. 1980).

- Consider more extensive decompression, especially if imaging studies suggest lateral or foraminal stenosis not addressed by the original surgery; consider performing the Wiltse approach for far lateral herniation.
- Back-dominant pain complaints may represent discogenic pain from degenerative disk disease. Consider provocative lumbar discography if the patient is a candidate for lumbar fusion surgery, although this test is less informative following discectomy. Consider that 40% of patients will have a positive result from discography following even a successful discectomy (Carragee et al. 2000).
- Multiply revised patients have better results with inclusion of a fusion procedure. Consider that symptomatic epidural fibrosis may also be caused by persistent root irritation from instability (Fritsch et al. 1996).

- Severe dysesthetic pain from permanent root injury or chronic radiculopathic pain in the setting of epidural scar or adhesions may respond to placement of a spinal cord stimulator (Devulder et al. 1997).
- Consider referral to a pain clinic for the development of a chronic pain management strategy, including medication such as antidepressants, amitriptyline, transcutaneous electrical nerve stimulation unit application, and various nerve ablation therapies.

Lumbar Spinal Stenosis

History and Physical

Type I

- Much less common than failed back syndrome following disk herniation

Type II

- Vascular claudication and neurogenic ("pseudo") claudication are symptomatically similar and often confused.
- Neurogenic claudication is relieved by lumbar flexion (e.g., sitting down or leaning over a grocery cart); vascular claudication may be relieved by standing still.
- Check lower extremity pulses.

Type III

- This is a less common cause.
- Relatively advanced stenosis on MRI or myelogram may be asymptomatic. Appropriate candidates for surgery should have significant lower extremity complaints, including claudication, radiculopathy, or both. Patients with radiographic stenosis and predominant back pain are not good candidates for laminectomy.

Type IV

- Compare preoperative and postoperative imaging studies to confirm surgery at the correct level.

Type V

- Segmental instability (i.e., spondylolisthesis) often coexists with stenosis, and most surgeons recommend instrumented or noninstrumented fusion in conjunction with decompression.
- Check preoperative radiographs for L4-L5 or L3-L4 (usually degenerative) or for L5-S1 (usually isthmic) spondylolisthesis.

Type VI

- Type VI has inadequate decompression.
- The most common cause of failed back following decompression surgery may be failure to decompress the lateral recess, foramen, or both.
- Review the preoperative MRI, CT, or CT myelogram and the operative note.
- Dural tears occur in up to 13% of cases and do not compromise the outcome if they are repaired immediately (Jones et al. 1989).

Type VII

- Epidural fibrosis

Radiography

- Plain films—Assess the extent of laminectomy on an anteroposterior view. Minimal laminectomy defect suggests possible inadequate decompression, especially of the lateral recess and foramen; overly wide laminectomy without fusion may cause segmental instability (Fig. 9–3) from excessive facet resection or iatrogenic pars interarticularis fracture (lateral view).
- MRI or CT myelogram—Directly assess the adequacy of decompression of the canal, lateral recess, and foramen; check for stenosis at adjacent levels.

Treatment

- Conservative management is less effective; patients often have limited ability to participate in physical therapy.
- Medication

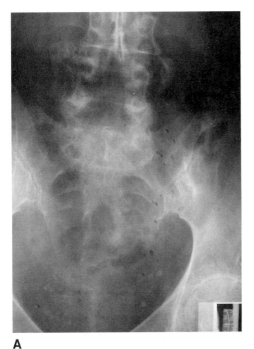

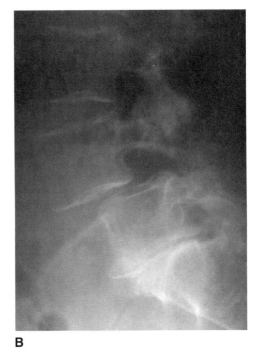

A   **B**

Figure 9–3: A, Wide laminectomy for spinal stenosis with bilateral facetectomies, pars interarticularis resection, and attempted noninstrumented posterolateral fusion. B, Development of postoperative segmental instability and grade II or III iatrogenic spondylolisthesis at the level of decompression.

- Antidepressants may be effective in patients with symptoms or signs of depression.
  - Amitriptyline or other membrane stabilizers can be used, particularly in the setting of dysesthetic pain.
  - Avoid narcotics.
  - Consider referral to a pain center for the management of medication.
- Consider epidural steroid injections or selective nerve root blocks under fluoroscopic guidance.
- Revision surgery
  - Consider revision decompression only if a clear site of residual stenosis or root compression can be identified on MRI or CT myelogram.
  - Consider posterior instrumented fusion if there is radiographic evidence of postoperative instability from preoperative spondylolisthesis, iatrogenic instability, or pars interarticularis fracture (Markwalder et al. 1993, Parts 1 and 2).

Following Fusion Surgery

- This is the most challenging subgroup of failed back patients. It is essential to review the preoperative history and diagnostic testing to determine the indication for fusion surgery. Lack of appropriate indications for fusion surgery may be an explanation for persistent pain. If the indication was appropriate, the next and often most difficult steps are to determine whether the fusion is solid and to rule out the development of a pseudarthrosis.

History and Physical

- Any period of postoperative symptomatic improvement and the length of time are informative. Particularly with instrumented fusions, initial symptomatic relief for several months followed by recurrent back pain suggests possible pseudarthrosis.
- Patient reports of painless "cracking" or "shifting" in the back with trunk motion are common and do not indicate pseudarthrosis or instrumentation failure.
- Cracking or shifting sensations associated with pain are concerning for pseudarthrosis or complications associated with instrumentation (Box 9–2).

Radiographic Signs of Pseudarthrosis

- Plain films
- Posterolateral fusion—Check for bridging bone between transverse processes on an anteroposterior view. The use of

Box 9–2:	Risk Factors for Postoperative Pseudarthrosis

- Revision procedure
- Postoperative wound infection
- Cigarette smoking
- Poor nutrition
- Systemic illness
- Steroid and nonsteroidal anti-inflammatory medication

certain bone graft substitutes, such as coralline hydroxyapatite, can result in persistent radio-opacity, obscuring the interpretation of fusion. Look for a transverse radiolucent line with a sclerotic margin suggesting pseudarthrosis, most commonly at the proximal or the distal level of multilevel fusion. Compare lateral flexion and extension views to identify motion (more than 5 degrees of angulation or 2 mm of motion suggests pseudarthrosis).

- Anterior interbody fusion—Such fusion is more easily assessed on a lateral view. Check for bridging trabecular bone crossing the interbody space. If an interbody device is in place, examine the space anterior to the device. Compare flexion and extension views to identify any "gapping" anteriorly with extension. The fracture of a structural allograft or the subsidence of an interbody spacer does not necessarily indicate pseudarthrosis.
- Instrumentation—Check for disengagement of components, implant breakage, haloing around pedicle screws, and screw back out. Examine the quality of bone fusion at the level of any instrumentation failure (Fig. 9–4).
- CT scan
- In the presence of radiculopathy, obtain CT myelogram to identify possible root impingement from a misplaced pedicle screw.
  - To evaluate the quality of fusion, obtain thin cut (1.5-2 mm) axial images with sagittal and coronal reformatted images. For posterolateral fusion, examine coronal images for bridging intertransverse process bone; for anterior fusion, examine sagittal and coronal images for bridging trabecular bone, most commonly anterior to or through an interbody device (Box 9–3).

Postoperative Infection

- Early acute postoperative wound infections are typically easily recognized with fever, chills, systemic signs and symptoms, local wound erythema and drainage, and increased back pain. Late postoperative infections, especially in the presence of implanted instrumentation, can be less apparent and should be considered when other causes for failed back are not present (Box 9–4).

History and Physical

- Fevers, chills, systemic complaints, weight loss, fatigue, and anorexia
- Swelling, tenderness, and erythema around the surgical wound on examination

Radiography

- MRI is usually diagnostic for significant osteomyelitis of vertebral bodies or discitis (Fig. 9–6). It is less useful for following the treatment of known infection because of the delay of several months between successful treatment and improvement of MRI changes. MRI obtained too early in the course of infection can sometimes lead to missed diagnosis.
- Nuclear medicine bone scan is less informative because of the increased metabolic bone activity associated with recent surgery.

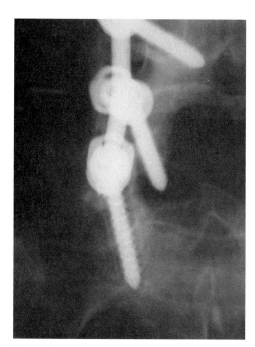

Figure 9–4: Haloing around the S1 pedicle screw suggesting loosening and possible pseudarthrosis.

Box 9–3:	**Junctional Degeneration**

Successful spinal fusion creates a lever arm proportional to the number of segments fused and transmits increased biomechanical forces to adjacent unfused segments. Although difficult to prove, most surgeons believe that this accelerates the degeneration of spinal segments adjoining the fusion. Look for evidence of junctional degeneration on plain films, CT, and MRI when patients have been asymptomatic for several years and then develop recurrent mechanical back pain (Fig. 9–5).

Box 9–4:	**Risk Factors for Postoperative Infection**

- History of any infectious condition occurring in the preoperative or postoperative period (e.g., skin infections, tooth abscess, urinary tract infection, or open sores)
- History of prolonged drainage from surgical wound
- Diabetes mellitus or history of immune disorder
- History of steroid use or chemotherapy
- Revision surgery
- Lengthy surgery
- Morbid obesity

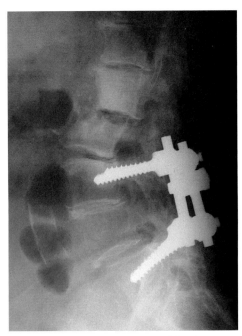

Figure 9–5: Junctional degeneration resulting in segmental instability proximal to successful instrumented lumbar fusion.

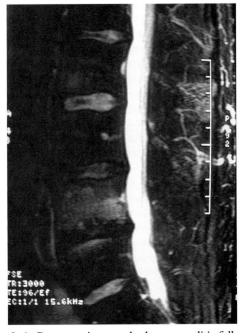

Figure 9–6: Postoperative vertebral osteomyelitis following lumbar microdiscectomy. Note the diffusely increased intramedullary signal on the T2-weighted MRI.

Laboratory Tests

- Complete blood count, erythrocyte sedimentation rate, and C-reactive protein
- Blood cultures insensitive
- Consider CT or fluoroscopic biopsy for culture (Box 9–5)

General Principles

- Avoid unnecessary surgery; in most patients with failed back syndrome, repeat surgery is of limited benefit and can result in clinical worsening (Goupille 1996).
- The success rate of revision surgery decreases with the number of revisions performed (Waddell et al. 1979).
- Fusion is associated with better results in patients undergoing multiple revision decompressive surgeries (Fritsch et al. 1996).

References

Benoist M, Ficat C, Baraf P et al. (1980) Postoperative lumbar epiduroarachnoiditis. Spine 5: 432-436.

This study reviewed 38 patients with the finding of postoperative epiduroarachnoiditis at the time of revision surgery. Results of scar excision were considered good in 13, fair in 8, and failed in 17.

Carragee EJ, Chen Y, Tanner CM et al. (2000) Provocative discography in patients after limited lumbar discectomy: A controlled, randomized study of pain response in symptomatic and asymptomatic subjects. Spine 25: 3065-3071.

This prospective observational study compared results of provocative lumbar discography in a group of 20 patients who were asymptomatic following lumbar discectomy with those of a group of 27 patients who had intractable low back pain following discectomy. "Positive" injections were found in 40% of the asymptomatic group and 63% of the symptomatic group. Psychometric testing of the symptomatic group revealed a 43% positive rate in patients with normal psychometric scores compared with a 70% rate in patients with abnormal scores. [Note: The data from this study has been reexamined by other investigators using alternative protocols for discography interpretation with significantly different results.]

Cauchoix J, Ficat C, Girard B. (1978) Repeat surgery after disk excision. Spine 3: 256-259.

This retrospective review of 60 patients undergoing revision surgery following lumbar discectomy identified a 5.9%

reoperation rate. The most common findings in patients with recurrent sciatica were perineural fibrosis and recurrent herniation, with the latter patients responding most favorably to revision surgery.

Devulder J, De Laat M, Van Bastelaere M et al. (1997) Spinal cord stimulation: A valuable treatment for chronic failed back surgery patients. J Pain Symptom Manage 13: 296-301.

This study reviewed the results of spinal cord stimulation in 69 patients with failed back surgery syndrome. Of the patients, 26 had stopped using the treatment. There were 43 who experienced good pain relief. The study found that 16 continued to require narcotic pain medication, but a synergistic effect was reported in 11. Of the patients, 11 returned to work.

Fager CA, Froidberg SR. (1980) Analysis of failures and poor results of lumbar spine surgery. Spine 5: 87-94.

This retrospective study of 105 patients attempted to identify the cause of failure in postoperative patients following lumbar spine surgery. Two thirds of patients had suffered work-related or vehicular accidents. Most patients did not have evidence of significant nerve root compression on preoperative imaging studies.

Fritsch EW, Heisel J, Rupp S. (1996) The failed back surgery syndrome: Reasons, intraoperative findings, and long-term results— A report of 182 operative treatments. Spine 21: 626-633.

This retrospective study presents the results of 182 revision surgeries performed over a 25-year period. Short-term results were satisfactory in 80% but declined to 22% with long-term follow-up (2-27 years). Multiple revision patients were associated with rates of epidural fibrosis and instability exceeding 60%. Laminectomy, as the index procedure, was associated with a higher rate of revision surgery. Fusion may be more successful than multiple fibrinolyses in severe "discotomy syndrome."

Goupille P. (1996) Causes of failed back surgery syndrome. Rev Rheum 63: 235-239.

This topical review describes the evaluation and treatment of various causes of failed back surgery syndrome.

Herron LD, Turner J. (1985) Patient selection for lumbar laminectomy and discectomy with a revised objective rating system. Clin Orthop 199: 145-152.

This prospective study of 275 patients evaluated a rating system for selecting patients with lumbar disk herniation for surgery. Among the patients with compensation or litigation issues, good outcomes were observed in 58% and fair or poor outcomes were seen in 42%. Among the patients without such issues, good outcomes were observed in 94% and fair or poor outcomes were seen in 6%.

Jones AAM, Stambough JL, Balderston RA et al. (1989) Long-term results of lumbar spine surgery complicated by unintended incidental durotomy. Spine 14: 443-446.

Incidental durotomy was reported at a rate of 0.3%-13%. This retrospective review of 17 patients undergoing primary repair of incidental durotomy revealed no adverse effect on the outcome at a mean follow-up of 25 months.

Kramer J. (1987) The discectomy syndrome. Z Orthop 125: 622-625.

This review describes the "postdiscectomy syndrome," attributing it to epidural scar formation. Patients experience

back and leg pain and demonstrate bilateral, positive straight leg raise testing. Proposed treatments include steroid injections or lumbosacral distraction spondylodesis.

Markwalder T, Battaglia M. (1993) Failed back surgery syndrome— Part 1: Analysis of the clinical presentation and results of testing procedures for instability of the lumbar spine in 171 patients. Acta Neurochir (Wien) 123: 46-51.

This review of 171 patients with failed back surgery syndrome suggests methods for identifying specific types of postoperative instability and the selection of patients for instrumented fusion using facet blocks and plaster immobilization.

Markwalder T, Battaglia M. (1993) Failed back surgery syndrome— Part 2: Surgical techniques, implant choice, and operative results in 171 patients with instability of the lumbar spine. Acta Neurochir (Wien) 123: 129-134.

Using the protocols described in the preceding study, excellent or good results were obtained in 89%, satisfactory in 14%, and moderate or poor in 7%.

Ross JS. (2000) Magnetic resonance imaging of the postoperative spine. Semin Musculoskelet Radiol 4: 281-291.

This review describes the use of MRI evaluation of the postoperative spine in patients with persistent or recurrent symptoms. Standard imaging protocols and MRI characteristics of the most common postoperative conditions are presented.

Spengler DM, Freeman C, Westbrook R et al. (1980) Low back pain following multiple lumbar spine procedures: Failure of initial selection? Spine 5: 356-360.

This retrospective study evaluated 30 patients who had failed multiple lumbar surgeries. All patients had acceptable indications for surgery preoperatively. The most common cause of poor results was thought to be poor patient selection in terms of psychosocial problems such as drug abuse, alcoholism, marital discord, and personality disturbance.

Waddell G, Kummell EG, Lotto WN et al. (1979) Failed lumbar disk surgery and repeat lumbar surgery following industrial injuries. J Bone Joint Surg [Am] 61-A: 201-207.

This retrospective study examined 103 Workmen's Compensation Board patients who underwent revision lumbar spine surgery with a 1-2 year follow-up. Of the second operations, 40% were considered successful. Multiply revised patients [AU3]demonstrated progressively worse percentages of successful results, with more patients experiencing clinical worsening as opposed to improvement. Revision surgery was more successful if patients experienced at least 6 months of relief from the index surgery, if the primary complaint was sciatica, and when a recurrent herniation was found.

Waddell G, McCullough JA, Kummel E et al. (1980) Nonorganic physical signs in low back pain. Spine 5: 117-125.

This classic paper won the 1979 Volvo Award in clinical science. Five nonorganic physical signs in low back pain patients are succinctly described. These signs serve as a screen for patients who require more detailed psychological assessment.

Williams KD, Park AL. (2003) Lower back pain and disorders of intervertebral disks. In: Campbell's Operative Orthopaedics (Canale ST, ed.), 10th edition. Philadelphia: Mosby.

CHAPTER 10

Kyphosis of the Cervical, Thoracic, and Lumbar Spine

Roberto Lugo★, Jonathan N. Grauer §, John M. Beiner †, Brian K. Kwon ‡, Alexander R. Vaccaro ‖, and Todd J. Albert ¶

★ M.D., Medical Student, Yale University School of Medicine, New Haven, CT

§M.D., Assistant Professor, Co-Director Orthopaedic Spine Surgery, Yale-New Haven Hospital; Assistant Professor, Department of Orthopaedics, Yale University School of Medicine, New Haven, CT

†M.D., B.S., Attending Surgeon, Connecticut Orthopaedic Specialists, Hospital of Saint Raphael; Clinical Instructor, Department of Orthopaedics, Yale University School of Medicine, New Haven, CT.

‡ M.D., Orthopaedic Spine Fellow, the Rothman Institute at Thomas Jefferson University, Philadelphia, PA; Clinical Instructor, Combined Neurosurgical and Orthopaedic Spine Program, University of British Columbia; and Gowan and Michele Guest Neuroscience Canada Foundation/CIHR Research Fellow, International Collaboration on Repair Discoveries, University of British Columbia, Vancouver, Canada

‖ M.D., Professor of Orthopaedic Surgery, the Rothman Institute at Thomas Jefferson University, Philadelphia, PA

¶ M.D., Professor and Vice Chairman, Department of Orthopaedics, Thomas Jefferson University Medical College and the Rothman Institute, Philadelphia, PA

Introduction

General

- The spine is normally lordotic in the cervical and lumbar regions and kyphotic in the thoracic and lumbosacral regions (Fig. 10–1). Together, these curves allow the occiput to be held in a balanced fashion over the pelvis.

- Kyphosis, from the Greek word *kyphos,* means "bowed or bent." When used clinically, this term often implies an increased curvature of the spine causing angulation with an excessive posterior convexity and anterior concavity.

- Increased kyphosis is, by far, the most common sagittal plane deformity. Many etiologies for this have been described (Table 10–1). Furthermore, increased kyphosis is less tolerated clinically than increased lordosis.

- Most of the causes of kyphosis can be explained in terms of a shortening of the anterior column, a weakening or lengthening of the posterior column, or both.

- Once kyphosis is initiated it may progress because of increased loading of the anterior vertebral structures and weakening or lengthening of posterior ligamentous structures.

- As the deformity increases, neurologic compromise may occur.

History and Physical Examination

- A thorough history should be obtained from any patient who has a spinal deformity. The nature of a deformity and any noted progression should be documented. Comorbid diseases such as osteoporosis, inflammatory

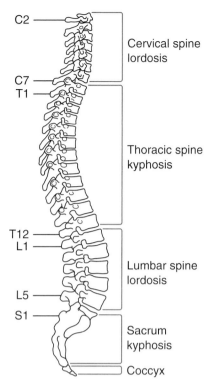

Figure 10–1: Normal spinal curvature with cervical and lumbar lordosis. Note that the plumb line dropped from the odontoid passes through the cervicothoracic, thoracolumbar, and lumbar sacral junctions.

disorders, and a history of infection bear specific mention. Furthermore, any prior spinal surgeries should be defined. Family history of spinal deformity is important as well.

- It is crucial to understand a patient's complaint because it will often dictate treatment. Patients with kyphosis generally have with pain, a neurologic deficit, or a cosmetic deformity.
- Axial pain is often related to muscle fatigue or instability.
- If a focal, sharply angulated kyphosis is seen in the thoracolumbar spine, it is referred to as a *gibbus deformity.*
- In the setting of kyphosis, range of motion in extension will be most limited.
- Compensatory deformities may develop when patients try to maintain forward gaze. For example, thoracic kyphosis may lead to a compensatory cervical or lumbar hyperlordosis. Additionally, compensatory hip and knee flexion may be seen.
- A neurologic examination will identify abnormalities if there is compression of the neural elements. There may be signs and symptoms of radiculopathy if there is nerve root compression or of myelopathy if there is spinal cord compression.

Diagnostic Evaluation (Table 10–2)

- Plain radiographs are useful in defining the nature of sagittal plane deformities. These should be taken with the patient standing and should include standing anteroposterior and lateral films of the entire spine on 36-inch cassettes.
- In addition to static films, dynamic films are useful to characterize the flexibility of a deformity.
- Cobb measurements are used to quantify deformities in the coronal or sagittal planes. Lines are drawn parallel to the endplates of the vertebrae at the borders of a curve. A second set of lines is drawn perpendicular to the first lines, and the angle of their intersection is the Cobb measurement (Fig. 10–2).
- The plumb line is a vertical line dropped from the odontoid or C7 vertebral body. In both the sagittal and coronal planes, this should fall through the L5-S1 disk space. Any other alignment suggests decompensation in the sagittal or coronal plane.
- Bone scans are sensitive but not specific for detecting subtle abnormalities that may contribute to spinal deformities.
- Computed tomography (CT), CT myelogram, and magnetic resonance imaging (MRI) are imaging modalities that can be used to further define bony, soft, or both types of tissue anatomy comprising a sagittal plane deformity.

Table 10–1:	Etiologies of Spinal Kyphosis
CATEGORIES	**SPECIFIC CAUSES**
Traumatic	Single-event trauma
	Microtrauma
Iatrogenic	Postlaminectomy
	Postirradiation
Inflammatory disorders	Rheumatoid arthritis
	Ankylosing spondylitis
Infectious	Pyogenic infection
	Tuberculosis
Postural	N/A
Scheuermann's kyphosis	See Table 10–3
Degenerative conditions	Cervical disk disease
	Osteoporotic fractures
	Paget's disease
Congenital	Defect of formation
	Defect of segmentation
Neoplastic	Primary tumors
	Metastatic tumors
Skeletal dysplasias	Achondroplasia
	Pseudoachondroplasia
	Diastrophic dysplasia
Developmental	Idiopathic scoliosis
Neuromuscular	Myelodysplasia
	Cerebral palsy

Table 10–2: Diagnostic Evaluation of Spinal Kyphosis

DIAGNOSTIC MODALITY	MEASUREMENTS	CLINICAL UTILITY	COMMENTS
Plain radiographs	Cobb measurement C7 plumb line	Anteroposterior films determine coronal plane abnormalities (scoliosis)	Should be taken in standing position
			May focus on cervical, thoracic, or lumbar spine
		Lateral films determine sagittal plane abnormalities (kyphosis or lordosis)	Full-length (36-inch) films are better to assess overall alignment and to measure deformity
Dynamic radiographs	Change in Cobb angles	Reveal spinal instability	Excursion may be limited if painful
		Define the flexibility of the deformity	
Bone scan		Assessment of blood flow associated with increased bone turnover as seen in infection, fracture, malignancy	Can distinguish between old and new compression fractures
			Cannot differentiate between lesions; therefore should be followed by CT or MRI for characterization
CT		Defines bony anatomy	Soft tissue visualization limited
CT myelography		Demonstrates bony anatomy, compression of neural elements	Can pick up subtle lesions
			Disadvantage is the invasiveness of the procedure
			If the patient has spinal hardware, the image will be attenuated and visualization will be impaired
MRI		Defines soft tissue structures	
MRI		Compression of neural elements may be identified	
MRI		Ligamentous disruption can be determined	

Treatment

- Nonoperative treatment is generally the initial treatment for any spinal deformity. Such treatments generally involve anti-inflammatory medications and physical therapy with an emphasis on extension exercises.
- Consideration can be given to bracing. However, in the skeletally mature population, this is not a lasting cure, and the use of bracing risks deconditioning of spinal musculature. Nevertheless, bracing has demonstrated efficacy in the treatment of certain types of kyphosis in the skeletally immature patient.
- Surgery is generally considered when deformities are progressive, cause neurologic compromise, or lead to pain unresponsive to conservative treatment.
- Anterior surgery should be considered with significant kyphotic deformities that are not corrected on dynamic extension radiographs. In these cases, anterior releases and, possibly, anterior column reconstructions should be performed.
- Posterior-only surgery can be considered for flexible deformities. Segmental compression is generally applied to several levels above and below the apex of the pathology being addressed.
- Alternatively, posterior surgery can be used to improve correction or further stabilize a sagittal plane deformity following an anterior release and reconstruction.
- Complications specifically common in deformity surgery include pseudarthrosis, neurologic deterioration, implant failure, and progression of deformity.

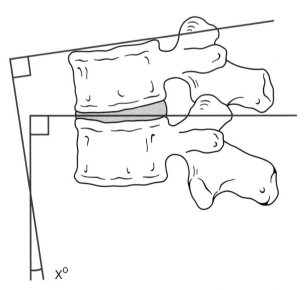

Figure 10–2: Calculation of the intervertebral angle in the sagittal plane using the Cobb technique.

Cervical Kyphosis

General

- The cervical spine is normally lordotic, with an average lordosis of 34-42 degrees (Harrison et al. 1996). A line dropped from the odontoid should pass behind C3 to C6 and through the cervicothoracic junction.

- Developmentally, cervical lordosis is a secondary curvature. Therefore the vertebral bodies have similar anterior and posterior heights, and the disks have greater height anteriorly than posteriorly (Moore et al. 1999).
- If surgical intervention is required, this region of the spine is well suited to preoperative or intraoperative traction to allow gradual deformity correction. This technique offers the advantage of allowing serial examinations of the awake patient to ensure that neurologic worsening does not develop.
- Postoperative immobilization with a collar or halo is possible if necessary.

Degenerative Kyphosis

- The cervical spine, which allows significant mobility, is prone to spondylosis (degenerative changes).
- As explained in Chapter 6, this can lead to the loss of normal lordosis or kyphosis when intervertebral disk height is lost and forward settling or flexion occurs.
- The mainstay of treatment for cervical radiculopathy and axial neck pain is conservative treatment.
- If the previously noted symptoms are resistant to conservative treatment, or if myelopathy is present, restoration of alignment and decompression is recommended.
- In general, correction is best achieved from anterior approaches where the anterior column can be reconstructed. Constructs longer than three levels may require additional posterior stabilization (Fig. 10–3).

Post-traumatic Kyphosis

- Traumatic injuries to the cervical spine can cause deformity acutely or subacutely if inadequately treated (Vaccaro et al. 2001).
- Cervical spine trauma is covered in Chapter 21. Flexion–distraction and flexion–compression injuries are most prone to post-traumatic kyphosis.
- Injuries to the posterior ligamentous structures are associated with post-traumatic deformities if aggressive management is not instituted. Particular attention should be given to such injuries in the lower cervical spine.

Postlaminectomy Kyphosis

- Laminectomy involves the decompression of the neural elements by the removal of the posterior bony arch. In the degenerative cervical spine, this may be performed for the treatment of spondylotic myelopathy or spondylotic radiculopathy.
- As introduced in Chapter 7, laminectomy may be predisposed to kyphosis because of the disruption of the posterior ligamentous and facet structures.
- Risk factors for the development of postlaminectomy instability include young age, lack of preoperative lordosis, and disruption of facet joints.

- Early in the postlaminectomy period, there is often good resolution of radicular or myelopathic symptoms because of the decompression of the neural elements. However, if kyphosis develops, the patient may begin to complain of recurrent or new neurologic symptoms. Axial neck pain caused by muscle fatigue and loss of forward gaze may follow.
- Because of the instability of this situation, combined anterior and posterior approaches are most commonly performed if conservative measures fail (Albert et al. 1998) (Fig. 10–4).
- The risk of kyphosis may be avoided by performing a fusion at the time of the laminectomy. This can be done with lateral mass (C3-C6) and isthmus or pedicle screw (C2, C7, or below) fixation. The disadvantage of this technique is the associated loss of motion.
- Cervical laminaplasty is another potential means of avoiding postlaminectomy kyphosis. This procedure uses one of several techniques to elevate, but not remove, the posterior bony arch. In doing so, the area for the neural elements is expanded, but the integrity of the interspinous ligaments is maintained. Matsunaga et al. (1999) reported a significantly lower incidence of postlaminectomy kyphotic after laminaplasty than after laminectomy.

Inflammatory Disorders

- Inflammatory disorders, such as ankylosing spondylitis, may lead to spinal kyphosis.
- As explained in Chapter 14, signs and symptoms of ankylosing spondylitis may range from loss of flexibility to fixed gross sagittal plane deformities. Eventually, a "chin on chest" deformity may result in the face pointing toward the floor.
- The chief complaint in patients with loss of forward gaze is generally restriction of their activities of daily living.
- Ankylosing spondylitis is initially managed with nonsteroidal anti-inflammatory medications and with routine exercises.
- Extension osteotomies can be considered for ankylosing spondylitis patients with severely limiting deformities (Fig. 10–5).
- Patients with cervical kyphosis secondary to ankylosing spondylitis are predisposed to extension distraction fractures. If such fractures occur, consideration should be given to fixing patients in their newly extended posture if they are neurologically stable. If neurologic compromise occurs, they may have to be returned to their previously flexed posture.

Skeletal Dysplasias

- The most common form of skeletal dysplasia manifested in the cervical spine is diastrophic dysplasia. This autosomal recessive disorder may be associated with

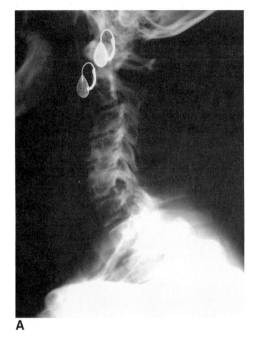

A

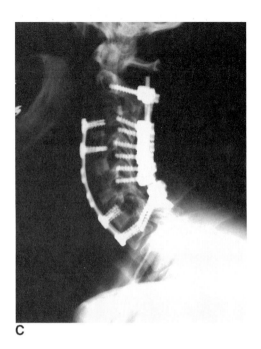

C

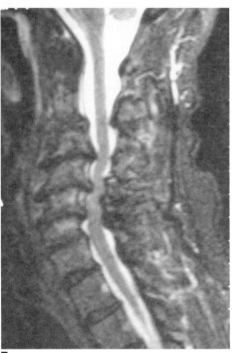

B

Figure 10–3: A 59-year-old woman with degenerative kyphosis of the cervical spine. She had radiculopathy and myelopathy. Radiograph (A) reveals kyphosis; MRI (B) reveals spinal cord compression. Follow-up radiograph (C) reveals the restoration of lordosis after the reconstruction of the anterior column with supplemental posterior stabilization.

severe cervical or thoracolumbar kyphosis that is generally self-limiting.

- Radiographs of patients with this disorder may demonstrate anterior wedging of the apical vertebrae.
- If the deformity is progressive, bracing may be considered.
- Surgery is considered only if a deformity is refractory to bracing or if neurologic deterioration is observed.
- Posterior fusion in situ can be considered for the younger patient. This allows continued anterior growth to partially correct the deformity.

Congenital Kyphosis

- Although congenital cervical kyphosis is uncommon, it may result in significant deformities, progressive disability, and neurologic deterioration.
- Congenital kyphosis usually arises from a vertebral segmentation defect (termed Klippel-Feil syndrome). This may be associated with other congenital abnormalities, most commonly in the heart or kidneys. Therefore patients should be counseled to rule out

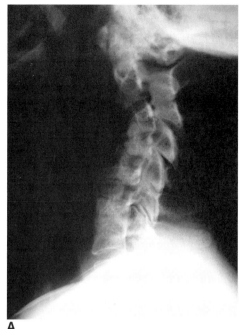

A

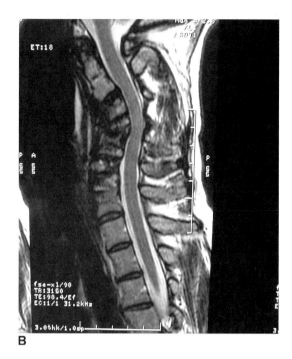

B

Figure 10–4: A 52-year-old woman with progressive postlaminectomy kyphosis. She underwent C3 and C4 corpectomies with a strut allograft packed with local bone and an antikick plate followed by a posterior C2-C7 instrumented fusion.

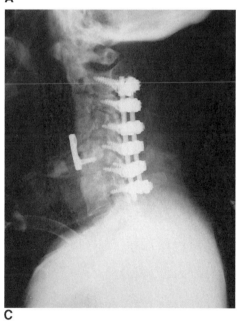

C

these abnormalities if Klippel-Feil syndrome is diagnosed.

- The classic triad of Klippel-Feil syndrome includes a short neck, a low posterior hairline, and limitations in neck motion. This syndrome is associated with scoliosis more than with kyphosis.

Thoracic Kyphosis
General

- The thoracic spine is normally kyphotic within a range of 20-45 degrees (Canale 1998). An average has been quoted at 31 degrees (Stagnara et al. 1982).

- Developmentally, thoracic kyphosis is a primary spinal curvature. Therefore the vertebral body heights are larger posteriorly than anteriorly, and the disks have similar anterior and posterior heights (Moore et al. 1999).

- The thoracic spine is unique in that it is stabilized by the rib cage.

- Patients with increased thoracic kyphosis may have back pain (often in the low back, neck, or periscapular area), fatigue, or a round back deformity.

Postural Thoracic Kyphosis

- Thoracic kyphosis may simply be postural. This is most common in adolescents and young adults.

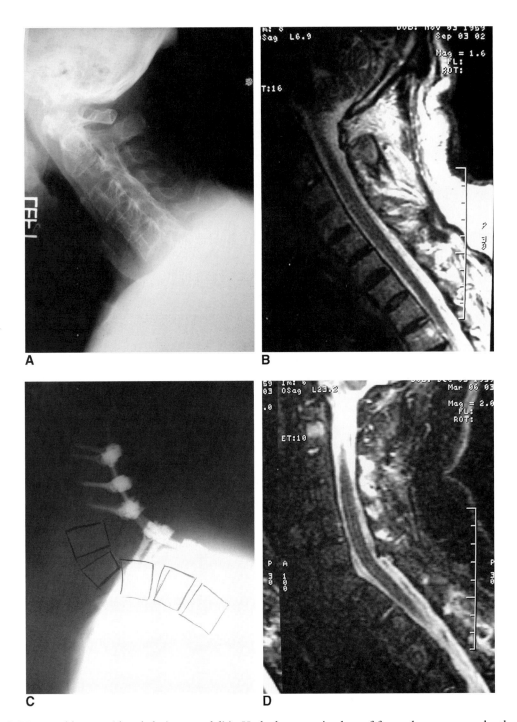

Figure 10–5: A 56-year-old man with ankylosing spondylitis. He had progressive loss of forward gaze as seen by the lateral radiograph (A) and the sagittal MRI (B). He underwent a cervicothoracic corrective extension osteotomy (C and D).

- Such deformities are generally smooth, flexible, and measure less than 60 degrees.
- These deformities are rarely progressive. Improvements of posture and extension exercises are recommended.

Scheuermann's Disease

- Along with postural round back, Scheuermann's disease (SD) is one of the most common causes of adolescent

kyphosis. Although usually a thoracic deformity, SD may be found in the lumbar spine.
- Patients usually complain of back pain or cosmetic deformity.
- Because this disease is common in athletes and laborers, a mechanical etiology is likely. However, several potential causes of SD have been proposed (Table 10–3).

Table 10–3:	Multifactorial Potential Causes of Scheuermann's Kyphosis*	
THEORETICAL CAUSES		**AUTHORS**
Avascular necrosis of the ring apophysis of the vertebral body		Scheuermann 1921
Herniation of disk material into the vertebral body (Schmorl nodes) causing disturbances of endochondral bone formation with subsequent wedging		Schmorl 1930
Persistence of anterior vascular grooves in vertebral bodies creating a point of structural weakness		Ferguson 1956
Osteoporosis		Bradford 1976
Mechanical stresses causing tightness of the anterior longitudinal ligament		Lambrinudi 1934
Abnormal collagen and matrix of vertebral endplate cartilage, including a decreased ratio between collagen and proteoglycan		Aufdermaur 1981

* (Canale 1998.)

- Pain generally localizes to the region of the deformity and stops with growth.
- If pain is primarily in the lumbar area and the deformity is in the thoracic region, the presence of a spondylolysis should be considered.
- Neurological abnormalities are not usually present.
- Measurements and findings necessary for a diagnosis of SD include the following (Canale 1998):

- More than 5 degrees of anterior wedging in three or more vertebrae at the apex of the kyphosis (also known as Sorenson's criteria)
    - Cobb angle of more than 45 degrees
    - Irregular vertebral endplates and narrowing of the disk spaces in the kyphotic region of the spine
- Thoracic kyphosis of less than 50 degrees with no evidence of progression should be followed with lateral films until growth is complete. An exercise program can also be instituted.
- Lumbar kyphosis (loss of lumbar lordosis) patients should avoid heavy lifting.
- Bracing may be useful in skeletally immature patients. It has been shown that teenagers with SD treated with a Milwaukee brace have better kyphosis correction than older patients with more excessive wedging.
- The primary indication for surgery in the skeletally immature is less than 75 degrees of kyphosis in spite of brace treatment.
- In skeletally mature patients, the presence of back pain, kyphosis more than 75 degrees, and possibly unacceptable cosmetic appearance are all relative surgical indications.
- If surgery is required, anterior release with posterior instrumentation and fusion is recommended (Fig. 10–6).

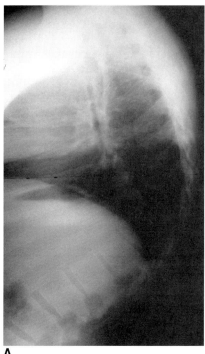

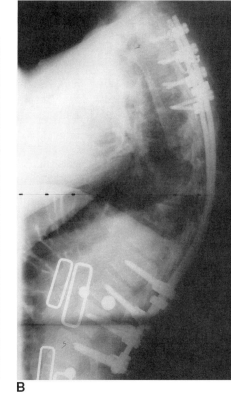

Figure 10–6: An 18-year-old boy with thoracic kyphosis. The patient has thoracic kyphosis of 75 degrees and vertebral wedging consistent with Scheuermann's disease (A). Back pain persisted despite conservative treatment. The patient underwent anterior releases and posterior instrumented correction and fusion (B).

A   **B**

Neoplastic Spinal Kyphosis

- Spinal tumors are covered in Chapter 17. In decreasing order, such lesions appear in the thoracic, sacrococcygeal, lumbar, and cervical regions (Weinstein et al. 1987).
- Metastatic tumors are, by far, the most common tumors in the spine.
- Metastatic and other malignant primary lesions have a predilection for the anterior spinal column. When anterior destruction occurs, kyphosis can result.
- Metastatic lesions are often treated with radiation with or without chemotherapy. However, instability, neurologic compromise, pain, or a combination of these may prompt the consideration for surgical intervention.
- The surgical approach for metastatic lesions depends on their location, but anterior column reconstruction with posterior stabilization has been associated with overall improved outcomes.
- Primary malignant lesions are ideally excised marginally but are often limited to intralesional excision secondary to anatomic constraints. Adjuvant therapy is tailored to the type and the stage of a lesion and to the extent to which it can be excised.
- Benign primary lesions require excision only if associated with structural compromise, neurologic impingement, or pain unresponsive to conservative modalities.

Postinfectious Kyphosis

- Spinal infections are covered in Chapter 16.
- Two types of infection bear description—bacterial infections and tuberculosis infections (Pott's disease).
- Bacterial infections generally begin in the disk space as discitis and can then progress to involve the vertebral bodies as osteomyelitis.
- Initially, attempts may be made to identify an organism in bacterial infections of the spine, especially in the adult. Antibiotic and brace immobilization are initiated.
- Infections that are identified late in their course or that fail noninvasive treatments may progress to kyphotic collapse. If this occurs, open debridement, reconstruction, and stabilization must be considered (Fig. 10–7).
- Similar to bacterial infections, Pott's disease is associated with the narrowing of disk spaces and kyphotic collapse. This affects the thoracic spine most frequently, followed by the cervical and lumbar regions (Al-Sebai et al. 2001).
- Initially, medical and brace treatments are initiated.
- In a study by Wimmer et al. (1997), conservative treatment was found to be a reasonable alternative to surgery in kyphotic deformities measuring less than 35 degrees.
- However, surgical treatment is advocated for the treatment of resistant infection or progressive deformity. This involves debridement and stabilization.

Osteoporotic Fractures

- Osteoporosis is a systemic skeletal disorder characterized by a decrease in bone mass and the deterioration of bone tissue with an increase in bone fragility and in the susceptibility to fractures.
- As described at greater length in Chapter 13, the spine is the most common site of such fractures. In fact, each standard deviation decrease in bone mass density is associated with a twofold increase in spine fractures.
- Major sequelae of osteoporotic compression fractures are back pain, vertebral height loss, and kyphosis.
- Kyphotic deformities in the thoracic and lumbar spine can precipitate a decrease in lung capacity that further increases functional impairment.
- Noninvasive treatment alternatives include the following:
  - Temporary narcotics
  - Bed rest or orthotics (however, these are associated with accelerated bone loss and deconditioning of spinal musculature)
  - Medical management of the underlying cause for the osteoporosis
- Continued progressive deformity, neurologic deterioration, and pain are indications for more aggressive treatment methods.
- Open fracture repair is fraught with difficulties because of poor bone quality and the frequently compromised medical status of this patient population.
- Minimally invasive methods to restore sagittal balance and decrease spinal pain are gaining popularity.
  - Vertebroplasty involves the percutaneous injection of polymethylmethacrylate (PMMA) into a fractured vertebral body.
  - Kyphoplasty involves the insertion of a balloon that is inflated in the vertebral body prior to the percutaneous injection of PMMA.
- The relative merit of these two procedures remains a topic of significant debate.
- Overall, kyphoplasty and vertebroplasty lead to 95% improvement in pain and functional status for patients not responding to conventional therapy (Garfin et al. 2001).

Skeletal Dysplasias

- Achondroplasia is a skeletal dysplasia associated with thoracolumbar kyphosis. This autosomal–dominant genetic disorder is the most common dwarfing condition.
- Kyphosis can be categorized as rigid or flexible with the latter being more likely to spontaneously resolve, as would be expected.
- Although brace treatment is often sufficient, surgical therapy has been recommended for the following situations (Kornblum et al. 1999):
  - Triangular apical vertebrae
  - Thoracolumbar kyphosis of more than 30 degrees
  - Thoracic kyphosis of more than 50 degrees

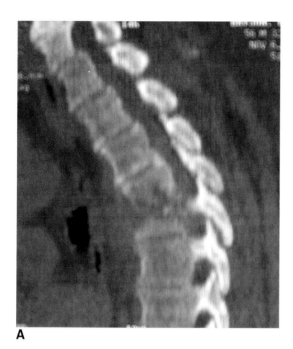

A

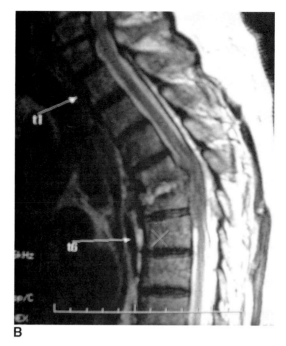

B

Figure 10–7: A 64-year-old man with thoracic pain and fevers. Workup revealed him to have discitis or osteomyelitis, thoracic kyphosis, and myelopathy. CT (A) and MRI (B) reveal focal kyphosis and cord compression. The patient underwent T4 and T5 corpectomies with iliac crest bone grafting and posterior T1-T8 instrumented fusions. Antibiotics were started.

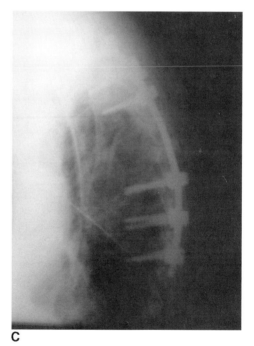

C

- Pseudoachondroplasia, an autosomal dominant disorder characterized by short-limbed dwarfism, is associated with gradual kyphotic deformities that are not sharply angular like in achondroplasia.

Lumbar Kyphosis

General

- The lumbar spine normally has 30 to 50 degrees of lordosis (Canale 1998).

- Developmentally, lumbar lordosis is a secondary curvature similar to the cervical curvature. As such, lordosis develops from an anterior-greater-than-posterior disk space height rather than from trapezoidal-shaped vertebral bodies (anterior-greater-than-posterior vertebral body heights) (Moore et al. 1999).

- Because of the large compressive loads experienced by the lumbar spine and the long moment arm of the body above this region, there is a risk of progression of sagittal plane deformities in this region of the spine.

Post-traumatic Kyphosis

- As noted previously, trauma can lead to kyphosis acutely or subacutely. Initial, deformity is largely based on the injury pattern. Later deformities are generally seen only if treatment is inadequate in providing stability during healing.
- Fractures with significant comminution of the anterior spinal column or disruption of the posterior column are most likely to progress to kyphosis (flexion compression and flexion distraction injuries are particularly prone to such deformities).
- The kyphotic deformity is best measured by comparing the superior and inferior endplates of the vertebrae directly above and below the fractured segment, respectively (Kuklo et al. 2001).
- Indications for surgical intervention include the following (Vaccaro et al. 2001):
    - Progression of kyphotic deformity
    - New or progressive neurologic deficit
    - Localized kyphotic deformity of greater than 30 degrees
    - Unacceptable cosmetic appearance with a rigid deformity
- Goals of surgery are neural decompression, spinal reconstruction, and stabilization to restore lumbar lordosis (Fig. 10–8).

Figure 10–8: A 31-year-old woman. She sustained a T12 burst fracture (A) with splaying of the posterior elements (B). She underwent a T12 corpectomy with an expandable cage and anterior rod fixation.

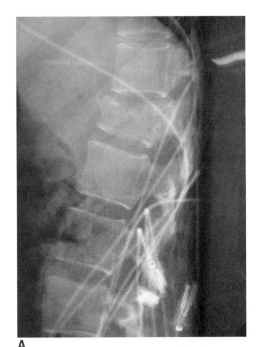

A

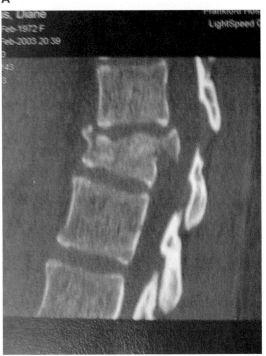

B

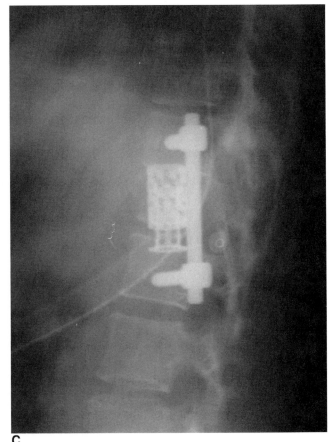

C

- In the setting of a chronic lumbar deformity, Smith-Peterson or pedicle subtraction osteotomies are alternatives to combined anterior and posterior reconstruction procedures.

Degenerative Kyphosis

- As with the cervical spine, the lumbar spine is prone to spondylosis.
- As degenerative changes progress, lumbar kyphosis or scoliosis may develop.
- Conservative treatment is the mainstay of treatment for such conditions.
- If conservative treatment fails and the lumbar deformity is progressive, surgical intervention may be considered.
- In addition to the anterior and posterior surgical options described for other regions of the spine, transforaminal lumbar interbody fusion and posterior lumbar interbody fusion are additional posterior surgical alternatives for focal deformities in this region of the spine.
- The method of surgical correction must be tailored to the patients' symptoms and underlying pathology.

References

Albert TJ, Vaccaro A. (1998) Postlaminectomy kyphosis. Spine 23: 2738-2745.
  Review of risk factors, biomechanics, workup, and surgical treatment of postlaminectomy kyphosis. This review promotes understanding of biomechanical principles to prevent and surgically treat postlaminectomy kyphosis.

Al-Sebai MW, Al-Khawashki H, Al-Arabi K et al. (2001) Operative treatment of progressive deformity in spinal tuberculosis. Int Orthop 25(5): 322-325.
  Report on 14 patients with spinal tuberculosis treated surgically. All had progressive kyphotic deformity. The report states that anterior and posterior debridement with fusion and instrumentation can improve correction in deformity in patients with progressive deformity, disease of three or more vertebrae, or destruction of anterior and posterior columns.

Bradford DS. (1977) Juvenile kyphosis. Clin Orthop 128: 45.
  Review of SD as a cause of juvenile kyphosis. The article describes the use of bracing for successful therapy. Surgery may be necessary with severe kyphosis, pain, neurologic compromise, or a combination of these.

Canale ST. (1998) Scheuermann's disease. In: Campbell's Operative Orthopaedics, 9th edition. St. Louis: Mosby, pp. 2942-2947.
  This chapter provides a detailed review of literature and modern approaches to treatment and surgical intervention in SD. It provides an overview of etiology and comprehensive review of diagnosis and treatment. The chapter also provides a range of lumbar lordosis and thoracic kyphosis.

Dai LY. (2002) Low lumbar spinal fractures: Management options. Injury 33(7): 579-582.
  Retrospective review of 54 patients with low lumbar spinal fractures. The article reviews the management options for low lumbar fractures, stating that most compression fractures can be managed conservatively. Denis classification of lumbar fractures was drawn from this article.

Garfin SR, Yuan HA, Reiley MA. (2001) New technologies in spine: Kyphoplasty and vertebroplasty for the treatment of painful osteoporotic compression fractures. Spine 26(14): 1511-1515.
  Literature review providing useful facts and the results of the use of vertebroplasty and kyphoplasty in the treatment of osteoporotic compression fractures.

Harrison DD, Janik TJ, Troyanovich SJ et al. (1996) Comparison of lordotic cervical spine curvatures to a theoretical ideal model of the static sagittal cervical spine. Spine 21(6): 667-675.
  This article is useful in providing an average measurement of cervical lordosis.

Kornblum M, Stanitski DF. (1999) Disorders of the pediatric and adolescent spine: Spinal manifestations of skeletal dysplasias. Orthop Clin N Am 30(3): 501-520.
  This article provides a comprehensive review of different etiologies in spinal deformity caused by skeletal dysplasias. Pertinent information is provided in specific cases of skeletal dysplasias that cause eventual spinal kyphosis, such as in achondroplasia and diastrophic dysplasia.

Kuklo TR, Polly DW, Owens BD et al. (2001) Measurement of thoracic and lumbar fracture kyphosis: Evaluation of intraobserver, interobserver, and technique variability. Spine 26(1): 61-65.
  Statistical analysis of various measurement techniques for thoracolumbar burst fracture kyphosis on lateral radiographs to determine the most reliable measurement technique. Fifty lateral radiographs were studied and reviewed by three spine surgeons. Of the five methods used, measuring from the superior endplate of the vertebral body one level above the injured vertebral body to the inferior endplate of the vertebral body one level below showed the best interobserver and intraobserver reliability overall.

Matsunaga S, Sakou T, Nakanisi K. (1999) Analysis of the cervical spine alignment following laminaplasty and laminectomy. Spinal Cord 37: 20-24.
  Comparative retrospective study involving patients who had undergone either laminaplasty or laminectomy to assess the incidence of the buckling-type alignment that follows these procedures. The purpose was to know the mechanical changes in the alignment of the cervical spine in these patients. Results favor laminaplasty over laminectomy from the aspect of mechanics.

Moore KL, Dalley AF. (1999) Curvatures of the vertebral column. In: Clinically Oriented Anatomy, 4th edition, pp. 434-435. Philadelphia: Lippincott Williams and Wilkins.
  This section includes embryologically relevant information about the development of the different spinal curvatures. It provides useful information for anatomic background.

Stagnara P, Mauroy JC, Dran G et al. (1982) Reciprocal angulation of vertebral bodies in a sagittal plane: Approach to references for the evaluation of kyphosis and lordosis. Spine 7: 335-412.
  This article is useful in providing an average measurement of thoracic kyphosis.

Vaccaro AR, Silber JS. (2001) Post-traumatic spinal deformity. Spine 26(24S): 5111-5118.

Review article that provides useful information about the etiology, diagnosis, and treatment of cervical, thoracic, and lumbar post-traumatic deformity. The article focuses on the importance of reestablishing integrity of compromised spinal columns so that spinal stability can be restored when considering surgical management.

Weinstein JN, McLain RJ. (1987) Primary tumors of the spine. Spine 12: 843-851.

Review of 82 cases of primary neoplasms of the spine in an attempt to identify common diagnostic and prognostic features.

The series justifies an aggressive surgical approach in the treatment of spinal tumors with prolonged survival.

Wimmer C, Ogon M, Sterzinger W et al. (1997) Conservative treatment of tuberculous spondylitis: A long-term follow-up study. J Spinal Disorders 10(5): 417-419.

Retrospective follow-up study of 40 tuberculosis patients treating spondylitis with orthotic supports for an average of 16 months and with antituberculous agents. Conservative treatment is proposed as an alternative to surgical intervention in kyphotic angles of less than 35 degrees.

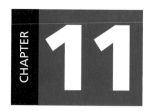

Spinal Scoliotic Deformities
Adolescent Idiopathic, Adult Degenerative, and Neuromuscular

Daniel J. Sucato

M.D., M.S., Assistant Professor, Department of Orthopaedics, University of Texas at Southwestern; and Staff Orthopaedist, Texas Scottish Rite Hospital for Children, Dallas, TX

Adolescent Idiopathic Scoliosis

Anatomy and Pathophysiology

- The etiology of adolescent idiopathic scoliosis (AIS) has not been elucidated; however, several theories have been studied and developed.

Genetics

- A familial predisposition has been accepted.
- Studies of monozygous twins demonstrate a concordance rate of 73%.
- The mode of inheritance is debated.

Effect of Connective Tissue

- Collagen and elastic fibers are the principal elements supporting the spine.
- An abnormal collagen/proteoglycan ratio of the intervertebral disks has been demonstrated.
- Elastic fiber abnormalities have been demonstrated in patients with AIS.

Skeletal Muscle

- A decrease has been seen in type II (fast twitch) fibers in the paraspinous muscles.
- Others have demonstrated normal fibers on the convexity but low frequency of type I (slow twitch) fibers on the concavity.
- A decrease has been found in the muscle spindles of the paraspinous muscles.

Muscle Contractile Mechanisms

- The contractile systems (actin and myosin) of platelets and muscle are similar and are partially regulated by calmodulin. This has been studied in AIS patients.
- Platelet calmodulin levels are higher in progressive curves.
- Melatonin (the antagonist of calmodulin) is lower in progressive curves.
- Contractile mechanisms have been studied in pinealectomized rats (produces decreased melatonin levels).

Neurology

- Inconsistent data
- Impaired peripheral, visual, and spatial proprioception

Role of Growth and Development

- Hypokyphosis has been seen in AIS. It may be a result of imbalance of anterior and posterior growth.
- Some authors have found patients with scoliosis to be taller with less kyphosis.

- Accelerated spinal growth starts earlier when compared with controls.

Diagnostic Tools

History

Pain

- Occurs in 30% of patients with AIS
- Uncharacteristic pain (awakens from sleep, continuous, radiating, or severe)—unusual and requires further study

Age at Onset

- Patients may present symptoms in the adolescent period; however, they may have had earlier onset. It is important to determine the etiology—it may be juvenile or infantile onset.

Growth Potential

- Age—Girls peak growth occurs from 11 to 12 years; boys peak from 13 to 14 years.
- Menarcheal status—Premenarcheal girls are a greater risk for progression and may crankshaft following posterior-only surgery.

Family History

- It is important to determine sibling occurrence to allow evaluation.

Physical Examination

Assessment of Deformity

- Standing examination
  - Coronal imbalance assessment
  - Coronal curve assessment
  - Shoulder height or asymmetry
- Adams forward bend test
  - Patient bends at the waist until the trunk is at 90 degrees
  - Rotational deformity assessment of the upper thoracic, thoracic, and thoracolumbar or lumbar curves
  - Assessment for symmetry of movement with flexion (absence of list to one side may denote nonidiopathic scoliosis)

Neurologic Examination

- Motor and sensory examination—Usually intact even with intracanal pathology
- Deep tendon reflexes—Knees and ankles
- Abdominal reflexes
  - A lateral-to-medial gentle stroke of the abdomen, which elicits movement of the umbilicus
  - Should be symmetric (absent or present)
  - If asymmetric, then high correlation with neural axis pathology (syringomyelia, tethored cord)—obtain magnetic resonance imaging (MRI)

Other Examination

- Lower extremities
  - Ensure no asymmetry in leg circumference, size, or length
  - Look for asymmetric foot deformities (intracanal pathology)

Radiographic Examination

Posteroanterior–Anterior Standing

- Measure upper thoracic, thoracic, and thoracolumbar or lumbar curves (Cobb method)
- Determine the deviation of C7 plumb line from the center–sacral–vertical line (CSVL)
- Trunk shift—Deviation of the mid-distance of the rib margins to CSVL
- Risser stage—See Fig. 11–1
- Status of triradiate cartilage (acetabular physis)—Open or closed

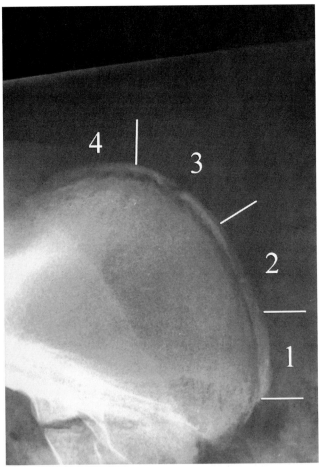

Figure 11–1: Risser stages to determine skeletal maturity. Risser 0 = No ossification of the iliac apophysis. Risser 1-4 = Ossification beginning laterally and finishing medially when the iliac wing is divided into four sections. Risser 5 = Fusion of the ossified iliac apophysis to the ilium.

Lateral Radiograph

- Thoracic kyphosis and lumbar lordosis (Cobb method)
- Junctional kyphosis
  - Between the structural upper thoracic and middle thoracic curves
  - Between the structural middle thoracic and the thoracolumbar or lumbar curves
- Sagittal balance—C7 plumb normally falls at the posterior edge of L5-S1
- Presence of thoracic hypokyphosis or apical lordosis is normal in AIS; absence may indicate neural axis pathology

Bend Films

Purpose

- Determine the curve type—more than 25 is structural (Lenke et al. 2001)
- Determine the flexibility index for each curve:
  - Subtract the bend Cobb angle from the posteroanterior–anterior (PA) Cobb angle and divide by PA Cobb × 100
- Determine fusion levels in the lumbar spine:
  - Flexibility of the disk below the distal fusion vertebra, which helps determine the distal extent of fusion
  - Ability of the planned distal fusion level to center over the sacrum

Types of Bend Films

- Supine anteroposterior best-effort bend
  - Patient lies supine on a table and bends to the right and the left
  - Most commonly used
- Push-prone test—Patient is prone and the examiner pushes medially and anteriorly on the rotational prominence
- Fulcrum bend film
  - Patient lies in a lateral position with the apex of curve on a large roll
  - May be better for the assessment of thoracic curve flexibility
- Traction films
  - Supine patient has manual traction applied (more common)
  - Standing patient has halter traction applied

Magnetic Resonance Imaging (Fig. 11–2)

- Absolute indications
  - Neurologic abnormalities
  - Juvenile and infantile onset
  - Congenital vertebral abnormalities
  - Cutaneous manifestations of dysraphism

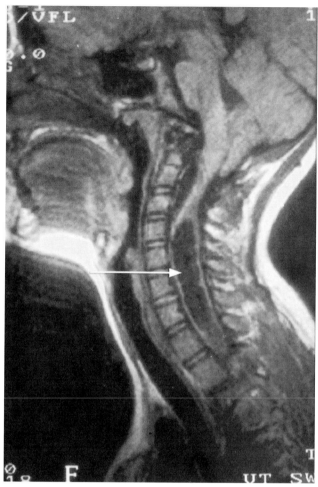

Figure 11–2: Magnetic resonance image of the cervical spine in a patient with a left thoracic curve. **Note the large cervical syrinx.**

- Relative indications
  - Atypical curve pattern, i.e., left thoracic curve or thoracic kyphosis
  - Rapidly progressing curve
  - Painful scoliosis—Often difficult to sort out the pain

Bone Scan

- Indications
  - Painful scoliosis without known etiology

Natural History

- The prevalence of AIS is 2% in the normal population with curves greater than 10 degrees. Of these patients, 5% will demonstrate progression greater than 30 degrees.

Gender Distribution

- Small curves—Girls equal boys
- Larger curves—8 times more common in girls than in boys

Risk Factors for Progression

- Skeletal immaturity (open triradiate cartilage, Risser sign 0-1, and premenarcheal)
- Curve location—Thoracic curves progress less often than lumbar curves
- Curve magnitude
  - Larger curves progress more often than smaller ones
  - At maturity, thoracic curves greater than 50 degrees progress into adulthood (average one per year) (Table 11–1)
  - Thoracolumbar/lumbar curves greater than 40 degrees progress into adulthood (especially with coronal decompensation)

Curve Classification

- Based on the apex of the curve
  - Cervical—Apex between C1 and C6
  - Cervicothoracic—Apex between C7 and T1
  - Thoracic—Apex between T2 and the T11-T12 disk space
  - Thoracolumbar—Apex between T12 and L1
  - Lumbar—Apex between the L1-L2 disk space and L4

Table 11–1:	Curve Progression Risk*	
	CURVE MAGNITUDE (10-19 DEGREES)	**CURVE MAGNITUDE (20-29 DEGREES)**
Risser sign 0-1	22%	68%
Risser sign 2-4	1.6%	23%

* (Lonstein JE et al. 1984.)

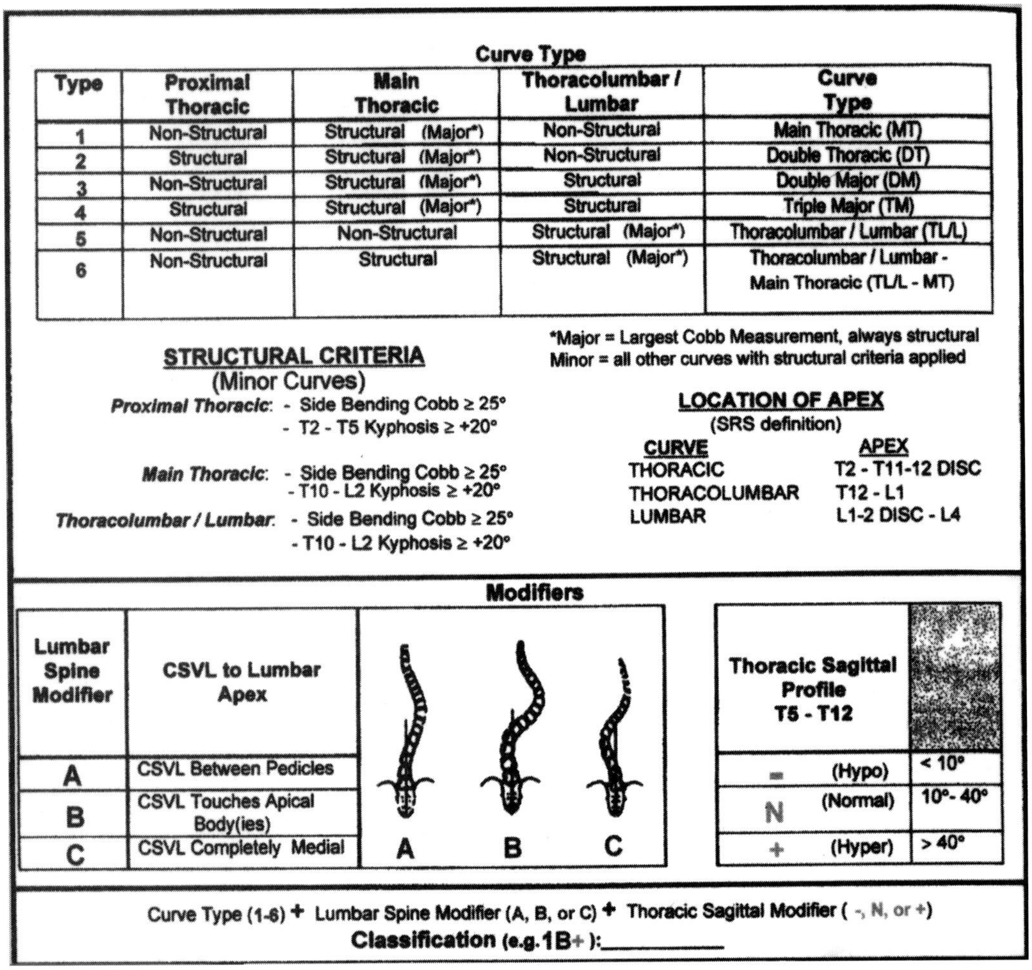

- Lumbosacral—Apex between L4 and S1
- King classification—Traditional classification of thoracic curves
  - King I—Lumbar curve greater than the thoracic curve
  - King II—Thoracic curve with a compensatory lumbar curve that crosses the midline
  - King III—Thoracic curve with a lumbar curve that does not cross the midline
  - King IV—Long thoracic curve in which L4 is tilted into the curve
  - King V—Double thoracic curve
- Lenke et al. (2001) classification—A more comprehensive and newer classification (Fig. 11–3)

Curve Type

Type	Proximal Thoracic	Main Thoracic	Thoracolumbar / Lumbar	Curve Type
1	Non-Structural	Structural (Major*)	Non-Structural	Main Thoracic (MT)
2	Structural	Structural (Major*)	Non-Structural	Double Thoracic (DT)
3	Non-Structural	Structural (Major*)	Structural	Double Major (DM)
4	Structural	Structural (Major*)	Structural	Triple Major (TM)
5	Non-Structural	Non-Structural	Structural (Major*)	Thoracolumbar / Lumbar (TL/L)
6	Non-Structural	Structural	Structural (Major*)	Thoracolumbar / Lumbar - Main Thoracic (TL/L - MT)

*Major = Largest Cobb Measurement, always structural
Minor = all other curves with structural criteria applied

STRUCTURAL CRITERIA
(Minor Curves)

Proximal Thoracic: - Side Bending Cobb ≥ 25°
- T2 - T5 Kyphosis ≥ +20°

Main Thoracic: - Side Bending Cobb ≥ 25°
- T10 - L2 Kyphosis ≥ +20°

Thoracolumbar / Lumbar: - Side Bending Cobb ≥ 25°
- T10 - L2 Kyphosis ≥ +20°

LOCATION OF APEX
(SRS definition)

CURVE	APEX
THORACIC	T2 - T11-12 DISC
THORACOLUMBAR	T12 - L1
LUMBAR	L1-2 DISC - L4

Modifiers

Lumbar Spine Modifier	CSVL to Lumbar Apex
A	CSVL Between Pedicles
B	CSVL Touches Apical Body(ies)
C	CSVL Completely Medial

	Thoracic Sagittal Profile T5 - T12	
−	(Hypo)	< 10°
N	(Normal)	10°- 40°
+	(Hyper)	> 40°

Curve Type (1-6) + Lumbar Spine Modifier (A, B, or C) + Thoracic Sagittal Modifier (−, N, or +)
Classification (e.g.1B+):_____

Figure 11–3: Lenke et al. (2001) curve classification. The three-part classification consists of curve type, lumbar modifier, and thoracic sagittal profile.

- Reliability has been tested with varying results
- Three components of the spine analyzed to produce the classification

Six Curve Types

- The larger curve is always considered structural; smaller curves are structural if the patient fails to bend to less than 25 degrees.
- 1—Single thoracic
- 2—Double thoracic
- 3—Double major
- 4—Triple major
- 5—Lumbar curve without thoracic curve
- 6—Lumbar curve with compensatory thoracic curve

Lumbar Modifier

- Based on where the CSVL falls in relation to the **apical** lumbar vertebra
- A—CSVL falls between the pedicles
- B—CSVL falls on the pedicle or lateral to the pedicle within the vertebral body
- C—CSVL falls outside of the vertebral body

Thoracic Kyphosis Modifier

- Measured from T5 to T12
- "−"—Kyphosis less than 10
- "N"—Kyphosis between 10 and 40
- "+"—Kyphosis greater than 40

Nonoperative Treatment

Observation

- Most patients who have AIS do not progress to the point of treatment.
- Radiographs should be performed every 4-6 months depending on the risk of progression.
- PA radiographs are used to determine the curve magnitude (Cobb method).

Bracing (Table 11–2)

Indications

- Curve progression to 25-30 degrees but less than 45 degrees
- Potential for growth (Risser sign less than 4)

Goal of Bracing

- Maintain the present curve magnitude or prevent it from progressing to a level that means surgery is required

Effectiveness

- Still questioned today despite many studies (limited by the ability to measure compliance)
- SRS 1995 publication: Braced versus nonbraced patients—Progression was seen in 64% of nonbraced patients compared with 26% of braced patients
- Unpublished data from Texas Scottish Rite Hospital by Katz et al.
  - Measured compliance with heat sensor
  - Preliminary results demonstrate the dose response to bracing; more than 12 hours in a brace was more effective in the skeletally immature patients

Operative Treatment

Indications

- Thoracic curves
  - Immature patients—Curve magnitude greater than 40-50 degrees
  - Mature patients—Curve magnitude greater than 50 degrees
- Thoracolumbar/lumbar curves
  - Curve magnitude greater than 40 degrees with significant coronal decompensation

Goals of Operative Treatment

- Halt curve progression with fusion
- Curve and deformity correction using instrumentation

Fusion Techniques

- Complete facetectomies at all instrumented levels

Bone Graft

- Autologous iliac crest
  - Most commonly used
  - Relatively high morbidity because of pain
- Rib—From concomitant thoracoplasty

Table 11–2: Types of Braces for Adolescent Idiopathic Scoliosis			
TYPE OF BRACE	**INDICATIONS**	**WEAR SCHEDULE**	**COMPLIANCE**
TLSO (Boston overlap)*	All curve types	16-22 hours	Middle compliance
Bending brace (Charleston)	Thoracolumbar, lumbar curves (25-35 degrees)	8-10 nighttime hours	Best compliance
CTLSO (Milwaukee) §	Thoracic curves with apex above T7	16-22 hours	Least compliance

* *TLSO*, Thoracolumbosacral orthosis.
§ *CTLSO*, Cervical thoracolumbosacral orthosis.

- Allograft—Fusion rates similar to autologous
- Local only—Rare

Fixation

- Modern segmental spinal instrumentation uses multiple fixation points and dual rods posteriorly and single or dual rods anteriorly.

Hooks

- Pedicle
  - Up-going hooks under the lamina or inferior facet engaging the pedicle
  - Can be placed in thoracic spine to T10
- Sublaminar—Can be up-going or down-going
- Transverse process—can be placed as up-going or down-going weakest hook
- Wires
  - Sublaminar—Excellent for translation (laterally and posteriorly)
  - Through the spinous process: Wisconsin (Drummond) wires
- Pedicle screws
  - Provide optimal fixation of all three columns

- Generally used in the lower thoracic and the lumbar spine
- Becoming used more often in the thoracic spine
- Anterior structural support
  - Mesh cages or ring allografts
  - Provides improved structural stiffness when performing anterior instrumentation and fusion

Posterior Correction Maneuvers

- All correction maneuvers attempt to translate the spine posteriorly and laterally and to derotate the spine in the axial plane
- Rod rotation
  - Popularized by Dubousset
  - Rod contouring and placement on the concavity are followed by a counterclockwise rotation (for a right thoracic curve)
- Translation or cantilever—Distal attachment of a contoured rod and then translation of the spine to the rod
- In situ contouring—The rod is attached to the contour of the spine and then shaped to improve spinal deformity

Figure 11–4: Preoperative and postoperative radiographs following anterior fusion from T9 to L2 using a single 0.25-inch rod and anterior structural support at the T12-L1 and L1-L2 levels for a 53 degree curve. Restoration of coronal and sagittal balance is achieved.

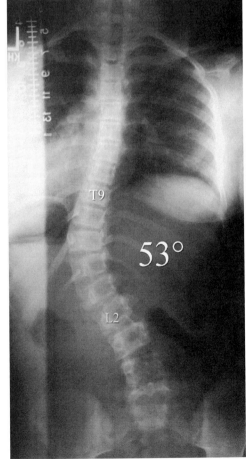
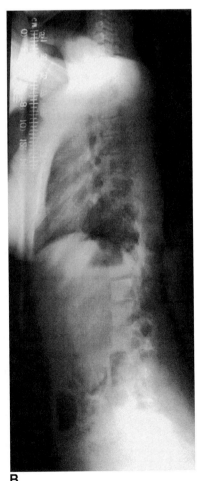

A   B

Anterior Correction Maneuvers

- Rod rotation (usually for thoracolumbar or lumbar curves)
  - The rod is contoured to the convexity of the spine, and rod rotation is performed to improve the coronal plane and restore or maintain lumbar lordosis.
- Compression (usually for thoracic curves)
  - The rod is seated completely or more often distally initially or proximally initially followed by compression.
  - A cantilever maneuver can be used (for the partially seated rod) followed by compression at each level.

Treatment Options

Anterior Instrumentation and Fusion (Fig. 11–4)

- Most common method used to treat thoracolumbar or lumbar curves
- Single thoracic curves can be treated either through an open thoracotomy or thoracoscopically (Fig. 11–5)

Fusion Levels

- Nearly always proximal end vertebra to distal end vertebra

Posterior Instrumentation and Fusion (Fig. 11–6)

- All curves may be treated
- Always indicated for double or triple curves

Fusion Levels

- Single thoracic curves
  - Proximal end vertebra to one level proximal to the stable vertebra with hook fixation
  - Proximal end vertebra to one or two levels proximal to the stable vertebra; may often stop at the distal end vertebra with pedicle screw
- Double thoracic curves
  - As for single thoracic curves except proximal fixation is most often to T2
- Double major curves

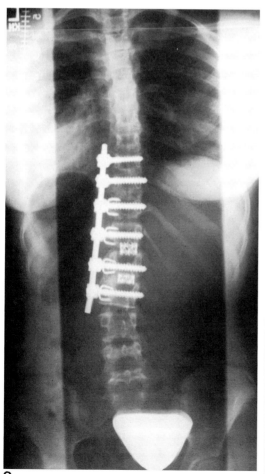

C

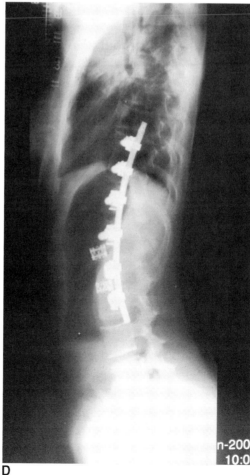

D

Figure 11–4: Cont'd

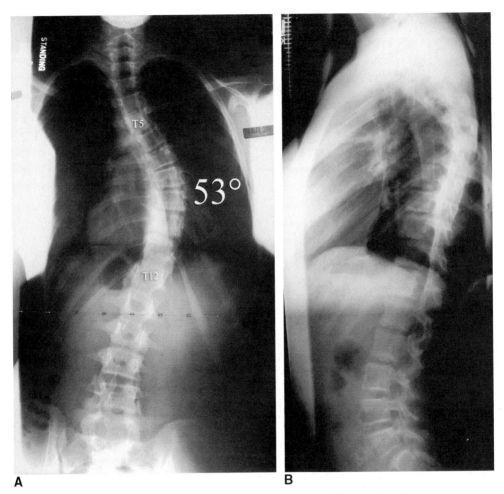

A **B**

Figure 11–5: Radiographs of a 12-year-old female who had a 53 degree thoracic curve. She underwent a thoracoscopic anterior spinal fusion and instrumentation from T5 to T12 with excellent correction of the coronal curve and restoration of coronal and sagittal balance.

- Proximal end vertebra
- Distal fixation most common to the lumbar distal end vertebra
- Distal fixation is best performed with pedicle screws for improved correction and maintenance of curve correction

Anterior Release or Fusion and Posterior Instrumentation or Fusion

- Anterior release required
- Stiff curves—More than 75 degrees that fail to bend to less than 50 degrees
- Skeletally immature
  - Open triradiate cartilage or Risser 0-1
  - Prevent crankshaft

- Performed open or thoracoscopically in the thoracic spine
  - Advantages of thoracoscopy include smaller incisions, less postoperative pain, less postoperative pulmonary problems, and improved cosmesis
  - Disadvantages of thoracoscopy are that it is technically demanding and more costly because of the use of disposable items

Aftercare and Follow-up

- Postoperative antibiotics, diet advancement, and walking while in the hospital
- Postoperative bracing is not required when using modern segmental instrumentation
- Activities are slowly advanced until patients are performing full activities between 6 and 12 months

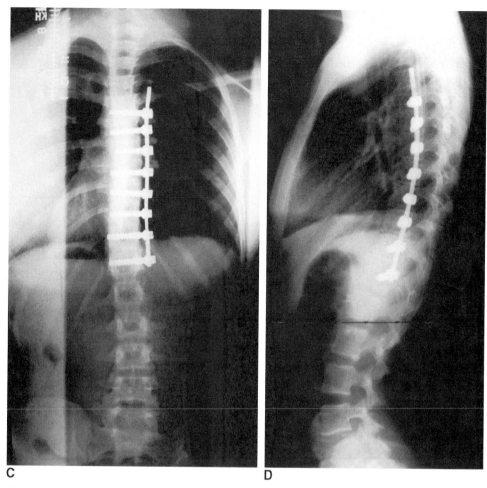

Figure 11–5: Cont'd

Outcome of Surgical Treatment

- Long-term follow-up only available for Harrington instrumentation
  - Average correction is approximately 50%
  - Distal fusion below L3 results in greater incidence of low back pain
- Midterm follow-up of segmental spinal instrumentation
  - Average coronal curve correction is approximately 60% with hook fixation
  - Improved maintenance and correction of sagittal plane
- Short-term follow-up using segmental pedicle screw fixation (Suk et al. 2000)
  - Average coronal curve correction is approximately 75%
  - Rare neurologic injury

Complications

- The reoperation rate for posterior spinal instrumentation is 5%-19% for all causes (Boxes 11–1 through 11–3) (Cook et al. 2000).

Adult Scoliosis and Deformity

Introduction

- Defined as a coronal plane Cobb angle greater than 10 degrees in a patient older than 20 years.
- The natural history of the curve in the mature patient is variable.
- De novo curves of the lumbar spine may progress rapidly.
- The rate of curve progression is not constant.
- Lumbar curves progress more rapidly than thoracic curves.
- Adult scoliosis more often presents symptoms of associated back pain, leg pain, or both.
- Treatment of adult deformity can be more challenging than that of adolescent deformity because of the following:
  - Greater curve stiffness
  - Presence of degenerative changes
  - Associated medical comorbidities
  - Need for neural element decompression, thus extending surgical time and removing areas for bony fusion

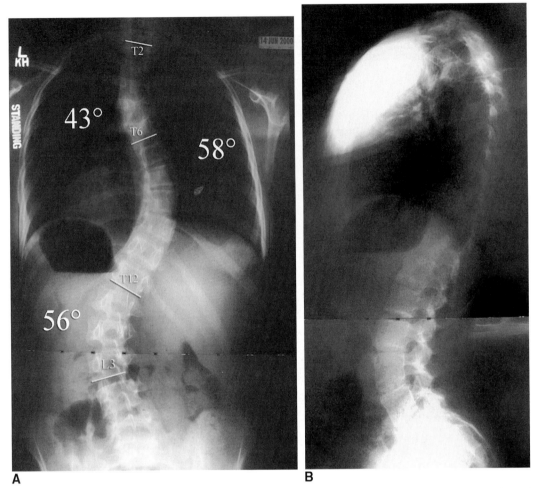

A   **B**

Figure 11–6: Radiographs of a 13-year-old female with a triple major curve (Lenke 4). She underwent a posterior spinal fusion and instrumentation from T2 to L3. Proximal hook fixation, apical sublaminar wire fixation, and distal pedicle screw fixation were used to achieve excellent correction with restoration of coronal and sagittal balance.

- Osteopenia
- Sagittal and coronal plane imbalance
- Difficulty in determining pain generators
- Frequent need for longer fusions and more common combined anterior or posterior procedures

Box 11–1:	Late Onset Surgical Pain

- Incidence—5%
- Treatment—hardware removal

Box 11–2:	Pseudarthrosis

- Incidence—3%
- Treatment—Compression instrumentation or bone graft

Box 11–3:	Delayed Infection

- Incidence—1%-7%
- Treatment—Hardware removal and short-term antibiotics

Classification

- See Box 11–4.

Pathophysiology and Natural History

Adult Scoliosis

- Curve progression is usually not seen if less than 40 degrees.
- Curve progression averages 1 degree per year if greater than 50 degrees.
- Risk factors for the progression of lumbar curves include the following:
  - Large apical rotation
  - Lateral and rotatory listhesis
- For double curves, the lumbar curve tends to progress more rapidly than the thoracic curve.
- There is no difference in pulmonary function among age-matched, normal patients.

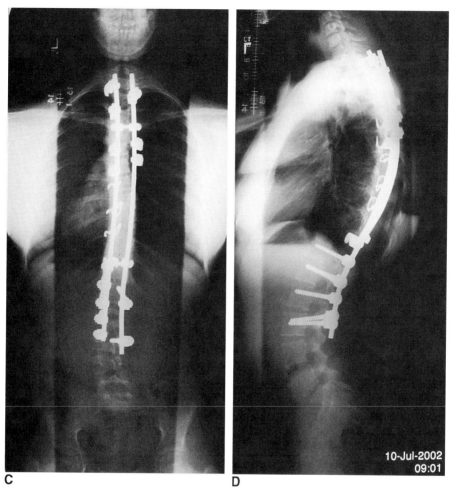

C   D

Figure 11–6: Cont'd

- Back pain incidence is similar; however, the severity is worse and more recurrent when compared with controls.
- The reasons for presenting symptoms to the physician could be as follows:
  - Pain at the location of the curve
  - Progression of the curve

De Novo Scoliosis

- Prevalence is approximately 6%.
- The average age at which symptoms are presented is the sixth and seventh decade of life.

Box 11–4:	Adult Scoliosis and Deformity Classification

- Adult scoliosis
  - Previous AIS
  - Without degenerative changes—Usually younger than 40 years
  - With degenerative changes—Usually older than 40 years
- De novo scoliosis (adult onset scoliosis)
  - Develops secondary to degenerative changes of the lumbar spine
  - Usually in elderly patients

- The average curve progression is approximately 3.3 degrees per year.
- A greater number of males are affected than in adult scoliosis (females are still more common in both).
- The reason for presenting symptoms is pain caused by one, or combinations, of the following:
  - Neurogenic claudication
  - Radicular symptoms
  - Back pain—**Not** usually the main complaint

Diagnostic Tools

Plain Radiographs

- Indications—All patients should have initial PA and lateral long-cassette radiographs.
- Long-cassette radiographs—PA and lateral radiographs should include the cervical spine down to the pelvis.
- Supine right-sided and left-sided bend films should be used to assess flexibility (especially when determining whether anterior surgery is necessary). They also are helpful when choosing fusion levels.

- Traction films are useful in assessing flexibility and choosing fusion levels.
- Ferguson view—An x-ray beam directed 30 degrees cephalad and focused on the lumbosacral junction provides an excellent view of the lumbosacral junction.

Assessment Parameters

Posteroanterior–Anterior Radiograph

- Cobb measurement of all curves (upper thoracic, thoracic, lumbar, and lumbosacral fractional curves)
- Coronal imbalance—Measured as a trunk shift from the CSVL or a deviation of a C7 plumb from the CSVL (most important in adult deformity)
- Rotatory listhesis or subluxation
- Disk height and wedging
- Osteophyte formation noted of the vertebral bodies and facet joints

Lateral Radiograph

- Cobb measurement—Thoracic kyphosis (T5 to T12) and lumbar lordosis (L1 to L5)—Loss of lumbar lordosis is usually seen.
- Sagittal balance—The C7 plumb line should fall on the posterior aspect of the L5-S1 disk level.
- Disk space height
- Osteopenia of the vertebral bodies
- Degree of degeneration the facet joints

Computed Tomography and Computed Tomography Myelography

- Indications—CT largely has been replaced by MRI, so indications today are as follows:
  - Inability to get MRI (presence of certain ferromagnetic implants or claustrophobia)
  - Assessment of central and lateral recess stenosis and presence of disk herniations in the setting of previous spine surgery
  - Best for assessment of the integrity of a spinal fusion
  - May be better for patients with large curves to assess canal stenosis
- Advantages—Still an accurate method of evaluating bone density and anatomy (osteophyte and facet arthropathy), canal and foraminal stenosis, and bony fusion
- Disadvantages—Radiation exposure and its invasive nature

Magnetic Resonance Imaging

- Technique
  - Usually T1- and T2-weighted axial and sagittal images
  - May add gadolinium in the face of previous surgery
- Indications—Assessment of central and lateral recess stenosis, presence of disk herniation, and morphology and degree of degeneration of the intervertebral disks when planning fusion levels

- Advantages—No radiation exposure and excellent visualization of osseous and soft tissue structures
- Disadvantages—Artifact and distortion in the presence of metal implants and claustrophobia for some patients

Nonoperative Treatment

- Aerobic conditioning
- Strengthening
- Stretching
- Nonsteroidal anti-inflammatory medications
- With associated lumbar radiculopathy or neurogenic claudication, nerve blocks or epidural steroid injections may be helpful.
- For lumbar curves, a lumbar corset may be beneficial in improving pain control.

Operative Treatment of Adult Scoliosis

- See Box 11–5.

Algorithm for Operative Treatment of Adult Scoliosis

Approach

- Based on curve type, magnitude, flexibility, and sagittal balance

Curve Type

- Thoracic curves
  - Posterior approach more commonly used
  - Only the thoracic curve is fused, leaving distal lumbar motion
- Thoracolumbar curves
  - Anterior (more common) or posterior approach
- Double major curves
  - Posterior approach to include both curves
- Indications to include an anterior (combined) fusion
  - Large stiff curves
  - Kyphosis (use structural anterior grafts)

Box 11–5:	**Indications for Operative Treatment of Adult Scoliosis**

- Documented curve progression
- Increased coronal imbalance, sagittal imbalance, or both
- Symptoms unresponsive to nonoperative treatment
- Relative indications
  - Pulmonary symptoms (rare)
  - Back pain—Not an indication alone for surgical intervention
  - Leg pain (with lumbar curves) because of objective nerve root compression

- Rotatory subluxation or listhesis
- Fusion to L5 or S1
- Performance of anterior and posterior surgery on the same day is dependent on the medical condition of the patient and the duration and clinical status of the patient at the completion of the initial stage of surgery

Fusion Levels

- Similar to AIS especially for the younger adult (younger than 40 years)
  - End-instrumented vertebra should be neutral (no rotation) and stable (bisected by the center sacral line)
  - For a patient older than 40 years with degenerative changes
  - Assessment of the distal lumbar disk levels below L3 with MRI is recommended to ensure that fusion does not require inclusion of these levels because of the presence of advanced degeneration
  - Levels of decompression for spinal stenosis are included in the fusion levels

Operative Treatment of De Novo (Degenerative) Scoliosis

- See Boxes 11–6 through 11–9.
- Anterior surgery accomplishes the following:
  - Anterior release improves correction and fusion rates

Box 11–6:	Indications for Operative Treatment of De Novo (Degenerative) Scoliosis

- Progressive deformity
- Spinal imbalance
- Neurogenic claudication unresponsive to conservative treatment

Box 11–7:	Decompression Only

- Mild scoliosis coronal curve less than 10 degrees
- No instability, lateral listhesis, or rotatory subluxation

Box 11–8:	Decompression, ASF and PSF, or Instrumentation

- Scoliosis >30 degrees
- Sagittal imbalance, coronal imbalance, or both

Box 11–9:	Decompression, PSF, or Vertebral Column Resection

- Scoliosis >30 degrees
- Fixed coronal imbalance

- Anterior surgery assists in creating lumbar lordosis
- Anterior structural grafting assists fusion and creates a ligamentotaxis effect
- Anterior surgery (structural support) of L4-L5 and L5-S1 increases fusion success, maintains or improves sagittal fusion success, and maintains or improves sagittal alignment when fusing to the sacrum

Internal Fixation

- Segmental internal fixation is always recommended
- Pedicle screw fixation
  - Improved three-dimensional correction when compared with hooks
  - Always used in the lumbar spine
  - Can be used in the thoracic spine safely when the morphology of the thoracic pedicle is of adequate size
- Sacropelvic fixation
  - Many implants available
  - Galveston, iliac screws, intrasacral rods, and S2 screws provide fixation to "backup" S1 screws

Treatment of Fixed Sagittal Imbalance

Indications for Treatment

- Fixed kyphosis with pain
- Significant sagittal imbalance—C7 plumb line falling anterior to the L5-S1 disk

Smith-Petersen Osteotomies

- Multiple osteotomies done posteriorly (may also need anterior surgery; see Fig. 11–7)
- Closes the posterior column and opens the anterior and middle columns (often requiring structural graft)

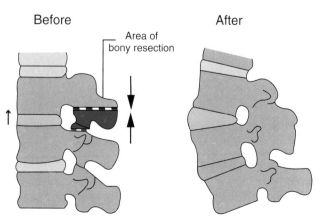

Figure 11–7: Smith-Petersen osteotomy. Correction is achieved by closing the posterior column (location of the osteotomy) and opening the anterior column. (Reprinted from Bridwell 2003.)

- Indications for posterior surgery only
  - Young patient
  - Fusing short of sacrum with mild or moderate correction needed in the setting of normal disks
- Indications for anterior and posterior surgery—Narrow disks that may not compensate for a significant correction of sagittal imbalance in a patient requiring greater than 30 degrees of correction

Pedicle Subtraction Osteotomy

- Technically more challenging (Fig. 11–8) (Bridwell et al. 2003)
- Closes the posterior and middle columns and hinges on the anterior column
- Should be done at L1 or distal (below the conus medullaris)
- Advantages over Smith-Petersen osteotomy
  - Done through the posterior approach alone, gains more than 30 degrees of correction, and does not lengthen the anterior column
  - Greater potential for healing without stretch on aorta or viscera
- Disadvantages—Technically difficult, increased blood loss, and greater potential for neurologic injury

Results and Complications following Adult Spine Deformity Surgery

- Pain (Ahlert et al. 1995, Grubb et al. 1994, Schwab et al. 2003)
  - A balanced patient with solid fusion usually has improvement in the severity of pain
  - The frequency of pain usually continues

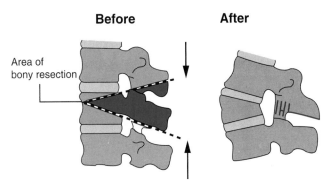

Before   **After**

Area of bony resection

Figure 11–8: Three-column pedicle subtraction osteotomy. **The osteotomy closes all three columns of the spine.** (Reprinted from Bridwell 2003.)

- Pseudarthrosis
  - The most common complication
  - Incidence—5% to 25%
  - Risk factors—Revision surgery, use of allograft bone, and use of nonsegmental hardware
- Infection
  - Incidence—0.5% to 8%
  - Risk factors—No perioperative antibiotics, poor nutrition (use total parenteral nutrition in staged surgery), poor soft tissue handling, and posterior surgery more common than anterior surgery
- Neurologic compromise
  - Incidence—Less than 1% to 5%
  - Risk factors—Combined anterior and posterior surgery, revision surgery, or osteotomy surgery
- Pulmonary embolism
  - Incidence—1% to 20%
- Spinal decompensation
  - Risk factors—Improper selection of fusion levels and possibility of error on longer fusions; ideally stop at neutral and stable vertebra

Neuromuscular Scoliosis

Introduction

- Scoliosis is common in patients with neuromuscular diseases.
- Larger curves cause difficulties with sitting or ambulation.
- Bracing generally does not affect the natural history of scoliosis in these patients.
- Progressive severe curves require operative treatment.
- The goals and treatment methods for neuromuscular scoliosis are slightly different than those for idiopathic curves.
  - Longer fusions, often to the pelvis
  - Fusions often for smaller curves
  - Complication rates high

Classification

- See Box 11–10.

Anatomy and Pathophysiology (of the more Common Diagnoses)
Cerebral Palsy (Fig. 11–9)

- Nonprogressive encephalopathy with varying degrees of severity
- Damage to the brain occurs prenatal, perinatal, or postnatal
  - Prenatal—Infections or toxins (drugs or alcohol)
  - Perinatal—Anoxic brain injury

Box 11–10:	Neuromuscular Scoliosis Classification

Neuropathic

1. Upper motor neuron
   - Cerebral palsy
   - Spinocerebellar degeneration
     - Friedrich's ataxia
     - Charcot-Marie-Tooth disease
     - Roussy-Lévy disease
   - Syringomyelia
   - Spinal cord tumor
   - Spinal cord trauma
2. Lower motor neuron
   - Poliomyelitis
   - Traumatic
   - Spinal muscular atrophy
     - Werdnig-Hoffmann
     - Kugelberg-Welander
     - Letterer-Siwe
   - Myelomeningocele
3. Dysautonomia (Riley-Day syndrome)

Myopathic

1. Arthrogryposis
2. Muscular dystrophy
   - Duchenne's
   - Limb-girdle
   - Fascioscapulohumeral
3. Fiber-type disproportion
4. Congenital hypotonia
5. Myotonia dystrophica

- Postnatal—Meningitis, near drowning, trauma, or child abuse
- Classifications
  - Muscle tone—Spastic, hypotonic, dystonic, athetosis, or ataxic
  - Geographic—Hemiplegic, diplegic, or quadriplegic
- Spine affected by abnormal tone and imbalance of the paraspinal muscles
- Spinal deformity more common in nonambulatory, quadriplegic, and spastic patients

Myelomeningocele

- Birth defect characterized by exposure of the meninges and dysplasia of the underlying neural elements, resulting in bowel, bladder, motor, and sensory paralysis distal to the malformation
- Incidence—1 in 1000 live births in the United States; 50% caused by dietary folate deficiency
- Clinically—Wide spectrum depending on the level of the lesion
  - Thoracic level—Sitter
  - Upper lumbar—Household or community ambulator with assistive devices

- Lower lumbar—Community ambulator with ankle foot orthoses (AFOs)
- Sacral—Community ambulator with or without AFOs
- Beware of the 15% incidence of latex allergy, which leads to anaphylaxis and subsequent death

Spinal Deformity

- Common and complex
- Causes of spine deformity
  - Congenital anomalies leading to scoliosis and kyphosis
  - Muscle imbalance
  - Hydrocephalus
  - Tethered cord

Duchenne's Muscular Dystrophy

- This is an X-linked recessive disorder.
- Encoding for dystrophin protein is abnormal, leading to complete absence.
- Becker muscular dystrophy has a decreased amount of dystrophin.
- The dystrophy is characterized by progressive weakness in boys who begin walking late (18 months) and eventually lose ambulatory ability by 12 years.
- The life span is shortened to less than 25 years because of pulmonary compromise.
- Histology includes muscle necrosis and fibrofatty muscle infiltration.
- Spinal deformity develops because of muscle imbalance and only appears following the loss of ambulatory status.
- Beware of the occurrence of malignant hyperthermia with anesthesia.

Spinal Muscular Atrophy

- This progressive muscular weakness is caused by a loss of anterior horn cells of the spinal cord.
- Type I (Werdnig-Hoffmann disease)
  - Severe weakness in the neonatal period and death by 2 years from respiratory failure
- Type II
  - Normal development until 5-6 months then failure to stand or walk
  - Spinal deformity is universal and can be rapidly progressive
- Type III
  - Onset before 3 years and progressive loss of ambulatory ability by 15 years
  - Spinal deformity is common
  - Type IIIb (Kugelberg-Welander syndrome)
  - Onset after 3 years
  - Weakness is often mild (foot drop) with limited endurance

Diagnostic Tools

Radiographs

- Standard PA and lateral radiographs—Assess curve severity (Cobb method) and the rate of progression
- Supine bending radiographs—Determine flexibility

Imaging Studies

- Specific imaging studies are diagnosis dependent.
- Myelomeningocele—MRI is used to identify tethered cord, syringomyelia, Chiari malformations, and hydrocephalus.

Laboratory Examination

- Laboratory examination is important to assess nutritional status.

Cerebral Palsy

- Good nutritional status is denoted by the following:
  - Albumin >35 g/L
  - Total lymphocyte count >1500 cells/mm^3

- Gastrostomy feedings are often necessary to improve nutritional status.

Duchenne's Muscular Dystrophy

- Pulmonary function tests ensure the following:
  - Forced vital capacity greater than 30%-40% of predicted capacity
- Cardiology referral for echocardiography of heart contractility

Nonoperative Treatment

Bracing

- The natural history of neuromuscular scoliosis is not affected by bracing.
- Thoracolumbosacral orthosis may be used in the skeletally immature child with cerebral palsy, myelomeningocele, and spinal muscular atrophy with a supple spine deformity to buy time prior to surgical treatment.

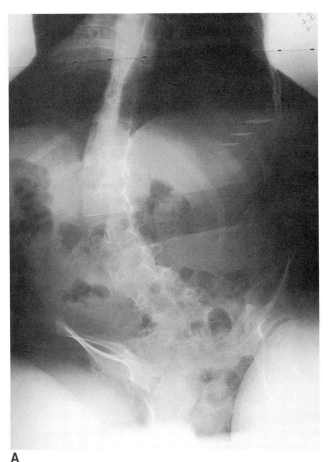

A

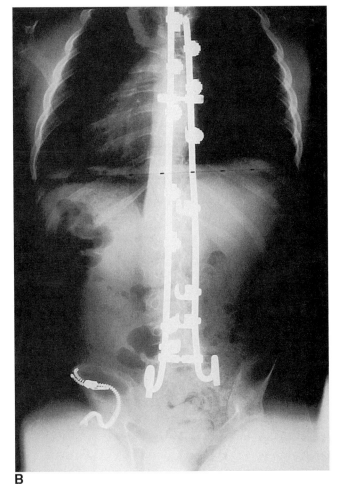

B

Figure 11–9: Scoliosis in a patient with cerebral palsy.

Modification of Seating Systems

- Significant improvements in sitting balance can be achieved with wheelchair modifications for the patient who is nonambulatory or partially ambulatory.
- It is difficult to achieve better sitting in stiff curves.

Operative Treatment

- In general, neuromuscular curves require longer fusions than idiopathic curves.
- For nonambulatory patients, fusion usually extends from T2 to the sacrum.
- Fixation
  - Traditionally segmental Luque wires have been used.
  - Hooks, screws are more often used today.
  - Pelvic fixation has many variations (Figs. 11–10 and 11–11, Table 11–3).

Cerebral Palsy

- Indications
  - Ambulatory patients—Curves greater than 50 degrees

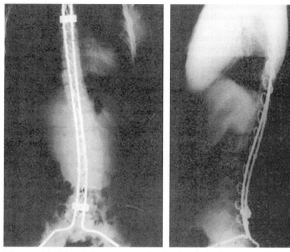

Figure 11–10: Galveston method of pelvic fixation with sublaminar Luque wires.

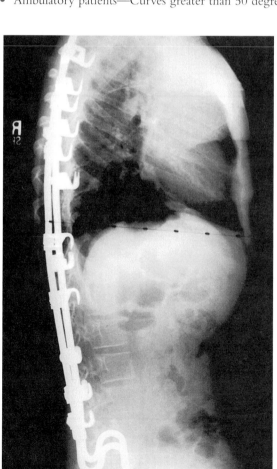

Figure 11–9 Cont'd:

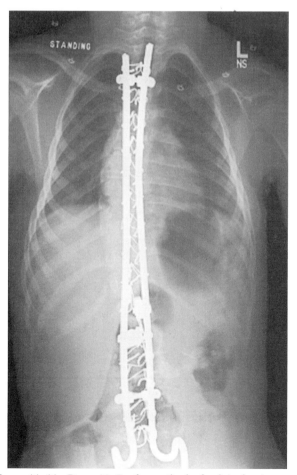

Figure 11–11: Dunn-McCarthy method of pelvic fixation.

Table 11–3: Types of Pelvic Fixation

TYPE OF PELVIC FIXATION	MODE OF FIXATION	ADVANTAGES	DISADVANTAGES
Galveston (Fig. 11–10)	Smooth rod in the iliac wing	Provides good initial fixation to the pelvis	Loosening over time Learning curve to bend the rod
Dunn-McCarthy (Fig. 11–11)	Smooth rods over the sacral ala	Technically easy	Smaller moment arm to correct pelvic obliquity Close to L5 nerve root
Iliosacral screws	Engages ilium and sacrum with a single implant	Single implant	Technically difficult Medium stability
Iliac screws	Threaded screw into the iliac wing	Excellent purchase into the hardest bone of the ilium Versatile—May be connected to any rod system	Occasionally difficult to make connection to rod

- Nonambulatory patients—Controversial; some affected early (greater than 50 degrees)
- Levels
  - Ambulatory patients—Proximal stable to distal stable vertebra
  - Nonambulatory patients—T2 to the pelvis
- Approach
  - Predominantly posterior
  - Anterior fusion may be necessary in very large (more than 100 degrees) stiff curves

Myelomeningocele

Scoliosis

- Indications—Progressive curves which limit sitting ability or lead to pressure sores.
- Levels
  - The level depends on the curve magnitude, ambulatory status, and pelvic obliquity.
  - The level is usually T2 to the sacrum in the older child.
  - In the growing child, the surgeon may instrument the thoracic curve without fusion to allow for growth.
- Approach
  - A combined anterior and posterior approach is necessary to ensure fusion because posterior elements are missing.
  - For select ambulatory patients with a thoracolumbar curve, an anterior approach and instrumentation may be sufficient.

Kyphosis

- Kyphaectomy indications
  - Significant soft tissue breakdown over the gibbus
  - Difficulty with sitting
- Levels—T2 to the sacrum
- Approach—All posterior with kyphus resection and ± spinal cord resection

Duchenne's Muscular Dystrophy

- Indications—Progressive thoracolumbar scoliosis of greater than 25-30 degrees
- Levels
  - T2 to the sacrum
  - Some advocate stopping at L5 for patients with little pelvic obliquity
- Approach—All posterior

Spinal Muscular Atrophy

- Indications—Progressive scoliosis
- Levels
  - Dependent on the ambulatory status, the age of the patient, and the pulmonary status
  - Stop short of the sacrum in ambulatory patients
- Approach
  - Anterior and posterior for the young patient with a large curve
  - All posterior for the older patient with a smaller curve

Complications

- The incidence of complications is generally higher following surgery for neuromuscular scoliosis.

Excessive Intraoperative Blood Loss

- Aggressive blood transfusion intraoperatively is necessary.

Infection

- Often dependent on the nutritional status of the patient
- Prevention
  - Good nutritional status prior to surgery
  - Preoperative and postoperative antibiotics
  - Intermittent irrigation of the soft tissues during surgery
  - Meticulous handling of the soft tissues

Pulmonary Compromise

- Prevention
  - Good preoperative assessment of pulmonary status
  - Aggressive postoperative pulmonary toilet

References

Adolescent Idiopathic Scoliosis

Cook S, Asher M, Lai SM et al. (2000) Reoperation after primary posterior instrumentation and fusion for idiopathic scoliosis. Spine 25: 463-468.

The authors analyzed a consecutive series of 182 patients who were treated with posterior spinal fusion for idiopathic scoliosis and demonstrated that the frequency for reoperation was 19%. The most common reason was late onset surgical pain in which the patients thought that the hardware was problematic. Removal of the hardware improved their symptoms. Other reasons for reoperation were pseudarthrosis, infection, and miscellaneous causes.

Lenke LG, Betz RR, Harms J et al. (2001) Adolescent idiopathic scoliosis: A new classification to determine extent of spinal arthrodesis. J Bone Joint Surg Am 83-A: 1169-1181.

The authors describe a new classification for AIS that is more comprehensive than the King classification using a two-dimensional analysis of curves. The classification defines three components of the spinal deformity: curve type (1 through 6), a lumbar modifier (A, B, or C) and a sagittal thoracic modifier (-, N, or +). The authors demonstrate greater intraobserver and interobserver reliability than the King classification.

Lonstein JE, Carlson JM. (1984) The prediction of curve progression in untreated idiopathic scoliosis during growth. J Bone Joint Surg Am 66: 1061-1071.

Richards BS. (1992) Lumbar curve response in type II idiopathic scoliosis after posterior instrumentation of the thoracic curve. Spine 17: S282-286.

The author reviewed 24 patients with King type II curves to determine whether preoperative assessment of lumbar curve flexibility could predict postoperative outcome when treated with segmental spinal instrumentation. Despite 73% lumbar curve correction on the preoperative supine bend films, the magnitude of the lumbar curve remained larger than the instrumented thoracic curve and was partially caused by the residual obliquity of the fourth lumbar vertebra.

Suk SI, Lee CK, Kim WJ et al. (2000) Segmental pedicle screw fixation in the treatment of thoracic idiopathic scoliosis. Spine 20: 1399-1405.

This retrospective clinical study compared the results of correction of AIS using pedicle screw fixation and hook fixation. The major coronal curve correction was 55% with hooks and 72% with screws. Patients who had hypokyphosis had better improvement and improved rotational correction when segmental screws were used.

Adult Scoliosis and Deformity

Albert TJ, Purtill J, Mesa J et al. (1995) Health outcome assessment before and after adult deformity surgery: A prospective study. Spine 20: 2002-2005.

This prospective study analyzed 55 adult scoliosis patients following surgery using the SF-36 outcome instrument. It demonstrated significant improvement in self-reported health assessment and function without losing the beneficial effects over time. There were no differences in outcome related to age (older than 40 years versus younger 40 years), distal extent of fusion, or the occurrence of a complication. The authors suggest that a more disease-specific outcome measurement tool would be appropriate in future studies.

Bradford DS, Tay BK, Hu SS. (1999) Adult scoliosis: Surgical indications, operative management, complications, and outcomes. Spine 24: 2617-2629.

This excellent review article provides an up-to-date description of the treatment of adult scoliosis and a good explanation of some of the controversial issues.

Bridwell KH. (2003) Adult deformity: Scoliosis and sagittal plane deformities. In: Principles and Practice of Spine Surgery (Vaccaro AR et al., eds.). Philadelphia: Mosby.

Bridwell KH, Lewis SJ, Lenke LG et al. (2003) Pedicle subtraction osteotomy for the treatment of fixed sagittal imbalance. J Bone Joint Surg Am 85: 454-463.

The authors report on 27 consecutive patients treated at a single institution with lumbar pedicle subtraction osteotomy for fixed sagittal imbalance. A radiographic and functional outcome assessment was performed. The average increase in lordosis was 34 degrees with an associated improvement in sagittal balance of 13.5 cm. There was significant improvement in the Oswestry and pain scores, and most patients were satisfied with the procedure overall. There was one pseudarthrosis at the level of the osteotomy.

Grubb SA, Lipscomb HG, Sug PB. (1994) Results of surgical treatment of painful adult scoliosis. Spine 19: 1619-1627.

This study analyzed the outcome of spinal fusion in 20 patients with painful adult scoliosis and 25 patients with painful degenerative scoliosis. The follow-up was between 2 and 7 years. Pain rating; activity level related to standing, sitting, and walking tolerance; ability to work; and period of disability was assessed. The authors report a pseudarthrosis rate of 17.5% (all patients fused to the sacrum with posterior-only surgery). Pain relief was correlated with a solid fusion and was seen in 80% of patients with idiopathic scoliosis and 70% with degenerative scoliosis. Improvement in sitting, walking, and standing was seen.

Schwab F, Dubey A, Pagala M et al. (2003) Adult scoliosis: A health assessment analysis by SF-36. Spine 28: 602-606.

The authors analyzed 22 patients with adult scoliosis and 27 patients with degenerative scoliosis (using the SF-36 outcome instrument) who had not had surgical treatment and compared them with norms for the US population. The results demonstrate that the patients with scoliosis had lower scores in all eight categories when compared with the general population and lower scores in seven of eight categories when compared with the US population 55 to 64 years old. The authors conclude that adult scoliosis is a medical condition with a significant effect in the fastest growing population in the US.

Neuromuscular Scoliosis

Comstock CP, Leach J, Wenger DR. (1995) Scoliosis in total-body–involvement cerebral palsy: Analysis of surgical treatment and patient and caregiver satisfaction. Spine 23: 1412-1424.

This retrospective review demonstrated that at a minimum follow-up of 2 years there was a 30% rate of late progression of the scoliosis, pelvic obliquity (>75°), and decompensation (>4 cm). Of the patients, 21% had revision surgery; however, 85% of the parents and caregivers were satisfied with the results of surgery.

Lintner SA, Lindseth RE. (1994) Kyphotic deformity in patients who have a myelomeningocele: Operative treatment and long-term follow-up. J Bone Joint Surg Am 76: 1301-1307.

The authors reviewed 39 patients who had myelomeningocele and resection of the kyphotic deformity. The average age at the time of surgery was 6 years and follow-up was 11 years. The correction of the kyphosis was from 111 degrees to 40 degrees postoperatively and 62 degrees at final follow-up. Of the 39

patients, 37 had an average increase of 3.2 cm in height of the lumbar spine.

Sponseller PD, LaPorte DM, Hungerford MW et al. (2000) Deep wound infections after neuromuscular scoliosis surgery: A multicenter study of risk factors and treatment outcome. Spine 25: 1461-2466.

This multicenter study analyzed 210 surgically treated patients and identified 21 patients who had a deep wound infection. Patients were analyzed and compared with 50 uninfected patients matched for age, diagnosis, and year of surgery. The risk factors for deep wound infection following spine surgery in these neuromuscular patients were severe cognitive impairment and the use of allograft. Identification of gram-negative organisms was common, and infection often led to the development of a pseudarthrosis.

Sussman MD. (1984) Advantage of early spinal stabilization and fusion in patients with Duchenne muscular dystrophy. J Pediatr Orthop 4: 532-537.

The author reports improved outcome when surgical stabilization and fusion of scoliosis is performed in patients with Duchenne muscular dystrophy. This improvement in outcome is seen as a lower complication rate, shorter hospital stay, improved curve correction and overall balance, and more rapid return to daily life. The author recommends surgical treatment when the curve progresses to between 30 and 40 degrees.

CHAPTER 12

Lumbar Spondylolisthesis

Bilal Shafi★, John M. Beiner §, Jonathan N. Grauer †, Brian K. Kwon ‡, and Alexander R. Vaccaro ‖

★M.D., M.S., Surgical Resident, Hospital of University of Pennsylvania, Philadelphia, PA
§M.D., B.S., Attending Surgeon, Connecticut Orthopaedic Specialists, Hospital of Saint Raphael; Clinical Instructor, Department of Orthopaedics, Yale University School of Medicine, New Haven, CT.
†M.D., Assistant Professor, Co-Director Orthopaedic Spine Surgery, Yale-New Haven Hospital; Assistant Professor, Department of Orthopaedics, Yale University School of Medicine, New Haven, CT
‡ M.D., Orthopaedic Spine Fellow, Department of Orthopaedic Surgery, Thomas Jefferson University and the Rothman Institute, Philadelphia, PA; Clinical Instructor, Combined Neurosurgical and Orthopaedic Spine Program, University of British Columbia; and Gowan and Michele Guest Neuroscience Canada Foundation/CIHR Research Fellow, International Collaboration on Repair Discoveries, University of British Columbia, Vancouver, Canada
‖ M.D., Professor of Orthopaedic Surgery, Thomas Jefferson University and the Rothman Institute, Philadelphia, PA

Introduction

Definitions

- Spondylolisthesis—Displacement of one vertebra on another
- From Greek
  - *spondylos*—vertebra
  - *olisthesis*—slippage
- Spondylolysis—Defect in the pars interarticularis, defined as the bone between the superior and the inferior articular processes

Anatomy (Fig. 12–1)

- The inferior articular process of each lumbar vertebra articulates with the superior articular process of the subjacent vertebra in an overlapping or shingle fashion.
- The pars interarticularis is the bony connection between the superior and the inferior processes.

Classification

- See Table 12–1.

Radiographic Measurements

- The severity of the spondylolisthesis is assessed by the magnitude of the slip and the slip angle using plain lateral radiographs.
- Taillard method (Wiltse et al. 1983)—The degree of the slip is expressed as a percentage of the anterior displacement of the inferior vertebral endplate of the cephalad body over the superior endplate of the caudal vertebra.

Congenital or Dysplastic Spondylolisthesis

Epidemiology

- Displacement occurs early, usually during the adolescent growth spurt (Newman 1963, Wiltse et al. 1976).

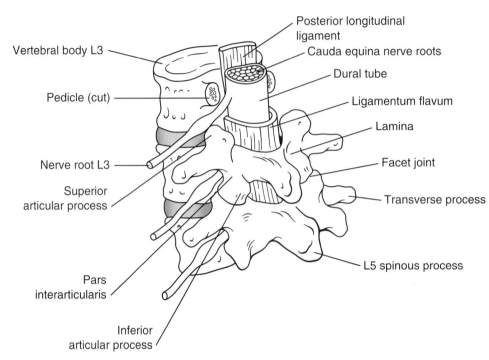

Vertebral body L3

Pedicle (cut)

Nerve root L3

Superior
articular process

Pars
interarticularis

Inferior
articular process

Posterior longitudinal
ligament

Cauda equina nerve roots

Dural tube

Ligamentum flavum

Lamina

Facet joint

Transverse process

L5 spinous process

Figure 12–1: Normal lumbar spinal anatomy. The superior articular process overlaps the inferior articular process with a variable angle to the coronal and sagittal planes, forming the facet joint.

Table 12–1:	Modified Wiltse Classification of Spondylolisthesis		
TYPE	NAME	DESCRIPTION	VERTEBRAL LEVEL
I	Congenital or dysplastic	Forward displacement because of dysplasia of the sacral or fifth lumbar arch, the facets, or both	Usually L5-S1
II	Isthmic or spondylolytic	Forward displacement because of a defect in the pars interarticularis	Usually L5-S1
III	Degenerative	Forward displacement because of segmental instability and degeneration of the disks and facets	L4-L5 (90%) L3-L4 or L5-S1 (10%)
IV	Traumatic	Forward displacement because of a fracture of the neural arch at a site other than the pars interarticularis	Usually L5-S1
V	Pathologic	Secondary forward displacement because of a pathologic lesion in the pars interarticularis, pedicle, or facet or a generalized metabolic disturbance	Any level
VI	Postsurgical	Iatrogenic disruption of facet, ligament, disk, or bone, which causes instability	Any level

- There is a 2:1 female-to-male ratio.
- This type represents 14%-21% of all spondylolisthesis cases (Newman 1976).
- Genetic component—There is an increased incidence of dysplastic lesions in affected first-degree relatives.

Etiology and Pathogenesis

- There is a congenital or dysplastic abnormality of the L5-S1 facet joint that prevents proper articulation. This allows the superior vertebra to slide forward over the inferior vertebra (Fig. 12–2).
- Displacement is early but limited based on the intact posterior neural arch.

- The pars interarticularis is intact but poorly developed, elongated, or lysed.
- In contrast to isthmic slips (described later in this chapter), this type of spondylolisthesis has an intact neural arch, which increases the chances that even low grade slips (25%-35%) will have associated compression of the cauda equina or exiting nerve roots (Fig. 12–3, Table 12–2).

Signs and Symptoms

- Pain radiating into lower extremities (rarely below the knee) with little or no back pain
- Cauda equina compression
  - Incontinence of bowel or bladder

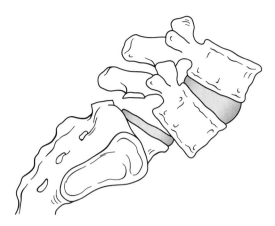

Figure 12–2: Illustration of a dysplastic spondylolisthesis showing a defect of the superior facet of S1 that prevents a true articulation between L5 and S1.

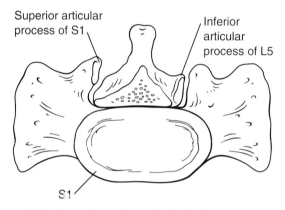

Figure 12–3: Illustration of type IB dysplastic spondylolisthesis, with sagittal orientation of the facet joints.

- Saddle anesthesia
- Fatigue or weakness in lower extremities

Diagnostic Evaluation

- Plain radiographs are anteroposterior (AP), lateral, and oblique x-ray films with lateral flexion and extension views.
- One should consider repeating these films every 4-6 months until skeletal maturity to follow slips considered stable.

Treatment

- Most congenital spondylolisthesis patients with progression of the slip require decompression and arthrodesis of the involved motion segment.

Isthmic Spondylolisthesis

Epidemiology

- This is the most common spondylolytic disorder among children and young adults.
- Of patients, 50% have spondylolysis alone (Wiltse et al. 1975).
- Males predominate in a 2:1 ratio. Males are twice as likely to have a pars interarticularis defect, but females are 4 times more likely to have a high-grade slip (Fredrickson et al. 1984).
- The disorder is related to the upright posture. It is absent in quadrupeds. In humans, it occurs after walking begins, most commonly from 7 to 8 years. It is absent in nonambulators and bed-ridden patients.
- The incidence is 5% in children from 5 to7 years, increasing to the adult level of 6%-7% by 18 years.

Etiology and Subtypes

- The isthmic defect is caused by hereditary dysplasia of the pars interarticularis.
- An erect posture, combined with the normal 40-60 degree of lumbar lordosis, produces a constant downward axial force combined with an anterior vector force or thrust, subjecting the pars interarticularis to repetitive trauma.
- This repetitive trauma causes microfractures, which heal incompletely; the basic defect is a fatigue fracture of the pars interarticularis (Wiltse et al. 1975) (Fig. 12–4, Table 12–3).
- The isthmic defect develops before skeletal maturity.
- Risk factors include vigorous exercise, participation in competitive sports involving repetitive lumbar extension, and Scheuermann's disease (Box 12–1).
- A strong genetic component is involved, with 28%-69% of family members affected. Certain ethnic populations are more commonly affected (e.g., Inuit, or Alaskan natives) (Wiltse et al. 1975).
- Four histopathologic patterns have been observed: thin fibrous bands, thick fibrous columns, a bony bridge, or a false joint (Lauerman et al. 1996).
- The abnormal pars interarticularis tissue is richly innervated and considered a source of pain during movement.

Table 12–2:	Subtypes of Congenital or Dysplastic Spondylolisthesis		
SUBTYPE	**DESCRIPTION**	**SIGNS OR SYMPTOMS**	**ASSOCIATED DEFECTS**
A	Dysplastic articular processes in a horizontal orientation	Severe hamstring spasm, early olisthesis	Spina bifida occulta (Fredrickson et al. 1984)
B	Dysplastic facet with an asymmetric sagittal malorientation and an intact neural arch (Fig. 12–3)	Leg pain, altered gait, back and hamstring spasm	Commonly cauda equina syndrome, nerve root compression
C	Other—Failed vertebral body formation, lumbosacral angular deformities	Congenital kyphosis	None

Figure 12–4: Illustration of the subtypes of isthmic (or Wiltse type II) spondylolisthesis. A, A stress fracture that does not heal normally. B, An elongated but intact pars interarticularis. C, An acute fracture of the pars interarticularis.

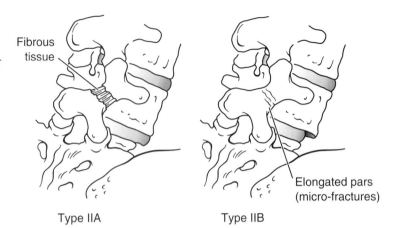

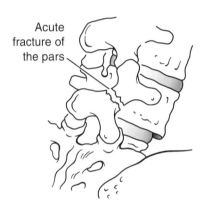

Table 12–3:	Isthmic Spondylolisthesis Subtypes (see Fig. 12–4)	
SUBTYPE	**DESCRIPTION**	**COMMENTS**
A	Early fatigue fracture that persists because of the constant motion of a poor mechanical environment	Fibrous tissue exists between the fracture edges
B	Elongated intact pars interarticularis because of repeated microfractures that heal	
C	Acute fracture because of trauma	Slippage is rare Heals with immobilization

Box 12–1:	Risk Factors for Isthmic Spondylolisthesis

- Repetitive extension activities (e.g., those of football linemen, gymnasts, divers, tennis players, and butterfly swimmers)— Increased loading of posterior elements of the spine
- Male gender—Possible increased level of high-risk athletic activity during adolescence
- Inuit race—Persistent stooped posture during common employment in harvesting seal blubber; high incidence (26%-50%) continues to increase in this population until individuals are 34 years old (Newman 1963)
- A known relative with the defect—Unclear but distinct hereditary "diathesis" that predisposes to the spondylolysis and olisthesis (Wiltse et al. 1975)

- Up to 40% of patients with isthmic defects have an accompanying spina bifida contributing to the added stress on the pars interarticularis.

Signs and Symptoms

- Most symptomatic patients present symptoms in late adolescence for evaluation.
- The most common complaint is a dull aching pain in the back, buttocks, or thighs beginning during the adolescent growth spurt and exacerbated by activity.

- Because many patients with spondylolysis or even low-grade slips are asymptomatic, other causes of the pain (infection, neoplasm, fracture, or disk herniation) should be explored before attributing symptoms to the spondylolisthesis.
- Of symptomatic children, 92% complain of recurrence during adulthood; 55% complain of sciatica at the affected nerve root or roots (Saraste 1987).
- True radicular symptoms are rare. Paresthesias and weakness are sometimes present in the distribution of the

affected nerve roots, reflecting compression of the root by the hypertrophic callus at the pars interarticularis defect. Higher-grade slips may have additional symptoms referable to the stretching of the superjacent nerve root as well.

• Pain appearing after patients are 40 years old is unlikely to be related to a pars interarticularis defect unless significant trauma has disrupted the stability of the fibrous union, if present.

• Disk degeneration starts at an earlier age in spondylolytic patients.

Physical Findings

• Deep palpation over the affected area may reproduce local and possibly radicular pain.

• Of symptomatic patients, 80% have spasm and foreshortening of the paraspinal and hamstring muscles as part of the body's attempt to stabilize the pelvis (Amundson et al. 1999).

• Limited forward flexion and decreased straight leg raise correspond to hamstring tightness.

• Lumbosacral kyphosis and trunk shortening is apparent with an absence of a waistline, abdominal, and flank skin folds with higher-grade slips.

• A posterior step-off along the spinous processes can be seen in patients with a grade II or higher slip.

• To stand erect, the hamstrings and iliopsoas contract to rotate the pelvis, arching the thoracolumbar spine into maximal lordosis. Sometimes the patient must also flex the hips and knees to attain an erect posture (Phalen-Dickson sign).

• The kyphotic deformity and thoracolumbar hyperlordosis leads to flat, square buttocks, a widened "sweetheart" pelvis, and a protruding inferior rib cage.

• Gait abnormalities are characterized by a waddle with limited hip flexion, shortened stride length, and a wide base of support.

• Physical findings correlate with the degree of slip and slip angle.

• Abnormal disks were found in 10% to 39% of patients with a pars interarticularis defect (Saraste 1987).

• A flexible scoliosis occurs in 5%-7% of all patients with spondylolisthesis (which usually corrects spontaneously following surgery for the slip).

Diagnostic Evaluation

• Plain radiographs should include AP and lateral views in the standing position.

• Oblique views increase the sensitivity of plain radiography by a small amount but at significantly increased gonadal radiation (Roberts et al. 1978).

• Dynamic lateral flexion and extension plain radiographs may illustrate the degree of instability of the olisthetic segment.

• Classically, the defect in the pars interarticularis can be seen as a collar on the "Scottie dog's neck" on oblique views (Fig. 12–5).

• In high-grade slips, the posterior body of L5 rests on the sacral promontory, concentrating the axial forces over a small area. This results in a trapezoidal or wedge-shaped L5 body and a rounded sacral dome, which can be seen on AP radiograph as the reverse "Napoleon's hat" sign (Fig. 12–6).

• Long-cassette AP and lateral radiographs are useful to evaluate coronal and sagittal balance and the presence of scoliosis.

• If no defect is visible on plain radiography but suspicion is high, a single-photon emission computed tomography (SPECT) is a sensitive modality that can detect and illustrate the metabolic activity at the region of a suspected pars interarticularis defect.

• A technetium bone scan, a component of a SPECT imaging study, can be used to assess acute injury or to document the healing process.

• Computed tomography (CT) can be used to define the bony anatomy more clearly; this can miss the defect in the pars interarticularis if the cuts or intervals are too large.

• Magnetic resonance imaging (MRI) is the study of choice for spinal stenosis because it allows visualization of soft tissue structures. It is also invaluable for demonstrating the presence of disk degeneration. The "wide canal sign" or ratio, measured as the AP diameter of the canal at the slip level divided by the AP diameter at the L1 level, has been offered as a means of detecting the presence of bilateral pars interarticularis defects with spondylolisthesis when the ratio is greater than 1.25 (Amundson et al. 1999).

• Provocative discography is a useful provocative study to assess the presence of coexisting symptomatic disk disease. If concordant pain is reproduced at the level of the spondylolysis or olisthesis, this contraindicates direct repair of the pars interarticularis defect in favor of arthrodesis in patients considering surgical intervention.

• Depending on the degree of slippage, patients should be followed every 3-6 months with plain radiographs (static and dynamic) until skeletal maturity to assess for the presence of progressive instability.

Radiographic Measurements (Fig. 12–7)

• Meyerding classification
  1. Grade I—0%-25% slip
  2. Grade II—26%-50% slip
  3. Grade III—51%-75% slip
  4. Grade IV—76%-99% slip
  5. Grade V—Spondyloptosis, or 100% slip

• The slip angle or angle of kyphosis is measured as the angle between the superior endplate of L5 and a line perpendicular to the posterior border of the sacrum.

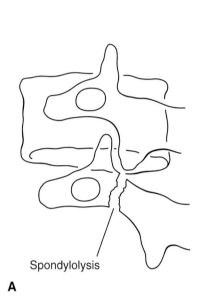

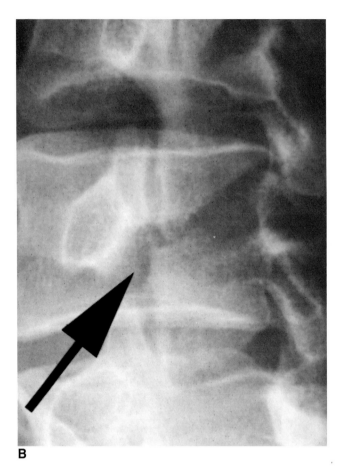

Figure 12–5: Illustration (A) and oblique radiograph (B) of a lytic pars interarticularis defect classically described as a collar on a Scottie dog.

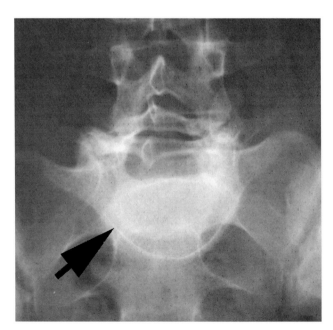

Figure 12–6: AP radiograph of a high-grade isthmic spondylolisthesis illustrating the inverted Napoleon's hat sign.

- The slip angle is the most sensitive indicator of potential instability and clinical symptoms (Boxall et al. 1979).
- Correction of the kyphotic deformity, as measured by the slip angle, is the most important goal of surgical reduction.
- The lumbar index is a measure of the wedging of the anterior L5 vertebral body, expressed as the quotient between anterior and posterior height of the slipped vertebra.
- Other measures include the percentage of rounding of the sacral dome, the degree of lumbar lordosis, and the degree of sagittal rotation (Box 12–2).

Treatment

- The truly asymptomatic patient with an incidental finding of a pars interarticularis defect without a slip can be followed on an as-needed basis if symptoms develop.
- If a spondylolisthesis is present, most authors advocate serial radiographs on a 3- to 6-month basis to determine the stability of the slip until skeletal maturity before discharging the patient.

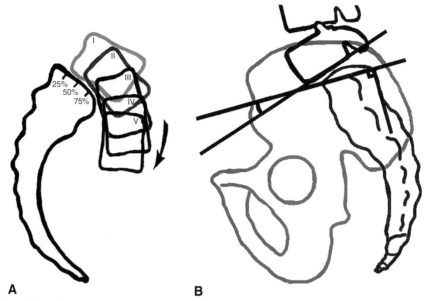

Figure 12–7: Schematic drawing illustrating the two most common radiographic measurements of spondylolisthesis. **A**, The percent slip. **B**, The slip angle. (Reprinted from Drummond et al. 2003.)

Box 12–2:	**Natural History of Isthmic Spondylolisthesis***

- In patients with lytic defects, 68% have a slip. If a slip is going to develop, it will develop by adolescence in most patients.
- Female patients with a documented slip often experience progression more than males.
- Of adults with a slip, the following percentages have been found:
  - 40% will not progress
  - 40% will progress less than 5 mm
  - Only 15% will progress more than 1 cm
- Isthmic progresses more than degenerative spondylolisthesis.
- Disk degeneration adds to the potential for slip progression (in isthmic not in degenerative slips).
- Some authors associate a high slip angle with a higher likelihood of progression.
- Traumatic pars interarticularis fractures are rare but usually heal well with conservative care.

* (Fredrickson et al. 1984, Saraste 1987.)

Nonoperative Treatment of a Symptomatic Patient

- Activity modification includes restriction of high-risk athletics, avoiding repetitive extension maneuvers.
- Physical therapy emphasizing flexibility and strengthening exercises should be employed.
- Immobilization with a lumbosacral orthosis or plaster jacket can be used for refractory cases.

- A positive bone scan or SPECT scan in a young child or adolescent implies the potential for possible healing at the pars interarticularis defect with external immobilization.
- A traumatic spondylolysis or olisthesis should be treated with brace or cast immobilization unless surgical intervention is required because of gross instability or symptomatic neural compression.
- Nonoperative treatment is effective in two thirds of patients with low-grade slips diagnosed early (Table 12–4).

Operative Treatment

- Goals of surgery include reduction in pain, prevention of further slip, stabilization of the spine, restoration of normal posture and gait, reversal and prevention of neurological deficit, and improved cosmetic appearance.
- Surgical procedures include direct repair of the pars interarticularis defect, posterolateral fusion with or without decompression, slip reduction or instrumentation, and possible interbody fusion (Table 12–5).
- Smokers have lower fusion rates (57% versus 95%) (Amundson et al. 1999).
- Pseudarthrosis or nonunion develops in approximately a third of patients with spondylolisthesis after posterolateral in situ arthrodesis without instrumentation because of the altered anatomy of the slip. Low surface area for fusion, increased stress across the fusion, and difficulty in exposing the L5 transverse process without exposing the L4 transverse process may

Table 12–4: Treatment Recommendations for Isthmic Spondylolisthesis

STATUS	RECOMMENDATION
Incidental pars interarticularis defect	Periodic observation, no restrictions
Grade I	Periodic observation, no restrictions
Grade II	If asymptomatic, observe with periodic radiographs; consider restriction of high-risk athletics.
	If symptomatic, restrict high-risk athletics and avoid heavy-labor occupations.
	Bracing or casting for acute symptomatic relief may be considered.
	If prolonged nonoperative measures fail, consider surgical intervention.
Grade III-IV or high slip angle	Surgical intervention should be considered in the symptomatic immature patient to correct deformity, prevent slip progression, and provide symptomatic relief.

motivate the surgeon to fuse from L4 to S1 in the setting of an L5-S1 slippage in anything other than a grade I spondylolisthesis.

- Slip progression (translation and angulation) occurs in 33% of cases regardless of the presence of a solid fusion (uninstrumented), especially in patients with high-grade slips, after a Gill laminectomy, or when no postoperative immobilization is used (Boxall et al. 1979).
- Gill laminectomy alone for decompression of the L5 or S1 nerve roots is controversial:
  - Rates of slip progression with decompression without fusion have been reported as high as 27% (Osterman et al. 1976).
  - Many nerve root symptoms (e.g., radicular pain, hamstring tightness, and weakness) will resolve after fusion without decompression (Wiltse et al. 1975), calling into question the need for decompression.
  - In adults with isthmic slips, the addition of decompression to a fusion procedure significantly increases the pseudarthrosis rate, leading to more unsatisfactory results in one study (Carragee 1997).
- The use of instrumentation (pedicle screw fixation) is not without potential drawbacks:

Table 12–5: Operative Treatment of Isthmic Spondylolisthesis

PROCEDURE	ADVANTAGES	DISADVANTAGES	RESULTS
Pars interarticularis defect repair	Preserves the motion segment	Does not address intervertebral instability Technically difficult	60%-90% success in selected patients (Dreyzin 1994)
Decompression (Gill laminectomy)	Avoids fusion	Residual back pain, increased instability with further slippage, increased lumbosacral kyphosis after surgery	Mostly unsuccessful
Posterolateral uninstrumented in situ fusion	Significantly improves pain, gait, hamstring tightness	Possible failure of fusion (pseudarthrosis) in up to 40% of patients	Variable; 60%-100% success
	Prevents slip progression	Need long-term postoperative bracing for improved outcomes	Improved outcome with a solid fusion in children
			Adults not as successful (Amundson et al. 1999)
Decompression with in situ fusion	Same as decompression alone but with the benefit of decreased slip progression and instability	Higher rates of pseudarthrosis reported than with fusion without decompression	Up to 100% success rates with solid fusion (Carragee 1997)
		Greater risk of slip progression than with fusion alone	Results poor if pseudarthrosis develops
In situ fusion with or without decompression and instrumentation	Improved fusion rates	Technical difficulty associated with instrumentation placement	Success rate correlates with patient selection, the presence of a solid fusion
			Some authors report no added benefit with internal fixation (Schnee et al. 1997)
Reduction and instrumented fusion	Adds stability to fusion, with higher fusion rates reported	Increased complication rate because of reduction maneuver	Results correlate with fusion rates, any presence of residual neurologic dysfunction
	Allows correction of deformity, restores body posture and mechanics, improves body image	Many instrumentation systems require fusion to L4 for reduction	

- Operative times are prolonged and blood loss may be increased.
- Clinical outcomes may be only minimally affected (Moller et al. 2000).
- Reduction of a high-grade slip is associated with a high complication rate (chiefly L5 radicular symptoms occurring at the final stage of reduction). Full correction of the olisthesis is not needed; correction of the kyphosis is most important.
- Reduction improves the fusion rate and outcome. Bradford (1988) offers the following indications for reduction in the adult patient with isthmic spondylolisthesis:
  - Vertebral slippage >60%
  - Slip angle >50 degrees
  - Age between 12 and 30 years
  - Symptoms uncontrollable by nonoperative means
- The addition of anterior column fusion (through anterior, posterior, or transforaminal lumbar interbody fusion) provides additional stability and decreases pseudarthrosis rates, improving clinical outcome (Table 12–6).

Degenerative Spondylolisthesis
Epidemiology

- Most often this type occurs at the L4-L5 level (Rosenberg 1975, Herkowitz 1995).
- It is often called "spondylolisthesis with an intact neural arch"; there is no pars interarticularis defect (Fig. 12–8).

- This type is more common in women (5-6 times more frequent than in men).
- Presenting symptoms usually appear after the patient is 40 years old.
- Black women are 3 times more likely to develop degenerative slips than the average population (as described later in this chapter).
- Approximately 10% of women older than 60 years have a degenerative slip (Frymoyer 1994).

Etiology

- Multiple factors contribute to the development of a degenerative spondylolisthesis, including disk degeneration, degenerative arthritis of the facet joints, and anatomic factors specific to the affected motion segment.
- The slip rarely exceeds 33% and progression occurs in only 30% of patients (Herkowitz 1995) (Box 12–3).

Signs and Symptoms

- Patients typically complain of low back pain radiating into the buttocks or lateral thighs.
- Stiffness is not a common finding; many patients are hyperflexible, reflecting a generalized ligamentous laxity. Hamstring tightness is not common, in contrast to isthmic slips.
- True radicular symptoms occur in approximately 50% of patients and when present are often referable to the L5 nerve root (Matsunaga et al. 1990). Tingling and numbness can occur down the lateral calf into the lateral toes.

Table 12–6: Approaches to Reduction and Internal Fixation of Isthmic Spondylolisthesis*				
PROCEDURE	**INDICATIONS**	**TECHNIQUE**	**RESULTS**	**COMPLICATIONS**
Posterior reduction and in situ fusion with extension casting	Young patients with a significant kyphotic deformity	Following L4-S1 in situ fusion, patients are placed in serial extension casts for three months	Two thirds reduction in slip angle but little change in trunk height or slip degree	Reported cases of transient L5 weakness, nonunion, partial loss of reduction in high-grade slips Up to 40% pseudarthrosis rates
Posterior instrumented reduction and fusion	Patients older than 10 years with high-grade spondylolisthesis	Nerve root decompression followed by posterior instrumented reduction through the application of gradual corrective forces	88% fusion with high patient satisfaction On average, 50% reduction in slip translation, slip angle	4% transient radiculopathy 1% neurological deficit 1.5% infection 2% hardware failure
Anterior and posterior reduction and fusion	Patients with high-grade deformities requiring additional stability or release to achieve fusion	Anterior L5 or S1 body partial resection, grafting, and fusion followed by posterior nerve root decompression and gradual instrumented reduction	Experienced surgeon can achieve 90% correction of slip angle with a residual grade I, II slip	Technically difficult surgery with high morbidity 30%-40% neurological deficit (unilateral foot drop most common) 10%-15% nonunion

* (Bradford 1988, Edwards 1990, Amundson et al. 1999.)

Figure 12–8: Drawing illustrating degenerative versus isthmic spondylolisthesis.

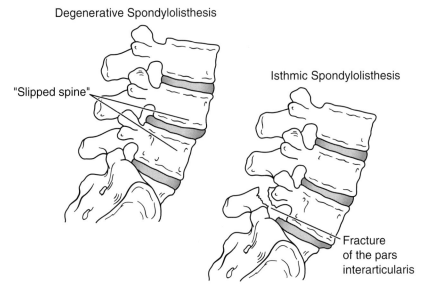

Degenerative Spondylolisthesis

Isthmic Spondylolisthesis

"Slipped spine"

Fracture of the pars interarticularis

Box 12–3:	Anatomy of the Degenerative Spondylolisthesis Motion Segment

- The normal lumbar lordosis of 40-60 degrees causes an anteriorly directed force vector across the middle lumbar vertebrae.
- The L5-S1 articulation is unusually stable because of coronally oriented facets, the strong iliolumbar ligaments, and frequent partial sacralization of L5 (more common in patients of African descent).
- The facet joints have a more sagittal orientation at the level of a degenerative spondylolisthesis (Grobler et al. 1993).
- These factors concentrate stresses most frequently across the L4-L5 and sometimes the L3-L4 motion segment.
- Degenerative disk disease shifts a larger part of the axial load to the facet joints.
- Generalized ligamentous laxity (greater in females) further reduces the resistance to forward slippage.
- Microinstability of the segment results in hypertrophic facet joints and osteophytes that stretch the joint capsules, leading to anterior and lateral olisthesis, rotary subluxation, and stenosis with root compression.

- Mild weakness exists in 15%-20% of patients in the L5 nerve root distribution (Herkowitz 1995), including the extensor hallucis muscle and sometimes the tibialis anterior or gastroc-soleus complex.
- The following symptoms of spinal stenosis are extremely common and are usually the reason these patients seek medical attention:
  - Proximal muscle weakness
  - Intolerance to walking or even standing, relieved by leaning over or sitting
  - Intermittent claudication
- Claudication must be differentiated between neurogenic and vascular causes (Table 12–7).

Diagnostic Evaluation

- Plain radiographs
  - A standing lateral radiograph is more sensitive than a nonweight-bearing film in detecting a spondylolisthesis.
  - An AP film is used to detect degenerative scoliosis, lateral olisthesis, or sacralization of L5.
  - Flexion and extension lateral x-ray films can reveal the rare case of translational or angular dynamic instability. Excessive translational motion is generally defined as greater than 4 mm of motion with flexion, and angular instability is considered present when there is a greater-than-10-degrees difference between flexion and extension radiographs.
- A CT myelogram may be ordered to delineate the extent of spinal stenosis in these patients. This also gives valuable information about the amount of osteoporosis present and a detailed view of the facet joint hypertrophy. The traversing nerve root is compressed by the superior articular process of the inferior vertebral segment (Fig. 12–9).
- Myelography has historically been the test of choice to evaluate spinal stenosis. Findings include traversing nerve root cutoff because of the facet hypertrophy and spondylolisthesis. Plain radiographs can be taken standing to accentuate the slip. However, complications of myelography include headache and nausea in up to 20% of patients.
- MRI has become the standard in evaluating these patients because it provides information about the nerve roots and about the soft tissue component of stenosis, such as hypertrophied ligamentum flavum or synovial cysts. Synovial cysts in the facet joint can be a source of compression of the nerves and an indicator of instability at the motion segment.

Table 12–7:   Comparison of Neurogenic and Vascular Claudication

CLINICAL CHARACTERISTICS	NEUROGENIC CLAUDICATION	VASCULAR CLAUDICATION
Location of pain	Back, thighs, calves, buttocks	Buttocks, calves
Quality of pain	Burning, cramping	Cramping
Aggravating factors	Erect posture, ambulation, extension of the spine	Any leg exercise, usually triggering calf pain at a reproducible interval
Relieving factors	Squatting, bending forward, sitting	Rest
Leg pulses and blood pressure	Usually normal	Blood pressure decreased
		Pulses decreased or absent
		Bruits, murmurs may be present
Skin or trophic changes	Usually absent	Often present (pallor, cyanosis, nail dystrophy)
Autonomic changes	Bladder incontinence (rare)	Impotence may coexist with other symptoms of vascular claudication

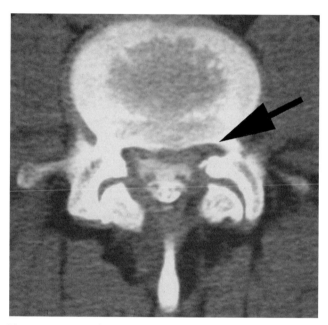

Figure 12–9: Axial CT scan revealing facet hypertrophy and lateral recess stenosis.

- MRI is used by some practitioners in place of myelography, though many surgeons still use both in preoperative planning for these patients.
- Electromyography and nerve conduction studies differentiate neuropathy from neurogenic claudication in diabetics.

Treatment (Box 12–4)

Nonoperative Treatment

- Short-term bed rest (1-2 days) followed by activity modification, combined with anti-inflammatory medication, is the mainstay of treatment.
  - Nonsteroidal anti-inflammatory drugs have no proven efficacy over aspirin or acetaminophen.
  - Oral steroid medications are best reserved for acute exacerbations of leg pain in the older patient. Gastrointestinal acid prophylaxis is important.

Box 12–4:   Natural History of Degenerative Spondylolisthesis*

- Of such patients, 25%-30% will experience progression of the spondylolisthesis.
  - In the postoperative patient, progression of the slip after an attempted fusion correlates with a poor outcome.
- It is rare for a degenerative spondylolisthesis to slip more than 30%.

Spinal Stenosis

- Nonoperative measures succeed in most patients.
- A progressive neurologic deficit is rare.
- Symptoms of cauda equina syndrome can be insidious. Urgent surgical decompression is often recommended in the presence of spinal stenosis and cauda equina syndrome.

*(Rosenberg 1975, Matsunaga et al. 1990, Frymoyer 1994, Herkowitz 1995.)

- Physical therapy—Isometrics followed by range of motion exercises followed by active flexion exercises, abdominal and low back strengthening, and weight reduction are used. Progression to aerobic conditioning is recommended.
- Epidural steroids and selective nerve root injections are valuable treatments for significant pain (leg pain is more reliably relieved than back pain).

Operative Treatment

- Goals
  - Pain relief
  - Improvement or prevention of neurological deficit
  - Increased tolerance to walking and standing
  - Improvement in quality of life
- Indications—Persistent or recurrent severe leg pain despite conservative treatment and progressive neurological deficit in the setting of confirmatory imaging studies demonstrating significant spinal stenosis (Herkowitz 1995) (Table 12–8, Box 12–5)

Table 12–8: Operative Treatment of Degenerative Spondylolisthesis

PROCEDURE	DESCRIPTION	ADVANTAGES	DISADVANTAGES	COMPLICATIONS
Decompressive laminectomy	Removal of lamina and part of medial facet joints	Least invasive surgery Provides rapid, substantial relief of pain Avoids morbidity of fusion	Does not address instability May cause iatrogenic instability	Slip progression occurs in 25%-50% of patients and may correlate with a poor clinical outcome (Mardjetko et al. 1994)
Decompression with posterolateral fusion	Full laminectomy and partial facetectomy with exposure and fusion of the transverse processes	Decreased slip progression and increased spinal stability if a solid fusion is obtained	Possible failure of fusion Bone graft harvest site morbidity Increased operative times and blood loss with some studies showing no effect on outcome	Longer operative times with attendant complications Persistent bone graft site pain in up to 20% of patients
Decompression with instrumented fusion	Decompression and fusion as described previously with segmental instrumentation	Most studies show increased fusion rates with improved functional outcomes Can allow partial reduction of deformity Allows more aggressive decompression	Loss of lumbar lordosis ("flatback" deformity) seen with older techniques that involve distraction Longer operative times are common Increased cost	Complications related to instrument placement including increased infection, problems related to implant migration or failure

Box 12–5: Fusion and Instrumentation—The Controversy

- Several randomized, prospective clinical trials and a meta-analysis examining the variables of fusion versus decompression alone and instrumented versus noninstrumented fusion support the following conclusions (Herkowitz et al. 1991, Bridwell et al. 1993, Zdeblick 1993, Mardjetko et al. 1994, Fischgrund et al. 1997):
  - Radical decompression fares poorly without the addition of fusion.
  - Fusion may not be necessary in all patients, but predicting which patients do not need the added procedure is elusive.
  - Pedicle screw instrumentation significantly increases the fusion rate in most studies.
  - Correlating the success of fusion with a better clinical outcome is complicated because many patients with a pseudarthrosis seem to be stable enough to enjoy a good outcome. Nevertheless, most studies demonstrate better outcomes with a solid fusion of the spondylolisthesis segment.
  - Device-related complications (such as screw breakage), as well as surgeon-related complications (such as incorrect instrumentation placement), have decreased in more recent studies with better instrumentation systems and increased surgeon familiarity with the techniques of insertion.

Traumatic Spondylolisthesis

- This acute fracture or dislocation of the facet or lamina creates instability.
- These are extremely rare injuries.
- Treatment should follow the guidelines for isthmic spondylolisthesis.
- A posterior fracture may be part of a much larger injury, including a fracture or dislocation of the spine that has spontaneously reduced; the clinician should be aware of this possibility and should initiate the appropriate diagnostic workup, including plain radiographs, CT, and MRI when appropriate.

Pathologic Spondylolisthesis

- Generalized bone disease
  - Osteoporosis and osteomalacia—Instability results from continuous fatiguing stresses applied to the osteoporotic pedicles and facet joints, which undergo microfractures. When the microfractures heal, they remodel in an elongated position leading to segmental instability (Tabrizi et al. 2001).
  - Other causes include Paget's disease and osteogenesis imperfecta (high-grade slips related to elongation of the pedicle).
- Tumors—Primary or secondary neoplasm can disrupt bony architecture leading to instability.

Iatrogenic Spondylolisthesis

- Spondylolisthesis can be caused by the surgical disruption of ligaments, bone, or the intervertebral disk.
- The most common cause is wide decompression without fusion. Discectomy further destabilizes the motion segment.
- Resection of more than 50% of each facet joint or an entire facet joint unilaterally predisposes the spine to increased instability (Abumi et al. 1990).
- Treatment should involve an instrumented posterolateral fusion with or without an interbody fusion depending on the degree of instability.

References

Abumi K, Panjabi MM, Kramer KM et al. (1990) Biomechanical evaluation of lumbar spinal stability after graded facetectomies. Spine 15: 1142-1147.

This was a serial sectioning study of cadaver lumbar spines with a stepwise increase in the amounts of the facets sacrificed followed by flexibility testing. When 50% of the facets, or 100% of a unilateral facet, were removed, instability developed (defined according to Panjabi's criteria).

Amundson G, Edwards CC, Garfin SR. (1999) Spondylolisthesis. In: The Spine (Rothman RH et al., eds.), 4th edition. Philadelphia: WB Saunders Co., pp. 835-885.

This is a detailed chapter on spondylolisthesis including congenital, isthmic, and degenerative types. The authors focus mostly on isthmic spondylolisthesis. They present the etiology, pathophysiology, presentation of symptoms, diagnosis, treatment options, and outcome data for each of these groups.

Boos N, Marchesi D, Zuber K et al. (1993) Treatment of severe spondylolisthesis by reduction and pedicular fixation: A 4-6-year follow-up study. Spine 18: 1655-1661.

Ten patients with severe spondylolisthesis were treated with reduction and pedicular screw fixation. The slip was reduced from 78.5% to 39.6%, and the slip angle was reduced from 43% to 17%. It was found that pedicular fixation was only successful in treating high-grade spondylolisthesis if it was combined with an anterior or posterior interbody fusion.

Boxall D, Bradford DS, Winter RB et al. (1979) Management of severe spondylolisthesis in children and adolescents. J Bone Joint Surg 61A: 479-495.

In this study, 43 patients with high-grade spondylolisthesis were treated nonoperatively and operatively. Operative treatments included fusion, decompression with fusion, and reduction with fusion. The slip angle was found to be a much better predictor of the severity of disease and the risk for slip progression. The authors indicate that postoperative extension casting reduced the risk of slip progression. Fusion alone had a successful outcome, but the risk of slip progression still existed.

Bradford DS. (1988) Closed reduction of spondylolisthesis: An experience in 22 patients. Spine 13: 580-587.

A technique is presented for a combined anterior and posterior reduction and fusion of an isthmic spondylolisthesis, and results are presented for 10 patients. The technique offered good success in terms of reduction, but 6 of 10 patients had major complications.

Bridwell K, Sedgewick T, O'Brien M et al. (1993) The role of fusion and instrumentation in the treatment of degenerative spondylolisthesis with spinal stenosis. J Spinal Disord 6: 467-472.

In this study, 44 patients were prospectively randomized (with exceptions and some bias) into three groups: decompression without fusion, decompression plus in situ posterolateral fusion, and decompression plus instrumented fusion. They were followed for a minimum of 2 years. Instrumentation significantly improved the fusion rate and prevented slip progression, which correlated with better clinical outcomes.

Carragee EJ. (1997) Single-level posterolateral arthrodesis, with or without posterior decompression, for the treatment of isthmic spondylolisthesis in adults. J Bone Joint Surg 79A: 1175-1180.

Here, 42 patients who failed nonoperative treatment for grade I or II spondylolisthesis without neurological deficit were treated with decompression with fusion, fusion alone, fusion with instrumentation, or decompression with fusion and instrumentation. The authors found that decompression increased the rate of pseudarthrosis and negatively affected the clinical outcome.

Dreyzin V, Esses SI. (1994) A comparative analysis of spondylolysis repair. Spine 19: 1909-1915.

Twenty patients with type IIA grade 0 or grade I spondylolytic defect were treated with one of two surgical techniques for pars interarticularis repair. Both techniques yielded a poor clinical outcome with a high failure rate.

Drummond DS, Scott AR. (2003) Pediatric spondylolisthesis. In: Principles and Practice of Spine Surgery (Vaccaro AR et al., eds.). Philadelphia: Mosby.

Edwards CC. (1990) Prospective evaluation of a new method for complete reduction of L5-S1 spondylolisthesis using corrective forces alone. Orthop Trans 14(3): 549.

The author describes a novel method of reducing a high-grade spondylolisthesis, explaining the surgical technique and complications.

Fischgrund JS, Mackay M, Herkowitz HN et al. (1997) Degenerative lumbar spondylolisthesis with spinal stenosis: A prospective randomized study comparing decompressive laminectomy and arthrodesis with and without spinal instrumentation. Spine 22: 2807-2812.

In this study, 76 patients with symptomatic spinal stenosis caused by degenerative spondylolisthesis were treated with posterior decompression and posterolateral fusion. Half the patients were randomized to receive internal fixation with transpedicular screws. Higher fusion rates were achieved in the instrumented group, but there was no difference in clinical outcome between the two groups.

Fredrickson BE, Baker D, McHolick WJ et al. (1984) The natural history of spondylolysis and spondylolisthesis. J Bone Joint Surg 66A: 699-707.

The authors studied 500 first-grade children radiographically to find the incidence of spondylolisthesis among children: 4.4% increasing to 6% in adulthood. The progression of olisthesis in adulthood was unusual. Spina bifida occulta and a trapezoidal L5 vertebra were found to be significantly associated with spondylolisthesis. The authors note a strong genetic factor contributing to the pars interarticularis defect. They also recommend no limitation to the lifestyle of children with spondylolisthesis.

Frymoyer JW. (1994) Degenerative spondylolisthesis: Diagnosis and treatment, JAAOS 2: 9-15.

This is a general review article addressing the epidemiology, etiology, pathophysiology, presentation of symptoms, diagnosis, and treatment options for degenerative spondylolisthesis. The most common complaint is back pain, which may progress to claudication-type leg pain. Of people who receive conservative treatment, 15% fail and require surgical treatment. The author suggests decompression and fusion as the ideal surgical option with careful selection of surgical candidates when morbidity increases with age.

Grobler L, Robertson P, Novotny J et al. (1993) Etiology of spondylolisthesis: Assessment of the role played by lumbar facet joint morphology. Spine 18: 80-92.

CT was used in this study to characterize the facet joint morphology in normal people and in patients with isthmic or degenerative spondylolisthesis. A gradually more coronal orientation was found from proximal to distal in the lumbar spine. Patients with degenerative spondylolisthesis had significantly more sagittal orientation to their facets at the L4-L5 level, leading to the conclusion that these patients are predisposed to the slip by a developmental abnormality of the facet joints.

Herkowitz H. (1995) Spine update: Degenerative lumbar spondylolisthesis. Spine 20(9): 1084-1090.

This is a review article on degenerative spondylolisthesis with an emphasis on associated spinal stenosis. The author outlines the epidemiology, presenting symptoms, physical examination findings, diagnostic findings, and treatment options. Treatment options addressed include fusion alone, decompression alone, decompression with fusion, and decompression with fusion and internal fixation.

Herkowitz HN, Kurz LT. (1991) Degenerative lumbar spondylolisthesis with spinal stenosis: A prospective study comparing decompression with decompression and intertransverse process arthrodesis. J Bone Joint Surg 73A: 802-808.

Fifty patients with spinal stenosis because of degenerative spondylolisthesis at L4-L5 or L3-L4 were treated with decompression (n = 25) or decompression and intertransverse process arthrodesis (n = 25) and followed for a mean of 3 years. Patients who underwent arthrodesis had a better clinical result with respect to pain relief and a decreased risk of slip progression than patients who underwent decompression alone.

Hu SS, Bradford DS, Transfeldt EE et al. (1996) Reduction of high-grade spondylolisthesis using Edward's instrumentation. Spine 21(3): 367-371.

Sixteen patients with high-grade spondylolisthesis underwent reduction and fixation using Edwards's instrumentation, reducing the degree of slip from 89% to 29% and the slip angle from 50% to 24%. Most patients reported good to excellent results, proving this technically demanding method to be effective for reducing severe deformity and pain.

Johnsson KE, Willner S, Johnsson K. (1986) Postoperative instability after decompression for lumbar spinal stenosis. Spine 11: 107-110.

Here, 45 patients were evaluated for slipping following decompression for spinal stenosis because of degenerative spondylolisthesis or acquired spinal stenosis. Patients with slip progression postoperatively demonstrated worse clinical outcomes.

Lauerman WC, Cain JE. (1996) Isthmic spondylolisthesis in the adult. JAAOS 4(4): 201-208.

This article addresses isthmic spondylolisthesis in the adult population. Adult patients usually have low back pain with or without radicular pain. Most patients improve with nonoperative treatment. If this fails, then fusion with or without decompression is the surgery of choice. Reduction and fixation are presented as surgical alternatives for severe cases of spondylolisthesis with their associated complications.

Mardjetko SM, Connolly PG, Schott S. (1994) Degenerative lumbar spondylolisthesis: A meta-analysis of the literature 1970-1993. Spine 10: 2256S-2265S.

The authors conducted a meta-analysis on an extremely varied set of papers dealing with the treatment of this disorder over several years, seeing vast changes in techniques and instrumentation options. Instrumentation was found to increase the rate of fusion, and fusion seemed to portend a better outcome, but there was no direct benefit of instrumentation on outcomes. There was no significant difference between anterior and posterior procedures in terms of outcome.

Matsunaga S, Sakou T, Morizono Y et al. (1990) Natural history of degenerative spondylolisthesis: Pathogenesis and natural course of the slippage. Spine 15: 1204-1210.

This was a retrospective observational study of 40 patients with degenerative slips followed for 5 years. Progression was noted in 30%, was greater (75%) in laborers, and was less in the presence of advanced degenerative disk disease. Notably, progression did not correlate with symptoms. The mean progression observed was 13%, leading to the conclusion that the innate mechanisms of spinal restabilization prevent progression of the disease.

Moller H, Hedlund R. (2000) Instrumented and noninstrumented posterolateral fusion in adult spondylolisthesis—A prospective randomized study (Part 2). Spine 25: 1716-1721.

A prospective randomized study was performed to determine whether transpedicular fixation improves the outcome of posterolateral fusion in patients with adult isthmic spondylolisthesis. At a 2-year follow-up assessment, the level of pain and functional disability were strikingly similar in the two groups, and there was no significant difference in fusion rate. The authors conclude that the use of supplementary transpedicular instrumentation does not add to the fusion rate or improve the clinical outcome.

Newman PH. (1963) The etiology of spondylolisthesis: With a special investigation by KH Stone. J Bone Joint Surg 45B: 39-59.

An excellent study of the contributing factors involved in the pathogenesis of spondylolisthesis, introducing many of the currently held theories from an observational study of cadavers and patients.

Newman PH. (1976) Stenosis of the lumbar spine in spondylolisthesis. Clin Orthop 115: 116-121.

The author describes the pathophysiology and treatment options of spinal stenosis for patients with congenital, isthmic, and degenerative spondylolisthesis.

Osterman K, Lindholm TS, Laurent LE. (1976) Late results of removal of the loose posterior element (Gill's operation) in the treatment of lytic lumbar spondylolisthesis. Clin Orthop 117: 121-128.

This study presents the late results of the Gill operation for the treatment of lytic lumbar spondylolisthesis in 75 patients. Follow-up averaged 12 years. Primary results were excellent, good, or fair in 83% at the end of the first year. However, the figures dropped to 75% when the cases were evaluated 5 or more years after operation. Progression of olisthesis was observed in 27% of the patients, usually in connection with progression of disk degeneration. This progression did not affect the clinical result of treatment. In nine patients, a fusion was later performed as a secondary operation. In these, the late result was still unsatisfactory in all but two cases. The operation is contraindicated in adolescents except in exceptional cases with signs of compression of the cauda equina. It is not recommended for patients younger than 30 years. The main indication for the Gill operation by these authors was painful spondylolisthesis with nerve root symptoms in patients older than 40 years.

Roberts FF, Kishore PR, Cunningham ME. (1978) Routine oblique radiography of the pediatric lumbar spine: Is it really necessary? Am J Roentgen 131: 297-298.

A series of 86 pediatric lumbar spine abnormalities was evaluated to determine the diagnostic benefit of radiography in the oblique projection compared with that of frontal–lateral projections alone. In only four patients was an abnormality apparent on the oblique view that had not already been demonstrated by the frontal–lateral series. Because the diagnostic yield was low at a patient cost of more than double the gonadal radiation dose, it is recommended that oblique views be eliminated in the routine radiography of the pediatric lumbar spine.

Roca J, Ubierna MT, Caceres E et al. (1999) One-stage decompression and posterolateral and interbody fusion for severe spondylolisthesis: An analysis of 14 patients. Spine 24(7): 709-714.

This was a retrospective study of 14 patients with severe spondylolisthesis (76% slip with 36% slip angle), severe radicular pain, and neurologic deficits treated with one-stage decompression and an anterior–posterior fusion. This procedure was found to be safe and effective in eliminating radicular pain in 13 of 14 patients with improvement in motor deficits and cosmetics.

Rosenberg NJ. (1975) Degenerative spondylolisthesis: Predisposing factors. J Bone Joint Surg 57A: 467-474.

The author studied 20 cadavers and 200 patients with degenerative spondylolisthesis to identify predisposing factors and common epidemiological traits. Causative factors included hemisacralization of L5, ligamentous laxity, and increased lumbosacral kyphosis. Slips never exceeded 30% and were not seen in patients younger than the fifth decade or concomitantly with an isthmic slip. Of those studied, 80% were treated successfully without surgery.

Saraste H. (1987) Long-term clinical and radiological follow-up of spondylolysis and spondylolisthesis. J Pediatr Orthop 7: 631-638.

Here, 255 patients with spondylolisthesis or spondylolysis were followed to correlate clinical findings with radiological findings over 20 years. Symptoms correlated with radiological findings of disk degeneration, low lumbar index, greater than 25% slip, and spondylolysis at L4. Progression of slip was not correlated to initial degree of slip or age at diagnosis, but patients were found to have early disk degeneration.

Schnee CL, Freese A, Ansell LV. (1997) Outcome analysis for adults with spondylolisthesis treated with posterolateral fusion and transpedicular screw fixation. J Neurosurg 86: 56-63.

A retrospective review of 52 adult patients with symptomatic low-grade spondylolisthesis treated with a posterolateral fusion

and pedicle screw fixation. In the absence of compensation claims, previous surgeries, and smoking habits, fusion with screw fixation resulted in 90% fusion rate and good clinical outcome.

Tabrizi P, Bouchard JA. (2001) Osteoporotic spondylolisthesis: A case report. Spine 26: 1482-1485.

The authors present a case report of spondylolisthesis caused by osteoporosis and a theory of the pathophysiology. They propose the slipping of the vertebra is caused by insufficiency of the bone structure causing elongation of the pedicles because of remodeling.

Wiltse LL, Jackson DW. (1976) Treatment of spondylolysis and spondylolisthesis in children. Clin Orthop 117: 92-100.

This article describes the two most common types of spondylolisthesis in children: isthmic and dysplastic. Most children do not develop symptoms; if they do, the authors outline initial nonoperative treatments and follow-up protocols. If this treatment fails or olisthesis progresses, the authors advocate fusion using a paraspinal approach.

Wiltse LL, Newman PH, MacNab I. (1976) Classification of spondylolysis and spondylolisthesis. Clin Orthop 117: 23-29.

The authors classify spondylolysis and spondylolisthesis into six groups based on etiology. For each classification, the anatomic findings and pathophysiology are explained.

Wiltse LL, Widell EH Jr., Jackson DW. (1975) Fatigue fracture: The basic lesion in isthmic spondylolisthesis. J Bone Joint Surg 57A: 17-22.

This was an observational study contending that all isthmic spondylolytic defects start as fatigue fractures. These occur earlier than other fatigue fractures, heal slowly or not at all, come with a hereditary "diathesis," and infrequently form the fluffy callus observed with other fractures of this type. Spondylolisthesis developed in 50% of cases.

Wiltse LL, Winter RB. (1983) Terminology and measurement of spondylolisthesis. J Bone Joint Surg 65A: 768-772.

This is an illustrated description of the various radiographic and clinical measurements of spondylolisthesis.

Wood KB, Popp CA, Transfeldt EE et al. (1994) Radiographic evaluation of instability in spondylolisthesis. Spine 19: 1697-1708.

The authors analyzed 50 patients with spondylolisthesis to determine if there was any difference in intervertebral motion during dynamic radiography (flexion and extension films) while standing or in the lateral decubitus position. The authors found that to maximize abnormal motion flexion and extension, films should be obtained in the lateral decubitus position. There was no difference in dynamic angulation based on patient position.

Zdeblick T. (1993) A prospective randomized study of lumbar fusion. Spine 18: 983-991.

This study evaluated the results of fusion for a multitude of diagnoses based on fusion without instrumentation, fusion with semirigid instrumentation, and fusion with rigid instrumentation. The success of fusion and clinical outcomes were related to the stiffness of the construct; more solid fusions and better outcomes were seen in the pedicle screw rigid fixation group. The study has several design flaws, including incomplete randomization and a high crossover rate.

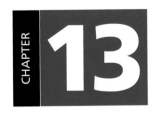

CHAPTER 13

Osteoporosis

Medical Management and Surgical Treatment Options

Eeric Truumees

M.D., Attending Spine Surgeon, William Beaumont Hospital, Royal Oak, MI; Adjunct Faculty, Bioengineering Center, Wayne State University, Detroit, MI

Introduction

- Populations worldwide, and especially in North America, are rapidly aging.
  - The prevalence of osteoporosis, already the most common metabolic bone disorder, is increasing.
  - Spine practitioners need to be aware of the risk factors for and the treatment of osteoporosis.
  - Spine practitioners will be called upon to treat the manifestations of osteoporosis itself (e.g., compression fractures) and to understand the ramifications of osteoporosis in the treatment of other spine diseases (e.g., placement of spinal instrumentation).
- Previously, osteoporotic vertebral compression fractures (VCFs) of the spine were thought to be benign, self-limited entities.
  - It is becoming clear that VCFs, like hip fractures, are part of a vicious spiral of increasing pain, dysfunction, and mortality.
  - Newer treatments, such as vertebroplasty and kyphoplasty, seek to stabilize these fractures and minimize physiologic decline (Box 13–1).
- Even in the best of circumstances, fixation of spinal and hip fractures may not return patients to previous levels of activity.

Box 13–1:	Spinal Manifestations of Osteoporosis

1. Hyperkyphosis with chronic spine pain
2. Loss of height
3. Acute VCFs
4. Sacral insufficiency fracture
5. Osteoporotic burst fracture
6. Poor spinal fixation in the treatment of degenerative instability of the spine

- Because lifestyle has a significant effect on its development, surgeons must recognize risk factors and help their patients prevent osteoporosis.
- Newer medical therapies are increasingly potent in halting the decline of bone load-bearing capacity.
- Even physicians who are uncomfortable managing osteoporosis should understand its natural history to be able to screen their patients and initiate referrals.

Pathophysiology

- Bone is a dynamic, well-organized, composite material composed of the following:

- Mineral (inorganic) phase
- Collagenous (organic) phase
- Cells and water
- The mineral phase, principally composed of hydroxyapatite $[Ca_{10}(PO_4)_6(OH)_2]$, is 60% to 70% of bone's dry weight.
- Organic matrix, of which 90% is collagen, makes up 30% of the dry weight.
- Osteoporosis causes both inorganic and collagenous phase bone loss.
  - Loss of bone crystal weakens the bone to compressive loading.
  - Loss of the organic matrix of bone makes it more brittle.
- The crystalline structure is regulated both at the molecular level by the strain patterns in the trabecular network and at the organ level by systemic (often hormonal) influences.
- Most adult bone is lamellar, characterized by highly organized, stress-oriented collagen. Stress orientation gives mature bone anisotropic properties wherein the mechanics of loading lamellar bone depend on the direction of force application.
  - Bone is strongest parallel to the collagen molecule long axis.
- In the mature skeleton, the architecture of lamellar bone takes two forms:
  - Trabecular (spongy or cancellous)
  - Cortical (dense or compact)
- In trabecular bone, internal spicules form a three-dimensional branching lattice aligned along areas of mechanical stress (Fig. 13–1). Trabecular bone is 8 times more metabolically active than cortical bone. Trabecular bone, 20% of the total bone mass, is found in long bone metaphyses and epiphyses and in the cuboid bones (e.g., vertebrae).

- Cortical bone, 80% of the bone mass, has a fairly uniform density. Cortical bone forms the "envelope" of cuboid bones and the diaphysis of long bones.
- Three cell types carry out bone metabolism—osteoblasts, osteocytes, and osteoclasts.
  - Osteoblasts and osteocytes differ in function and location but arise from the same lineage. Osteoblasts are found lining the bone surface and trailing osteoclasts in cutting cones, where they produce osteoid.
  - As bone is created, osteoblasts become encased in a mineralized matrix and are known as *osteocytes*. These cells remain in contact with the osteoblasts on the bone surface by cellular processes within canaliculi. Endocrine signals are typically transmitted by the osteoblasts, and strain-generated signals within the bone are regulated by osteocytes.
  - The major bone resorptive cell is the *osteoclast*, characterized by large size (20 to 100 μm) and multiple nuclei. These cells are derived from pluripotent cells of bone marrow and bind to the bone surface through cell attachment proteins (integrins).
- Throughout life, the body constantly remodels bone by removing old bone and creating new bone. Osteoporosis is a host of systemic regulatory changes that alter the normal balance between formation and resorption.
- In contradistinction, in osteomalacia, an osteoid is formed at an appropriate rate but is not normally mineralized (Table 13–1).
- With lower rates of bone formation in osteoporosis, the overall mineral density of the bone decreases. Increased osteoclast activity decreases connectivity among trabeculae. The combination of decreased mass and discontinuity of the normal latticework leads to decreased resistance to fracture (Box 13–2).

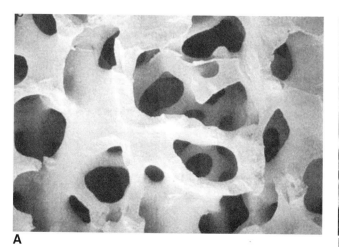
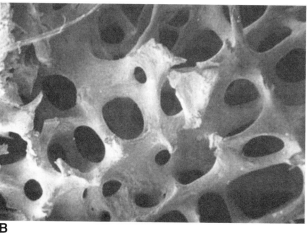

A   **B**

Figure 13–1: Scanning electron micrographs of normal (A) and osteoporotic (B) bone. Note both the thinner trabeculae and the lack of continuity among them in the osteoporotic specimen.

Table 13–1:   Comparison of Osteoporosis and Osteomalacia

	OSTEOPOROSIS	OSTEOMALACIA
Definition	Bone mass decreased	Bone mass variable
Mineralization	Normal	Decreased
Age of onset	Generally elderly	Any age
Etiology	Endocrine abnormality	Vitamin D deficiency
	Age	Abnormality of vitamin D pathway
		Idiopathic
		Renal tubular acidosis
		Hypophosphatasia
Symptoms	Pain referable to fracture	Generalized bone pain
Signs	Tenderness at fracture	Generalized tenderness
Laboratory findings		
Serum Ca++	Normal	↓ or nl (↑ in hypophosphatasia)*
Serum P	Normal	↓ or nl (↑ in renal osteodystrophy)
Alkaline phosphatase	Normal	↑ (not in hypophosphatasia)
Urinary Ca++	High or normal	↓ or nl (↑ in hypophosphatasia)
Bone biopsy	Normal	Abnormal

* nl, Normal.

- Several environmental, genetic, and pharmacologic factors affect the development of osteoporosis. Root etiology, although likely multifactorial, is not yet understood. Osteoporosis is grossly divided into three types based on presumed etiology.
  - Type I—Postmenopausal
  - Type II—Senile
  - Type III—Secondary
- Most individuals will increase bone mass until the early part of the fourth decade. Thereafter, bone mass is lost at a rate of approximately 0.5% per year.
  - The mechanism of bone loss resulting from normal aging is poorly understood, but its rate is equivalent in women and men.
  - Yet not everyone develops osteoporosis. The two most important determinants for the development of

Box 13–2:   Structural Changes in Osteoporotic Bone

- Material characteristics
  - Loss of bone mineral
  - Loss of bone collagen
  - Loss of tissue density
- Structural characteristics
  - Microarchitectural decay
  1. Loss of trabeculae
  2. Propagation of microcracks
  - Decrease in bone mass
  - Altered in bone geometry

osteoporosis are the peak bone mass and the rate of bone loss.
  - The most effective way to prevent the devastating complications of VCF is to increase peak bone mass. Eating disorders, exercise-induced amenorrhea, lack of weight-bearing exercise, and low dairy or calcium diets each contribute to the increasing rates of osteoporosis among young women.
- Several factors, such as genetic, environmental, and nutritional conditions and chronic disease, are associated with accelerated bone loss (Box 13–3).
- One of the most common causes of osteoporosis is decreased gonadal hormone levels (i.e., menopause). Bone-forming cells have estrogen receptors. Estrogen blocks the action of parathyroid hormone (PTH) on osteoblasts and marrow stromal cells.
  - Without estrogen, osteoblasts and marrow stromal cells secrete increased levels of interleukin 6, which stimulates the osteoclasts to resorb bone.
  - Estrogen deficiency accelerates bone loss up to 2%–3% per year for 10 years.
  - Although hypogonadic men may get type I osteoporosis, this form affects women more often than men.
  - Type I osteoporotics are typically in their 50s and 60s and are susceptible to fractures of trabecular bone (wrist and spine).
- Type II osteoporosis affects both men and women equally, arises when they are in their 70s and 80s, and increasingly affects cortical bone.
- Bone loss caused by various medications and disease states are termed *secondary*, or type III osteoporosis.
  - Endogenous or exogenous hypercortisolism is frequently implicated in type III osteoporosis. Cortisol negatively affects bone mass through decreased intestinal calcium absorption, increased renal calcium

Box 13–3:   Risk Factors for Osteoporosis

- Advanced age
- Endocrine abnormalities
  - Hypercortisolism
  - Hyperthyroidism
  - Hyperparathyroidism
  - Hypogonadism
- Other diseases
  - Tumors
  - Chronic disease
  - Expression of abnormal collagen or bone matrix genes
- Inactivity or immobilization
- Dietary issues
  - Calcium-deficient diet
  - Alcoholism
  - Body mass index <22 kg/m^2
- Smoking

loss, and direct inhibition of bone matrix formation. Alternate-day dosing of corticosteroids decreases bone damage.

- Bone mineral density (BMD) defines the severity of osteoporosis. With factors such as cardiovascular status, medications, neuromuscular disorders, and body habitus, BMD is the major determinant of fracture threshold.
    - T-score represents the number of standard deviations of mineral content in the patient's bone from the mean young adult value. For each standard deviation below the norm, fracture risk increases 1.5-fold to 3-fold. A T-score of −1 implies a 30% chance of fracture.
    - Z-score compares BMD with age-matched controls. Z-scores less than −1.5 should prompt a more extensive workup for osteomalacia or neoplasm.
- By World Health Organization criteria, a T-score of less than −1 is defined as osteopenia. Less than a 2.5 standard deviation from the mean defines osteoporosis. Patients with T-scores below a 2.5 standard deviation and with fragility fractures have severe osteoporosis (Fig. 13–2).
    - This definition of osteopenia differs from the radiographic term, which implies only decreased bone mineral and could represent other disease processes, such as bone loss from wear debris, osteomalacia, or neoplasm.
- Like hypertension, the bone loss of osteoporosis is usually gradual and silent. Unless carefully sought, the disease may manifest itself with an acute event—that is, a fracture.

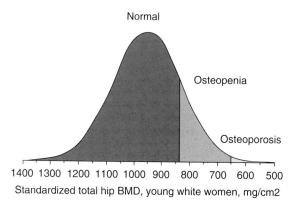

Figure 13–2: Bone mineral density exhibits a normal (bell-shaped distribution) in the population at large. Osteopenia is defined as BMD lower than one standard deviation (T = −1) from the mean for a same-gender young adult. By these World Health Organization criteria, osteoporosis exists when the BMD is more than 2.5 standard deviations below the norm. Severe osteoporosis exists when the T-score is less than −2.5 and the patient has sustained a fragility fracture.

- Three fracture types are common in the axial skeleton—VCFs, osteoporotic burst fractures, and sacral insufficiency fractures.
    - Also, osteoporosis complicates the treatment of other spine interventions, such as instrumented stabilization of a degenerative spondylolisthesis.
- Spinal fractures are classified morphologically.
- The most common injury is the VCF. There are a wide range of fracture patterns including failure of the superior, inferior, and both endplates. Furthermore, lateral compression deformities may worsen preexisting coronal plane deformities (Fig. 13–3).
    - In the lumbar spine, the central portion of both endplates collapses, resulting in a biconcave or codfish vertebra.
    - In the thoracic spine, maximal height loss occurs at the anterior portion of the superior endplate and leads to a wedge-compression fracture.
    - The senile burst fracture represents increased axial loading and failure of the middle column with retropulsion of bone into the spinal canal.

Incidence

- In North America today, 35 million people are at risk for osteoporosis. Over the next 3 decades, this number is expected to triple.
- The most common manifestation of spinal osteoporosis is the VCF, which will affect one third of all North Americans. The 700,000 VCFs per year in the United States outnumber hip and wrist fractures combined.
- In the United States alone, the annual direct medical costs associated with osteoporotic fractures exceed $13.8 billion. By 2030, these annual costs may exceed $60 billion, or $164 million per day. The indirect costs of early retirement, lost independence and productivity, and human pain and suffering are incalculable.

Clinical Features

- Osteoporosis per se is asymptomatic. The clinician should suspect osteomalacia in patients with radiographic osteopenia and bone pain.
- At risk populations should be screened (Box 13–4).
- Fragility fractures often involve the spine, ribs, hip, and wrist. The patient will report localized pain, dysfunction, and deformity.
- Evaluation of a suspected osteoporotic spine fracture begins with a careful history. Note the amount of energy sustained. Severely osteoporotic patients can fracture while sneezing or rolling in bed.
- Patients complain of focal, intense, deep midline spine pain. Diffuse, paravertebral pain often is a muscle spasm and may also be present, but it should not be the chief complaint.

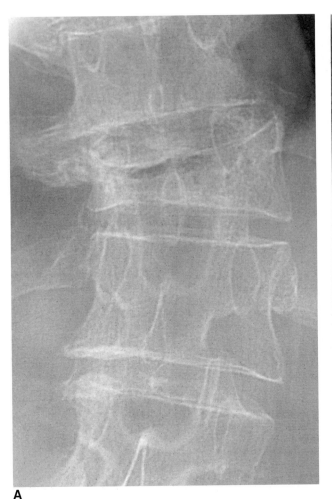

A

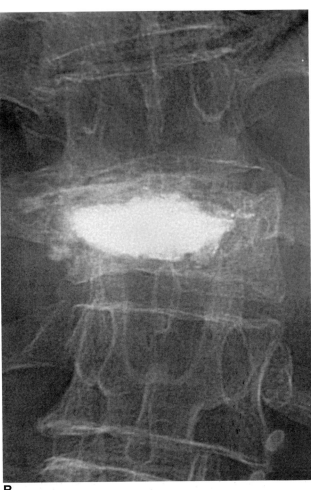

B

Figure 13–3: A 74-year-old man with degenerative scoliosis and secondary osteoporosis. He sustained a lateral compression vertebral fracture with progression of his coronal plane deformity (**A**). He continued to have focal pain at 12 weeks. A kyphoplasty afforded partial reduction of the fracture and improvement of his Cobb angle to the prefracture level (**B**).

Box 13–4:	Dual-Energy X-ray Absorptiometry Screening Criteria

- All patients
  - Sustained a low energy fracture
  - Have osteopenia on plain radiographs
  - Have diseases that place them at risk for osteoporosis
  - On medications that place them at risk for osteoporosis
- Women
  - Postmenopausal
  - Older than 65 years
  - Younger than 65 with one or more risk factors
  - On HRT for prolonged periods
  - Considering HRT if BMD will affect decision

- Pain symptoms are mechanical and worsen with loading. Although recumbency often relieves symptoms, patients with a prominent kyphosis will have a pain lying directly on their back.
  - Ask about associated thoracic or lumbar radicular problems.
  - Note the time course of the patient's current symptoms and the course of any previous fractures.
- Red flags such as night pain, fevers, chills, unusual weight loss, or bowel or bladder changes require thorough investigation.
  - Ensure that BMD testing has been performed and the appropriate antiosteoporotic regimen has been initiated.
  - Ask about a history of cancer, tuberculosis, systemic infection, or other fractures.
- Begin the physical examination by observing the patient closely, assessing general condition and comfort, sagittal spinal balance, body shape, difficulty in breathing, and obesity.

- Palpate the ribs. Coexisting and iatrogenic rib fractures are common.
- Acute fractures are typically point tender over the spinous process.
- Undertake a complete neurologic examination. Although major neurologic deficits are rare (0.05%), patients may have stenosis or neuropathy.
- Sacral insufficiency fractures may cause pain in the tailbone or sacroiliac (SI) joint regions. Patrick's test and other SI joint-loading maneuvers will increase pain.
- Laboratory evaluation is used to exclude other causes of osteopenia, such as osteomalacia.
  - Occasionally, serum blood tests alone are insufficient to exclude the diagnosis of osteomalacia, at which time a transiliac bone biopsy may be indicated.
  - Bone biomarker assays are being increasingly requested, as a complementary modality to densitometry, to monitor the effectiveness of treatment and assess fracture risk. Markers of bone formation include bone-specific alkaline phosphatase (an osteoblast enzyme) and osteocalcin (a bone matrix protein). Collagen degradation products (cross-linked telopeptides and pyridinolines) are markers of bone destruction.
  - In patients with unusual fracture patterns or histories suggestive of malignancy or infection, laboratory evaluation may include erythrocyte sedimentation rate, white blood cell count with differential, C-reactive protein, serum and urine protein electrophoresis, and prostate antigens.

Diagnostic Tools

- Although plain radiographs are appropriate in the evaluation of symptomatic patients, they are the least accurate and least precise method of assessing bone density. A 30% decrease in bone mass is necessary to detect osteopenia on plain films.
- On the other hand, a variety of noninvasive bone densitometry tests provide information about the density of bone at the measured site. Lumbar spine measurements correlate well with the incidence of spontaneous vertebral fracture.
  - Dual photon absorptiometry (DPA) measures axial skeletal BMD through the radioisotope soft tissue signal attenuation.
  - In the last decade, dual-energy x-ray absorptiometry (DEXA) has supplanted DPA and become the standard. DEXA's advantages are superior precision (1%-2% at the spine and 3%-4% at the femur), lower radiation dose, shorter examination time, higher image resolution, and greater technical ease.
  1. DEXA is used both to assess baseline bone density and to track response to therapy.
  2. Scoliosis, VCFs, osteophytes, extraosseous calcifications, and vascular disease may falsely increase DEXA scores.

- The cross-sectional image of the vertebral body generated by quantitative computed tomography (qCT) allows preferential measurement of trabecular bone density. The higher trabecular bone turnover makes qCT a sensitive indicator of bone density in these vulnerable skeletal areas. qCT is accurate to within 5% to 10%, but the radiation dose is higher than with DEXA.
- Ultrasound is attractive as a means of measuring bone density because it is rapid, is inexpensive, and does not expose a patient to ionizing radiation. However, it is not as precise as DEXA and is mainly for initial screening.
- In patients with known fractures, the goals of imaging are to determine the following:
  - Extent of vertebral collapse
  - Location and extent of any lytic process
  - Visibility and degree of pedicular involvement
  - Presence of cortical destruction
  - Presence of epidural or foraminal stenosis
  - Age or acuity of the fracture
- Standing radiographs reveal overall sagittal and coronal spinal balance.
- Thoracolumbar fractures are obvious, but sacral fractures may be difficult to see.
  - Comparison films, including chest radiographs, may reveal fracture age.
  - Apparent sclerosis may be healing or compressed trabeculae.
  - Consider spot films orthogonal to the fracture, particularly at the thoracolumbar junction.
  - Obtain serial lateral radiographs to assess for further collapse.
  - Signs of posterior cortical compromise include widened pedicles and more than 50% height loss.
  - Endplate erosion suggests infection.
  - Signs of neoplasm include pedicular destruction (the winking owl sign) and fractures above T6.
- Magnetic resonance imaging (MRI) allows more definitive assessment of canal involvement and fracture acuity. In acute fractures, fracture edema is reflected by increased signal on T2 or short T1 inversion recovery (STIR) sequences and decreased T1 signal (Fig. 13–4). Both T1 and T2 marrow signal changes normalize over time. Key features differentiating malignant from osteoporotic fractures include pedicular and soft tissue extension.
- Chronic, unhealing VCFs may be caused by avascular necrosis of the vertebral bone (Kummel's disease). Such continuing collapse of the vertebra after minor trauma is particularly common in patients with known risk factors for avascular necrosis such as previous radiation therapy or chronic corticosteroid use.
  - On MRI, these fractures demonstrate the "double line sign" of discrete fluid collections within a vacuum cleft with areas of diminished T2 signal surrounding the cleft (Fig. 13–5).

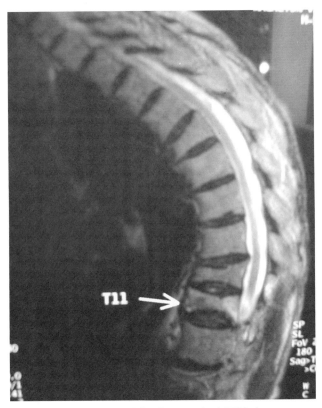

Figure 13–4: This T2-weighted parasagittal MRI demonstrates an acute fracture at T11 with edema in the vertebral body. T10 and T6 demonstrate healed fractures with height loss but a normalized marrow signal.

- In patients unable to undergo MRI, a CT scan offers high bone and soft tissue contrast and clearly delineates posterior cortical compromise. Fracture acuity may then be determined by bone scan (Fig. 13–6).
- Both MRI and CT demonstrate sacral insufficiency fractures. On bone scan, these lesions may have the classic "H" configuration or may appear as a linear band of increased uptake in the region of the sacral ala (Fig. 13–7).

Nonoperative Care

- Nonoperative care is divided between management of the underlying osteoporosis and management of any spinal fractures.
- Previously, successful management of osteoporosis was frustrated by delayed and inaccurate diagnosis, insufficient understanding of the disease process, and inadequate follow-up. *Before* the first fracture, at risk patients must be screened.
- For osteopenia, recommendations include oral calcium, physiologic vitamin D, and weight-bearing exercise. Increasingly, tai chi and other low-impact, balance-promoting exercises are recommended. These measures decrease bone resorption and help mineralize osteoid but do not increase total bone mass. Individuals taking

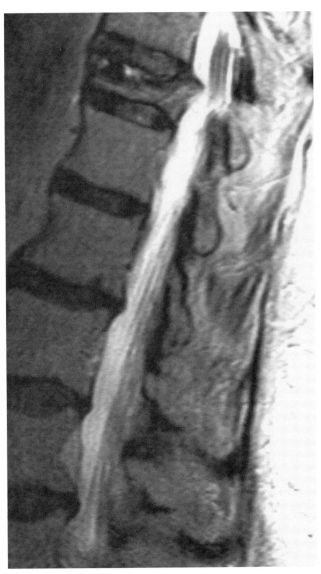

Figure 13–5: This T2-weighted parasagittal MRI (from the same patient as Fig. 13–3) demonstrates typical findings of Kummel's disease. Despite a 12-week interval, the fracture had not healed and edema remains apparent. An area of decreased T2 signal is seen just below the fracture plane representing avascular necrosis of bone. Fig.13–3, *A,* demonstrates a "vacuum" sign within the bone, also an indication of Kummel's disease.

calcium supplements sustain one quarter of the hip fractures of those with low calcium intake.

- In menopausal women, estrogen supplementation may be appropriate. Women on estrogen have fewer fractures. Estrogen does not increase bone formation; its primary effect lies in bone mass maintenance.
  - Recent studies appear to show increased rates of coronary artery disease, stroke, pulmonary embolus, and cancer in women on hormone replacement therapy (HRT).
  - These untoward side effects have increased interest in the selective estrogen receptor modulators such as

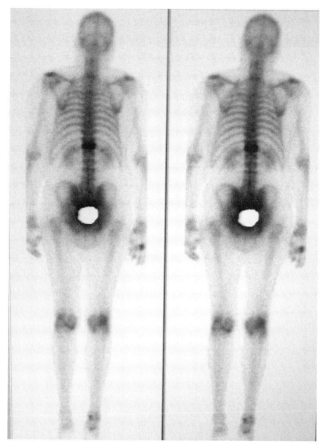

Figure 13–6: Bone scan. This bone scan demonstrates markedly increased uptake at the T12 level consistent with an acute VCF in a patient with a 10 week history of severe, midline thoracolumbar junction spine pain.

raloxifene (Evista). These agents appear to have bone preserving effects similar to those of estrogen without the cancer and coronary complications.

- Patients with true osteoporosis (femoral T-score below −2.5) or a history of fragility fracture should receive more aggressive pharmacologic management.
  - Calcitonin, administered through subcutaneous injection or nasal spray, decreases osteoclastic bone resorption. Over short-term treatment, calcitonin enhances bone formation, leading to a slight net bone accretion. Over long-term treatment, osteoblastic activity slows and bone mass stabilizes.
  - Bisphosphonates are recommended for their dramatic suppression of bone resorption and have been shown to prevent hip fractures and VCFs.
  1. First, bisphosphonates directly stabilize the bone crystal, making it more resistant to osteoclastic bone resorption.
  2. Second, they directly inhibit osteoclast activity, preserving bone architecture and overall density.
  3. Weekly administered forms of these agents are associated with similar efficacy, better compliance, and no increase in toxicity. Patients with severe osteoporosis unable to take oral bisphosphonates may benefit from intermittent intravenous therapy.
  - Parathyroid hormone (PTH) (Forteo) has recently been approved by the Food and Drug Administration for the treatment of osteoporosis. Although expensive, intermittent subcutaneous PTH administration leads to early dramatic increases in bone mass, especially in areas of trabecular bone.
- Most osteoporotic fractures may be managed nonoperatively. Goals include the following:
  - Decreased pain
  - Early mobilization

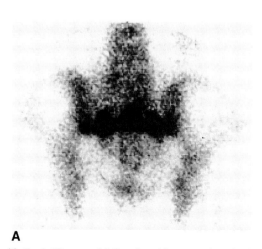

A

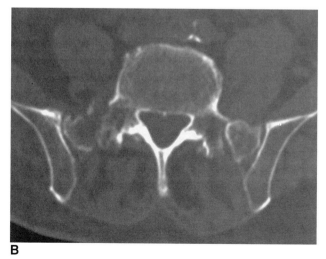

B

Figure 13–7: A 70-year-old female with severe low back pain. **A,** Bone scan demonstrating increased uptake consistent with sacral insufficiency fracture. **B,** Axial CT image of the same patient demonstrating bilateral, osteoporotic sacral ala fractures.

- Preservation of sagittal and coronal spinal stability
- Prevention of late neurologic compromise
- During the initial, painful interval, those patients presenting symptoms to their physicians are typically offered pain medications and braces. Narcotic pain medications may be continued until the patient can bear weight comfortably. Nasal calcitonin and bisphosphonates, useful in the treatment of osteoporosis, may be effective in decreasing fracture-related pain.
  - Limited activity and often bed rest are self-imposed.
  - A limited contact orthosis such as a tri-pad Jewett extension brace or a Cash brace is easy to fit and wear. But, compliance is typically poor. Elderly patients often have a body habitus that is not particularly easy to brace (a short, obese trunk). Furthermore, those patients with shoulder problems will have difficulty donning and doffing the brace.
  - Physical therapy may aid the patient's return to mobility.
- There are few appealing treatment options for sacral insufficiency fractures. A walker decreases painful loading. A concomitant pubic ramus fracture requires limited weight-bearing on the affected side and walker ambulation. Unfortunately, there is no effective bracing for these injuries.

Surgical Management

- The acute pain of a VCF usually lasts 4 to 6 weeks but in some circumstances persists beyond 3 months. In elderly patients, pain medications are not well tolerated and may cause as many functional problems as the underlying fracture. At least 150,000 compression fractures per year are refractory to outpatient management, leading to hospitalization, protracted bed rest, and intravenous narcotics.
- Fractures less likely to improve with standard medical management include the following:
  - Thoracolumbar junction (T11-L2)
  - Bursting patterns
  - Wedge-compression fractures with >30 degrees of sagittal angulation
  - Vacuum shadow in fractured body (ischemic necrosis of bone)
  - Progressive collapse in office follow-up
- Patients with these recalcitrant fractures or continuing collapse can be offered a vertebral body augmentation (VBA) procedure—that is, kyphoplasty or vertebroplasty (Boxes 13–5 and 13–6).
- Vertebral augmentation with polymethylmethacrylate (PMMA) variably restores strength and stiffness to a fractured body. Strength reflects the ability of the vertebral body to bear loads and may protect against future fracture of the treated segment. Stiffness limits micromotion

Box 13–5:	**Indications for Vertebral Body Augmentation**

1. Primary osteoporosis
2. Secondary osteoporosis
3. Multiple myeloma
4. Osteolytic metastasis

within the compromised vertebral body. Limitation of micromotion ostensibly relieves the fracture pain.

- For polyvinyl alcohol, a 1-cm incision and a transpedicular cannulation are used to gain access to vertebral body. A unipedicular or bipedicular needle placement can be performed during vertebroplasty. The vertebra is then filled with liquid PMMA.
- Kyphoplasty uses a bipedicular approach and balloon tamps to create voids in the bone. This balloon may partially reduce the fracture and theoretically allows placement of more viscous cement.
- These procedures may be performed under general anesthesia or with local anesthesia and intravenous sedation. Turn the patient prone on a radiolucent operating frame. Bolsters allow partial postural reduction of the fracture. Obtain true anteroposterior (AP) and lateral images with fluoroscopy. Typically, a transpedicular route to the vertebra is selected. In some thoracic cases, the narrow and straight pedicle precludes appropriate medialization and an extrapedicular approach is required.
- Beginning with AP fluoroscopy, an 11-gauge Jamshidi needle is positioned at 10 o'clock or 2 o'clock on the pedicular ring. Unlike pedicle screws, the goal is not to proceed "straight down the barrel" but rather to medialize through the cylinder of the pedicle. Start laterally and aim medially. Once in bone, verify your

Box 13–6:	**Relative Contraindications to Percutaneous Vertebral Body Augmentation**

- Neurologic symptoms
- Young patients
- Pregnancy
- High velocity fractures
  - Fractured pedicles or facets
  - Burst fracture with retropulsed bone
- Medical issues
  - Allergy to devices
  - Allergy to contrast medium
  - Bleeding disorders
  - Severe cardiopulmonary difficulties
- Technically not feasible
  - Vertebra plana
  - Multiple painful vertebral bodies
- Active infection

trajectory on the lateral image. If the AP and lateral images do not demonstrate a clearly intrapedicular position, check an en face or oblique view.

- Under lateral fluoroscopy, advance the Jamshidi midway point through the pedicle. Return to the AP view and verify tip position. Until the Jamshidi has passed through the posterior cortical margin of the vertebral body, it must be lateral to the medial pedicle wall on the AP image. If the needle has been medialized appropriately, return to lateral, and advance until 1-2 mm past the posterior vertebral body margin. Now the needle should be barely across medial pedicle border on the AP.

- Several needle and delivery systems are available for vertebroplasty. Typically, the cannulas are advanced into the central portion of vertebral body and PMMA is delivered under live fluoroscopy.

- In kyphoplasty, the Jamshidi is replaced with a working cannula and additional instruments are passed to allow introduction of the balloon. If well medialized, advance to within 2 mm of the anterior cortex.

- Better medialization allows more anterior placement.
- Live fluoroscopy is recommended when approaching the anterior cortex.
- Once both balloons are in place, inflate them in 0.5-cc increments until the following occurs:
  - Realignment of vertebral endplates
  - Maximum balloon pressure (>220 psi) without decay
  - Maximum balloon volume—4 cc for 15/3 and 6 cc for 20/3 balloon types
  - Cortical wall contact
- Currently, the void created by the intravertebral balloon tamp is filled with PMMA.
  - Newer calcium phosphate and hydroxyapatite cements are being tested.
  - Add sterile barium to the PMMA powder to increase radiopacity.
- For vertebroplasty, the PMMA is injected in to the body in a fairly liquid state to allow it to interdigitate between the crushed trabeculae of the fracture (Fig. 13–8).

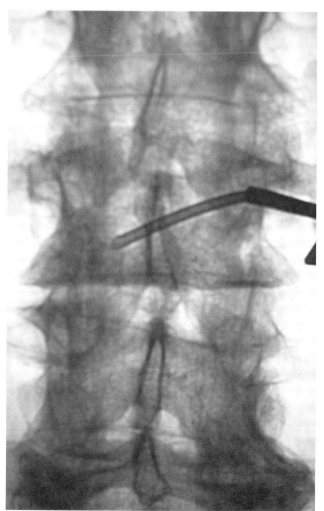

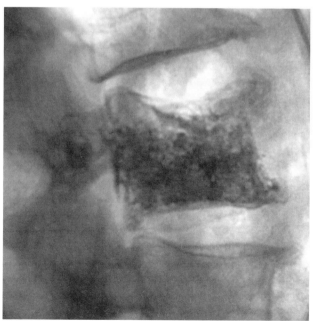

Figure 13–8: These are fluoroscopic images of a 78-year-old male with 3 months of intractable pain from an osteoporotic compression fracture with minimal collapse and no retropulsion. **A,** A 13-gauge, curved Cook needle was introduced using a unipedicular approach. **B,** PMMA was injected into the vertebral body with a good fill and excellent pain relief. Note the slight filling of the epidural veins.

A

B

- For kyphoplasty, the PMMA is placed into bone filler devices (BFDs). When a toothpaste consistency has been reached, the PMMA can be applied in a gradual and controlled manner (Fig. 13–9).
- Close the wound with a suture or Steri-Strip. No braces are needed.

- Osteoporotic burst fractures are more common than previously thought.
  - Middle column compromise may take the form of cortical buckling. If canal occlusion is less than 33%, consider VBA in select cases.

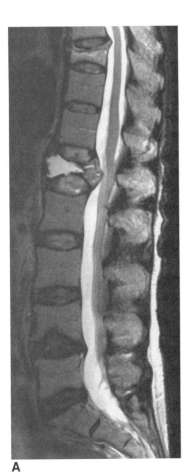

Figure 13–9: This 65-year-old female had a 3-week history of intractable pain and the inability to walk because of an osteoporotic burst fracture at L1. **A,** The T2 parasagittal MRI demonstrates an acute fracture with middle column buckling and canal compromise. This patient had no neurological symptoms. **B,** This sagittal reconstruction CT scan after kyphoplasty demonstrates good filling of the fracture without an increase in bone retropulsion or PMMA extravasation. The patient reported nearly immediate, marked pain relief. **C,** This lateral fluoroscopic image (of another patient) demonstrates the KyphX balloon tamp in position reducing a VCF.

A

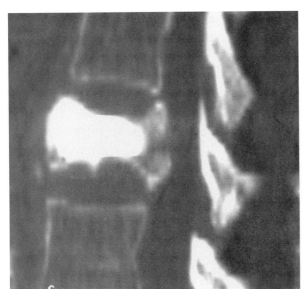

B

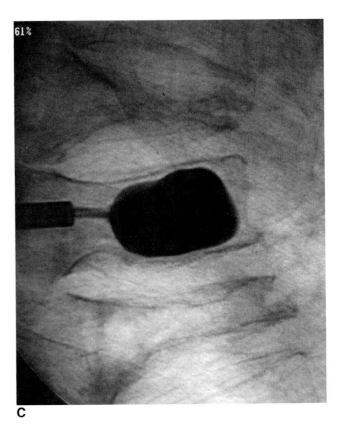

C

- VBA should not be undertaken if the fracture is significantly comminuted because of the increased risk of cement extravasation. In patients with neurologic injury, open surgery may be required.
- Open surgery is indicated for osteoporotic fractures only in the context of significant or progressive neurologic deficit or deformity.
- Operative fixation is associated with high morbidity and mortality in this frail patient population.
- Regardless of the indication, spinal instrumentation often fails in osteoporotic bone. Improved fixation may be achieved through AP surgery; PMMA augmentation of the screw tract; increased number of bony anchor points, including hooks; and maximized screw diameter.

Aftercare and Follow-up

- Patients undergoing VBA procedures are often more comfortable after the procedure than before. Currently, hospitals are not reimbursed unless the patient is admitted.
- Caution patients that additional fractures are common. Encourage exercise, especially walking.
- There are no particular postoperative restrictions, but all osteoporotic patients should avoid heavy lifting and bending to pick objects off of the floor.
- If significant functional disability, muscle spasm, or weakness remains, initiate a course of physical therapy.

Complications and Outcomes

- The primary complication of osteoporosis is fracture.
- VCFs were thought to be benign injuries with few, if any, significant long-term sequelae. This conception arose from the estimated two thirds of VCFs never reported by patients to their physicians. Furthermore, many of those cases brought to medical attention respond rapidly to simple nonoperative treatment.
- Based on recent populationwide studies, it is becoming increasingly evident that any VCF can have significant functional and physiological effects (Box 13–7).

Box 13–7:	**Consequences of Vertebral Compression Fractures**

- Intractable pain
- Physiological effect
- Increased mortality
- Recurrent fracture
- Kyphotic deformity
- Gastrointestinal dysfunction
- Pulmonary dysfunction
- Functional decline
- Increased hospitalization

- Acute VCFs are variably painful. Some patients note mild and transient symptoms, but others require hospitalization. Although most patients report significant symptomatic improvement in the first 4 weeks, acute pain can persist for months.
- Once the acute pain subsides, chronic pain disorders can develop. Many of these appear to arise from the change in the sagittal balance of the spine. For example, some patients report painful rubbing of their ribs on their ilium. The risk of developing chronic pain increases with the number of vertebral fractures.
- Typical daily activities, such as standing, sitting, or bending, intensify the pain. Standing tolerance may decrease to only a few minutes. Lying down relieves the pain, but bed rest only accelerates bone loss.
- VCFs and increased kyphosis are associated with decreased truncal strength, greater back-related disability, annual bed days, and annual limited-activity days. This weakness and inactivity increase the risk of additional fractures from 5 to 25 times baseline.
  - Similarly, the risk of hip fracture rises 5 times in patients sustaining a VCF.
- In one study of physical function, common tasks such as walking, bending, dressing, carrying bags, climbing stairs, rising from a supine position, and rising from a seated position were assessed. Only 13% of VCF patients were able to accomplish these activities without difficulty, 40% had difficulty, and 47% required assistance.
- The deformity associated with each of these fracture types may have multiple physiologic implications. Together, the osteoporotic body habitus is characterized by loss of height and thoracic hyperkyphosis (the dowager's hump). Abdominal protuberance and loss of lumbar lordosis may also be noted.
  - Many otherwise active elderly patients complain bitterly about the cosmetic effects of these changes.
  - Beyond the cosmetic effects, compression on the abdominal viscera by the ribcage or by loss of height through the lumbar spine leads to decreased appetite, early satiety, and weight loss.
  - Similarly, thoracic hyperkyphosis leads to compression of the lungs and, subsequently, decreased pulmonary function with an increased risk of pulmonary death. Lung function, as measured by forced vital capacity and forced expiratory volume, is significantly reduced in patients with thoracic or lumbar fractures.
- The precise risk of neurologic deficit after VCF is not known. Interestingly, a tardy neurologic decline may occur up to 18 months after the initial injury. These late neurologic changes are thought to show dysfunction of the spinal cord when it drapes over the apex of kyphosis.
- Women sustaining osteoporotic VCFs report several debilitating psychological effects including crippled body image and self-esteem, depression, and anxiety.

- The 5-year survival after osteoporotic spine fracture is significantly worse than for age-matched peers (61% vs. 76%) and is comparable with survival rates after hip fracture. Excess mortality increases with the number of fractures.
- VBA attempts to interrupt the cycle of decline. There are no randomized trials comparing nonoperative management with VBA. Vertebroplasty and kyphoplasty are well tolerated and associated with a 70%–95% rate of pain relief.
- In 2000, Grados and colleagues reported the first long-term outcomes of osteoporotic vertebral body compression fractures treated by percutaneous vertebroplasty. By 1 month, pain decreased significantly. Results were stable over time. There were no severe treatment-related complications. The vertebral deformity did not progress in any of the injected vertebrae. A slight, but significant, increase in adjacent segment fracture risk was reported.
- Garfin, Yuan, and Reilly note that 95% of patients treated with either kyphoplasty or vertebroplasty can expect significant improvement in pain and functional status (Table 13–2).
- VBA complications are categorized into medical, anesthesia, instrument placement, and PMMA problems.
  - More common than any of these groups, though, are additional fractures and failure to improve. Failure to improve, in most cases, is caused by inappropriate patient selection. Like any spine procedure, there must be close agreement among history, physical examination, and imaging findings. The more diffuse the patients' pain, the less likely they are to benefit from VBA.
  - The natural history of spinal osteoporosis includes a significant increase in the risk of additional fractures after the first fracture. Placement of PMMA into the

spine may *increase* the risk of adjacent segment fracture. The correction of the proper weight-bearing axis with kyphoplasty may *decrease* the risk of additional fracture.
- Although VBA procedures are not typically morbid or physiologically taxing, medical and anesthesia problems are not unusual in these elderly patients.
- Technical errors related to misplacement of the vertebroplasty needles or kyphoplasty instrumentation are more common but can be decreased with quality imaging and meticulous surgical technique.

Table 13–2:	Outcomes after Vertebral Body Augmentation				
AUTHOR	# PTS.	F/U (MON)	SIG PAIN RELIEF (%)	PARTIAL PAIN RELIEF (%)	NO RELIEF (%)
Barr	38	18	63	32	5
Cortet	16	6	94	6	0
Cyteval	20	6	75	15	10
Debussche	5	13	100	0	0
Gangi	4	9	100	0	0
Grados	25	48	96	0	4
Heini	17	12	76	0	24
Jensen	29	1	90	0	10
Kim	45	1	90	0	10
Martin	9	14	77	0	22
Mathis	1	9	100	0	0
Maynard	27	3	93	0	7
O'Brien	6	3	67	0	33
Ryu	159	3	87	0	13
Theoduru	15	6	100	0	0
Zoarski	30	15	96	0	4

#Pts., Patients; f/u, follow-up in months; sig, significant.

Table 13–3:	Complications after Vertebral Body Augmentation					
	# PTS.	RECURR FX (%)	COMP RATE (%)	LEAKS (%)	CLEAR ROOT INJ (%)	PE (%)
Study 1	38	5	8	?	2.6	0
Study 2	67	?	0	?	2	0
Study 3	16	0	0	65	2	0
Study 4	20	20	10	40	4.3	0
Study 5	5	?	0	?	0	0
Study 6	4	?	0	?	0	0
Study 7	25	52	16	32	0	4
Study 8	17	0	0	20	0	0
Study 9	29	3	10	41	0	7
Study 10	45	0	0	?	0	0
Study 11	9	?	?	Common	0	0
Study 12	1	0	0	0	0	0
Study 13	27	?	?	?	?	?
Study 14	6	0	0	33	0	0
Study 15	159	?	13	40	0	?
Study 16	15	20	0	0	0	0
Study 17	30	0	0	3	0	0

#Pts, Patients; recurr fx, recurrent fracture; comp rate, complication rate; inj, injury; PE, pulmonary embolus.

- The most devastating VBA complications come from PMMA extravasation. In vertebroplasty and kyphoplasty, up to a 6% leak risk per level has been identified. Many of these leaks are asymptomatic, but major neurologic compromise and PMMA pulmonary embolus (PE) have been reported. Avoiding fractures with marked cortical compromise and slow PMMA injection under live image intensification will decrease this risk. The placement of more viscous cement into a cavity of known volume with kyphoplasty also limits extravasation risk (Table 13–3).

References

Baba H, Maezawa Y, Kamitani K et al. (1995) Osteoporotic vertebral collapse with late neurological complications. Paraplegia 33(5): 281-289.

> One of several studies describing a series of patients with osteoporotic burst fractures and evolving neurologic symptoms. This paper reports 27 patients developed neurologic symptoms anywhere from 1 month to 1.5 years after spinal fracture.

Deramond H, Depriester C, Galibert P et al. (1998) Percutaneous vertebroplasty with polymethylmethacrylate: Technique, indications, and results. Radiol Clin North Am 36(3): 533-546.

> This paper, by one of the originators of the technique, reviews the history, development, indications, and technique of vertebroplasty.

Do HM. (2000) Magnetic resonance imaging in the evaluation of patients for percutaneous vertebroplasty. Top MRI 14(4): 235-244.

> This paper reviews the use of MRI in patient selection for vertebroplasty. The author notes that acute fractures are best demonstrated on STIR sequences (Tr/TE 4000/60, inversion time 150 msec). He reports that, with fracture healing, the abnormal signal normalizes over time. Useful characteristics to differentiate osteoporotic from malignant fractures are described.

Garfin SR, Yuan HA, Reiley MA. (2001) New technologies in space: Kyphoplasty and vertebroplasty for the treatment of painful osteoporotic compression fractures. Spine 26(14): 1511-1515.

Grados F, Depriester C, Cayrolle G et al. (2000) Long-term observations of vertebral osteoporotic fractures treated by percutaneous vertebroplasty. Rheumatology (Oxford) 39(12): 1410-1414.

> This is one of the major, long-term, retrospective outcomes studies of vertebroplasty conducted on 40 osteoporotic patients with a mean follow-up of 48 months. Visual analog pain scales significantly decreased (P < 0.05) from a mean of 80 mm before operation to 37 mm 1 month after operation and 34 mm at final follow-up. There were no severe complications and no progression of vertebral deformity in any of the injected vertebrae. A slight, but significant, increase in the risk of adjacent-level vertebral fracture was reported. The authors conclude that vertebroplasty is safe and effective in the treatment of focal back pain secondary to osteoporotic vertebral fracture when conservative treatment has failed.

Harrington KD. (2001) Major neurological complications following percutaneous vertebroplasty with polymethylmethacrylate: A case report. J Bone Joint Surg Am 83-A(7): 1070-1073.

> This was one of the first reports of PMMA extravasation during vertebroplasty with major neurologic consequences. Here, spontaneous VCFs of T10, T11, and L1 were treated under general anesthesia. Although the patient reported excellent relief of her mechanical thoracolumbar pain, she noted the new, severe radiating pain from the back to the lower abdomen, groin, buttocks, and thigh with hypoesthesia and pseudoclaudication. A postprocedural CT scan demonstrated extensive extravasation of the PMMA into the spinal canal from T10 to L2. Harrington strongly suggests using high-quality imaging and added barium in the PMMA to reduce the incidence of these problems. The PMMA should be applied under live fluoroscopy as slowly and in as viscous a state as possible.

Heaney RP. (1992) The natural history of vertebral osteoporosis: Is low bone mass an epiphenomenon? Bone 13: S23-S26.

> This was one of the first papers to describe the evolving concept of the VCF as part of a vicious cycle of functional decline. After fracture, physician mandated or self-imposed bed rest can lead to a further 4% loss of bone mass, thereby increasing the chance of further fracture.

Kado DM, Browner WS, Palermo L et al. (1999) Vertebral fractures and mortality in older women: A prospective study. Arch Intern Med 159: 1215-1220.

> This population-based prospective study of 9,575 women followed for more than 8 years demonstrated a 23%-34% increased mortality rate compared with patients without VCFs. The most common cause of death was pulmonary disease, including chronic obstructive pulmonary disease and pneumonia (hazard ratio 2.1).

Lieberman IH, Dudeney S, Reinhardt MK et al. (2001) Initial outcome and efficacy of "kyphoplasty" in the treatment of painful osteoporotic vertebral compression fractures. Spine 26: 1631-1638.

> This was the initial efficacy report on 70 consecutive kyphoplasty procedures performed in 30 patients with painful primary or secondary osteoporotic VCFs. There were no major complications related directly to the use of this technique or the use of the inflatable bone tamp. Cement leakage occurred at six levels (8.6%). Significant improvements were noted in the SF-36 scores for Bodily Pain 11.6-58.7 (P = 0.0001) and Physical Function 11.7-47.4 (P = 0.002). In 30% of the vertebral levels, little height restoration was achieved. In the other 70%, however, kyphoplasty restored 47% of the lost height.

Liebschner MA, Rosenberg WS, Keaveny TM. (2001) Effects of bone cement volume and distribution on vertebral stiffness after vertebroplasty. Spine 26: 1547-1554.

> This is one of several biomechanical studies into the effects of PMMA on vertebral strength and stiffness. Here, a finite-element model analysis found that vertebral stiffness recovery after vertebroplasty was strongly influenced by the volume fraction of the implanted cement. Only a small amount of bone cement (14% fill or 3.5 cm3) was necessary to restore the stiffness of the damaged vertebral body to the predamaged value. Use of a 30% fill increased the stiffness more than 50% compared with the predamaged value. Use of a unipedicular approach allowed a similar return of stiffness, but a medial–lateral "toggle" toward the untreated side occurred when a uniform compressive pressure load was applied. The authors recommend using lower cement volume with symmetric placement.

Lindsay R, Silverman SL, Cooper C et al. (2001) Risk of new vertebral fracture in the year following a fracture. JAMA 285(3): 320–323.

> This study collated fracture risk data from several osteoporosis drug trials and found that the overall risk of vertebral fracture in osteoporotic patients was 6.6%. Despite at least minimal calcium and vitamin D therapy in all patients, the presence of one or more fractures at baseline increased the chance of sustaining another fracture fivefold in the next year.

Maynard AS, Jensen ME, Schweickert PA et al. (2000) Value of bone scan imaging in predicting pain relief from percutaneous vertebroplasty in osteoporotic vertebral fractures. Am J Neuroradiol 21(10): 1807–1812.

> This patient studied the use of bone scan in predicting positive clinical outcomes after vertebroplasty. Overall, subjective pain relief was noted in 26 (93%) of the 28 procedures. In all 14 of the patients with quantifiable pain levels, pain improved at least 3 points on a 10-point scale. The authors conclude that increased activity on bone scan is highly predictive of positive clinical response to percutaneous vertebroplasty.

Metabolic and Inflammatory Diseases of the Spine

Victor M. Hayes★, Farhan N. Siddiqi★, Dmitriy Kondrachov★, and Jeff S. Silber§

★M.D., Chief Resident, Long Island Jewish Medical Center, Long Island, NY
§ M.D., Assistant Professor, Department of Orthopaedic Surgery, Long Island Jewish
Medical Center, North Shore University Hospital Center, Long Island, NY; Albert Einstein
University Hospital, Bronx, NY

Metabolic Spine Disorders

Disorders of Bone Density

- **Osteopenia**
  - Condition of low bone mass when bone resorption is greater than bone formation
  - A value for bone mineral density (BMD) more than 1 standard deviation below the young adult mean but less than 2.5 standard deviations
- **Osteoporosis** (World Health Organization definition)—Osteoporosis is a condition characterized by low bone mass (osteopenia) and microarchitectural deterioration of bone tissue, leading to enhanced bone fragility and a consequent increase in fracture risk. It is the most common disease of bone (Table 14–1). It must meet one of the following criteria:
  - A BMD measurement of more than 2.5 standard deviations below the young adult normal mean
  - A previous fragility fracture

Anatomy or Biomechanics of Fragility Fractures

- Most spine pathology caused by osteoporosis affects the vertebral body.
- Vertebral body bone strength is determined by cortical thickness, bone size, trabecular bone density, and microarchitecture.

- The cortical vertebral shell accounts for approximately 10% of vertebral strength in vivo, and the trabecular centrum is the dominant structural component of the vertebral body (Silva et al. 1997).
- Horizontal trabeculae are preferentially lost, leaving the vertically oriented trabecular struts unsupported and substantially weaker (Snyder et al. 1993).

Pathophysiology

- Fracture incidence is directly related to the degree of bone loss.
- Commonly encountered spine problems that relate to osteoporosis are described in the next subsections.

Compression Fractures

- There are 700,000 vertebral compression fractures annually in the U.S.
- Low-energy microfractures within the vertebral body cause a single (anterior) column injury.
- Compression fractures typically involve the midthoracic or thoracolumbar region.
  - The vertebral body bears greater loads in these regions, especially with increasing kyphosis.
- The pain symptoms have no correlation with radiographic findings. Although 65% of patients are asymptomatic, the following have been reported:
  - Spinal deformity caused by two or more compression fractures significantly affects overall health and the

Table 14–1: Subtypes of Osteoporosis						
OSTEOPOROSIS SUBTYPES	**AGE ONSET**	**FEMALE/MALE RATIO**	**CAUSE**	**CELL TYPE**	**BONE TYPE AFFECTED**	**COMMON FRACTURES**
Type I (postmetapausal)	50-65	6:1	Estrogen deficiency	Osteoclast	Trabecular bone	Vertebral body radius
Type II (sessile)	>70	2:1	Aging	Osteoblast	Cortical bone	Hip
			Calcium deficiency			Humerus
			Increased PTH			Pelvis

ability to perform activities of daily living, especially in the elderly.

- There is a 5% age-adjusted increase in mortality and a 9% loss in predicted forced vital capacity (FVC) for each osteoporotic vertebral compression fracture (Leech et al. 1990).
- Patients with one compression fracture have four times the risk of developing a compression fracture at another level.

Difficulty with Successful Placement of Spinal Internal Fixation

- Positive and linear correlation between BMD and pullout strength of pedicle screws
  - The use of polymethylmethacrylate (PMMA) during pedicle screw insertion can increase pullout resistance twofold in severely osteoporotic bone (Wittenberg et al. 1993).
- Increased risk of pedicle fracture with screw placement
  - Pedicle screw size should not exceed 70% of the outer diameter of the pedicle to avoid fractures in these patients (Hirano et al. 1998).

Diagnostic Tools

- Plain radiographs
  - 30% decrease in bone mass before it is detectable on plain radiographic films
  - Must assess the amount of compression, angulation, or kyphosis and the stage of healing (acute, subacute, or chronic)
- Dual-energy x-ray absorptiometry (DEXA) scanning
  - Used to assess BMD and to monitor the progress of treatment
  - Accurately reflects response to treatment
  - Does not provide information about bone turnover rate (formation vs. resorption)
- Laboratory workup
  - For an uncomplicated patient with osteoporosis, a laboratory workup would include a chemistry panel, a complete blood count, and 24-hour urine calcium.
  - The purpose is to check for secondary causes of osteoporosis, which include renal or hepatic failure, anemia, acidosis, hypercalciuria, and abnormalities of calcium or phosphate metabolism.

- Magnetic resonance imaging (MRI) with contrast
  - Suspicion of infection, neoplasm, or neural compromise because 15% of compression fractures are caused by secondary osteoporosis

Nonoperative Care of Compression Fractures

- Observation because most fractures heal within 6-12 weeks
- Bed rest initially, but avoid prolonged immobilization
- Pro re nata (PRN) pain medication (e.g., Tylenol or mild narcotics)
- Physical therapy to decrease bone loss
- Bracing, which may stabilize the fracture
  - However, bracing contributes to bone loss and is poorly tolerated (especially by the elderly).

Operative Care of Compression Fractures

Vertebroplasty

- Involves the injection of bone cement (PMMA) through the pedicles or directly into the vertebral body fracture to restore structural stability and therefore relieve pain (67%-100%)

Kyphoplasty

- Insertion of a bone "tamp" into the vertebral body to create a void to accept the injection of bone cement (PMMA)
  - May restore vertebral body height through the use of a bone tamp

Relative Indications for Vertebroplasty and Kyphoplasty

- Painful acute or subacute (most effective if the fracture is approximately 6 weeks old) primary or secondary compression fractures nonresponsive to conservative therapy
- Prophylactic augmentation of noncompressed osteopenic levels adjacent to an instrumented fusion in osteoporotic patients
- Anterior column support of an osteoporotic vertebral body following a posterior decompression

Complications of Vertebroplasty and Kyphoplasty

- Short-term complications
  - Cement extravasation
  - Pain and neural injury because of cement contact (thermal burn) with spinal cord or nerve roots
  - Cement emboli
- Long-term complications (not fully evaluated)
  - Local acceleration of bone resorption
  - Foreign-body reaction at the cement–bone interface
  - Increased risk of fracture in treated or adjacent vertebrae through changes in mechanical forces

Disorders of Bone Density

- **Increased osteodensity**—Increased bone mass caused when bone formation is greater than bone resorption

Osteopetrosis (Albers-Schönberg Disease)

- This rare disease is caused by decreased osteoclastic resorption but normal bone formation.
- The most common form (adult tarda) is autosomal dominant and mild.
- The congenital form is autosomal recessive and the most severe.

Pathophysiology

- Decreased osteoclastic resorption but normal bone formation results in increased bone density and bone marrow obliteration.
- Clinically significant spinal involvement is uncommon; however, case reports of spondylolysis and/or spondylolisthesis secondary to lesions in the lumbar spine have been reported.
- Disordered architecture also makes bones susceptible to fractures.

Diagnostic Tools

- Plain radiographs
  - Sclerotic bands underlying endplates result in the hallmark "rugger jersey" appearance of the vertebrae.

Treatment

- Use interferon alpha and nonoperative treatment of fractures.
- Fractures requiring surgical stabilization present unique challenges, and careful preoperative planning is necessary.

Disorders of Bone Mineralization

- **Osteomalacia**—Inadequate deposition of calcium and phosphorous in bone tissue matrix. The total bone amount is normal; however, newly formed bone is inadequately mineralized.
  - This causes 4%–15% of hip and spinal compression fractures.

Some of the Multiple Etiologies

Intestinal Malabsorption or Malnutrition

- These are secondary to changes seen with aging.
- Immobile malnourished elderly patients without access to sunlight develop vitamin D deficiency.
- Decreased renal and liver function in the elderly lead to decreased vitamin D production (Table 14–2).

Malignancy

- Causes osteomalacia through humorally activated demineralization with hypercalcemia and hypo-phosphatemic osteomalacia (Goranov et al. 2002)

Renal Osteodystrophy

- Severe renal disease leads to the loss of normal vitamin D production and calcium and phosphorous metabolism.
  - This leads to osteomalacia, bony lesions, fracture, and pain.
- Kidneys fail to produce active vitamin D, and this leads to decreased calcium absorption.
- Renal disease causes increased phosphate resorption and calcium excretion.
  - Excess phosphate binds the calcium in serum and leads to extraosseous calcification.
  - Increase in parathyroid hormone (PTH) secretion—The body produces excess PTH in response to

Table 14–2: Recommended Treatment for Different Types of Osteomalacia	
TYPE OF OSTEOMALACIA	**TREATMENT**
All patients	Calcium 1500 mg/day
Vitamin D$_2$ deficiency	Vitamin D$_2$ 50,000 IU 3-5 times per week, then 1000-2000 IU/day when stable serum levels
Intestinal malabsorption	25-hydroxivitamin D$_3$ 20-100 mg/day
Phenytoin induced	25-hydroxivitamin D$_3$ 20-100 mg/day
Type I vitamin D-dependent rickets (production)	1,25-hydroxivitamin D$_3$ 2-3 µg/day until treated, then 0.5-1 µg/day
Type II vitamin D-dependent rickets (receptor)	1,25-hydroxivitamin D$_3$ 35 µg/day
X-linked hypophosphatemic rickets	1,25-hydroxivitamin D$_3$ 2-3 µg/day until treated, then 0.5-1 µg/day Phosphorous 1-2 g/day
Renal osteodystrophy	1,25-hydroxivitamin D$_3$ 1-2 µg/day Restriction in phosphate Parathyroidectomy if PTH levels uncontrollable

elevated phosphate levels, leading to excessive bony calcium loss.
- Calcium loss from bone—Osteolytic brown tumors

Genetic Disorders

- Type I vitamin D-dependent rickets
  - Abnormal kidney development—Deficient 1-8-hydroxylase
- Type II vitamin D-dependent rickets
  - Abnormal vitamin D receptor
- X-linked hypophosphatemic rickets (Vera et al. 1997)
  - Mutation in the PHEX gene—loss of PO_4 in renal tubules
  - No PO_4 available for bone mineralization
  - Osteopenia secondary to abnormal osteoblasts

Therapeutic and Environmental Causes

- P-450 activation increased by certain drugs, which may inactivate vitamin D production (e.g., phenytoin or cadmium)

Heavy Metals

- Aluminum and iron ingestion inhibits the formation of hydroxyapatite crystals and inhibits osteoblast function.

Pathophysiology

- Natural history is bone pain, stress, and fragility fractures.
- Manifestations mimic osteopenic and osteolytic disorders.

Some of the Spine Manifestations

- Compression fractures
- Spinal stenosis—vitamin D-resistant rickets (Velan et al. 2001)
  - Seen in the Japanese population but less frequent in Western populations
  - Can affect any spinal level
- Lower back pain (Al Faraj et al. 2003, Videman et al. 1998)
  - Incidence high where vitamin D deficiency is endemic
  - Mandatory screening for serum vitamin D levels
- Bone pain mimicking ankylosing spondylitis (AS) (Akkus et al. 2001)
  - Resolves with oral vitamin D and calcium intake
- Cervical spondyloarthropathy (Kumar et al. 1997)
  - Debilitating neck pain from renal osteodystrophy
  - Surgical fusion may decrease pain and allow increased activity

Diagnostic Tools

- Plain radiographs
  - Indistinguishable on radiographs from osteoporosis.
  - Looser's transformation = radiolucent lines (microfractures)
- Laboratory levels
  - Hypocalcemia, hypophosphatemia, and elevated PTH

- Low serum and urine 25-OH vitamin D
- Urine calcium < 100 mg/24 hrs
- Iliac biopsy for confirmation

Medical Treatment

- Much more responsive to dietary vitamin D, calcium, and phosphate than causes of osteoporosis

Disorders of Bone Remodeling

Paget's Disease (Osteitis Deformans)

- It is the second most common disorder of bone.
- Focal disorder of bone affects all elements of skeletal remodeling (resorption, formation, and mineralization).
- One third of patients with Paget's disease have spinal involvement.
- Most patients are asymptomatic, and the diagnosis is usually made incidentally by routine chemistry or radiographs.

Pathophysiology

- The primary defect is an exaggeration of osteoclastic bone resorption, initially producing localized bone loss. This is followed by pronounced bone formation, resulting in enlarged and deformed bones.
- Spinal stenosis and back pain are common.
  - One third of these patients have symptomatic spinal stenosis.
  - Half of these patients have back pain.
  - Facet arthropathy may result in both back pain and symptoms of spinal stenosis.
- Nerve compression results from an expansion of pagetoid vertebral bodies.

Diagnostic Tools

- Plain radiographs
  - Bone diameter is expanded, cortices are thickened, and trabeculae are coarse and widely separated. Vertebrae may have a framed-picture appearance.
- Laboratory tests
  - Serum alkaline phosphatase (elevated) and calcium (normal)
  - Urinary hydroxyproline excretion (elevated)
- Bone scan
  - Most sensitive test in identifying pagetic bone lesions
  - Lesions with markedly increased uptake
- MRI
  - Only indicated when the disease causes suspected neural compression

Nonoperative Treatment

- Acetaminophen and nonsteroidal anti-inflammatory drugs (NSAIDs)

- Bisphosphonates
- Nasal calcitonin
  - Symptomatic spinal stenosis with neurological claudication responds well to medical therapy with calcitonin and bisphosphonates (Hadjipavlou et al. 2001).

Operative Treatment

- Decompression rarely is necessary.

Complications

- Decompression can lead to spinal instability.
- Increased intraoperative bleeding can occur.

Endocrinopathies Affecting the Spine

- Can lead to severe osteoporosis and osteomalacia

Glucocorticoid Excess

- Causes include Cushing's disease, iatrogenic steroid treatment, and adrenal tumors
- Mechanisms include the following:
  - Decreased calcium absorption across the intestinal wall through a decrease in calcium-binding proteins
  - Increased urinary calcium excretion
  - Increased bone resorption
  1. Resorption of bony matrix proteins
  2. Secondary elevated PTH in response to low serum calcium
- Spinal manifestations
  - Severe osteoporosis—even with Prednisone intake of 10 mg by mouth every day
  - Compression fractures resulting in thoracic kyphosis secondary to Cushing's disease in young adults (Angela et al. 1999).

Type I Diabetes

- Calciuria and negative nitrogen balance leads to osteoporosis through calcium and bony matrix resorption.
- Spinal manifestations include accelerated osteoporosis and increased susceptibility to disk herniation.
  - Undersulfated glycosaminoglycan in proteoglycans of lumbar disks leading to possible weakness in the anulus fibrosis (Robinson et al. 1998).

Hyperparathyroidism

- PTH is released in response to low serum, ionized calcium
  - PTH binds to osteoblast receptors, activating bone turnover and releasing interleukin-6 (IL-6).
  - IL-6 causes osteoclast activation and the net resorption of calcium.

- PTH increases renal calcium resorption, phosphate excretion, and vitamin D production.
- PTH can be elevated primarily or secondarily (i.e., renal disease or Cushing's disease).
- Laboratory values show elevated serum calcium.
- Severe skeletal calcium loss leads to osteomalacia and lytic bone lesions (Brown tumors).

Hyperthyroidism

- Causes include primary hyperthyroidism or iatrogenic from excessive thyroid hormone replacement.
- Elevated levels promote bone formation and resorption.
  - The net result is bone loss.
- Hyperthyroidism leads to progressive osteoporosis.
  - There is an elevated risk of hip and compression fractures in women.

Miscellaneous Disorders Affecting the Spine

Diffuse Idiopathic Skeletal Hyperostosis (Table 14–3)

- There is a generalized ossification of ligaments of unknown origin.
- The spine is the most commonly affected area.
- Prevalence in males older than 50 is 25% and in females older than 50 is 15%.
- This is less commonly seen in African-American and Native American populations.

Anatomy

- Longitudinal ligaments of the spine, in particular the anterior longitudinal ligament, are most often affected.

Pathophysiology

- The ligament ossification leads to an increased fracture risk. Fractures are commonly caused by a hyperextension force to the thoracolumbar spine; these patients have an increased incidence of spinal cord injury because of the presence of rigidly fused spinal segments. These segments produce long lever arms and are highly unstable.

Table 14–3:   Diagnostic Criteria for Diffuse Idiopathic Skeletal Hyperostosis*
Absence of apophyseal joint bony ankylosis and sacroiliac joint erosion, sclerosis, or intraarticular osseous fusion
Relative preservation of intervertebral disk height in the involved vertebral segment and absence of extensive disk disease
Flowing calcification and ossification along the anterolateral aspect of at least four contiguous vertebral body segments

* Thoracic vertebrae are involved in 100% of cases (T7-T11 most common), lumbar in 68%-90%, and cervical segments in 65%-78%.

Minimal trauma has been shown to produce unstable fractures.

Diagnostic Tools

- Plain radiographs
  - Used to help establish the diagnosis (Fig. 14–1)
- Plain x-rays, computed tomography (CT), MRI, or bone scan
  - Indicated in patients with back pain following any trauma, even minor, to rule out occult fracture
  - Difficult to demonstrate fractures because of the excessive bone formation or associated osteoporosis

Treatment

- Thoracolumbar fractures may benefit from surgical stabilization, especially when associated with neurologic compromise or instability.
- Displaced fractures, late diagnosis, nonunion, or osteolysis of the spine are potential indications for surgical stabilization.
  - Posterior segmental instrumentation and fusion without distraction or compression are often recommended.
  - Bracing tends to not work in these patients because the long lever arms are difficult to immobilize adequately.

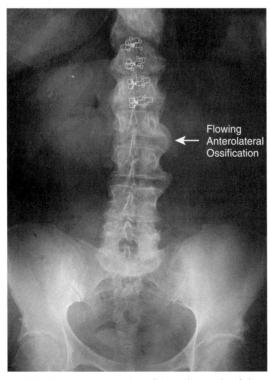

Figure 14–1: An anteroposterior plain radiograph of the thoracic spine in a patient with diffuse idiopathic skeletal hyperostosis demonstrating a flowing anterolateral "candle wax" ossification.

Inflammatory Spinal Disorders
Immune Mediated Disorders Affecting the Spine

Rheumatoid Arthritis

- Rheumatoid arthritis (RA) is a chronic, progressive, systemic, inflammatory disease primarily affecting synovial joints.
- Prevalence in the adult general population is about 1%.
- RA affects the cervical spine in up to 85% of individuals.
- Of those with cervical RA, 58% develop a neurologic deficit.
- Once a myelopathy develops, 75%-90% will progress.
- Patients at highest risk for progression are males with severe peripheral disease, on steroids, or both.

Anatomy and Biomechanics

- The intimate relationship among the facet joints, ligaments, vertebrae, and spinal cord in the upper cervical spine makes instability in this region potentially harmful.
- Cine-radiography motion studies of cervical motion in RA patients revealed abnormal kinematics that can lead to uncontrolled movement of the vertebrae, resulting in spinal cord compression (i.e., dynamic instability).

Pathophysiology

- Synovitis and pannus formation are the hallmarks of the disease that leads to bone, cartilage, and ligament erosion. The resultant ligamentous laxity can lead to subluxation, instability, and neural (cord or root) compression.
- The spectrum of neurologic symptoms is broad and can range from mild neck pain and occipital headaches to myelopathy, paralysis, and death.
- C1-C2 instability is the most common cervical abnormality seen.
- Of RA patients, 50%-61% develop one or a combination of the following three cervical spine instability patterns:
- Atlantoaxial instability
  - Most common instability (50%) pattern noted in RA
  - Translation of C1 on C2
  - Most subluxations are anterior and result from attenuation of the transverse and apical spinal ligaments
- Basilar invagination
  - Cranial migration of the odontoid above the transverse diameter of the foramen magnum
  - Caused by erosion and bone loss between occiput-C1 and C1-C2 articulations

- Neurologic symptoms caused by direct compression of the cervical medullary junction or ischemia from compression of the neural vasculature
  - Migration evaluated by measuring Chamberlain's line, Wackenheim's line, and the Ranawat measurement
- Subaxial instability
  - Least common and found in 20% of patients
  - Occurs as a direct result of facet, ligament, and disk destruction
  - May be seen at multiple levels causing a stepladder deformity frequently associated with kyphosis
  - Spinal canal diameter (SCD) is the best prognostic factor for assessing subaxial instability.

Diagnostic Tools

Physical Examination

- Gait, equilibrium, cervical range of motion, and motor and sensory testing
- Pathologic reflexes
  - Hoffman reflex—Upper motor neuron sign produced by applying a sudden hyperextension to the distal phalanx of the third finger, eliciting flexion of the metacarpal phalangeal and interphalangeal joints of the thumb and second finger.
  - Babinski sign, hyperreflexia, and clonus
- Patients with more severe disease in the peripheral skeleton (hands) usually develop worse disease involving the cervical spine.

Plain Radiographs

Assessing Stability

- SCD is measured from the posterior vertebral body to the spinolaminar line.
  - Cord compression occurs when SCD is less than 14 mm on the neutral lateral plain radiograph.
  - Posterior space available for the cord at the atlantodens junction is the most reliable indicator for risk of neurologic deterioration.
  - Posterior space available for the cord is measured from the posterior dens to the anterior aspect of posterior atlas arch.
- Atlantodental interval
  - Normally <3 mm (adults) and <5 mm (children)
  - Normal posterior atlantodental interval is >14 mm
  - Tip of odontoid should be inline with basion

Flexion or Extension Radiographs

- Such radiographs are used to assess for dynamic instability.
- Red flags for instability are subaxial vertebral translation more than 3.5 mm or an 11-degree angulation between adjacent vertebrae.

- These radiographs should be used as a preoperative screen in all rheumatoid patients to avoid complications that may occur during intubation.
- Such radiographs are helpful in assessing fusion levels if surgery is indicated.

Magnetic Resonance Imaging

- MRI has the advantage of being able to visualize spinal cord compression because of bone and **soft tissue pannus**.
- Two thirds of patients with RA have a soft tissue pannus of more than 3 mm not visualized on plain radiographs. This further reduces the SCD.
- Flexion or extension MRI is useful in evaluating dynamic instability.
- MRI is indicated if an SCD of less than 14 mm or an instability is seen on radiographs.

Laboratory Tests

- The Rhesus factor is negative in 15% of patients.
- C-reactive protein is frequently elevated (three times the normal amount) in patients with subluxations in the cervical spine.

Nonoperative Treatment

- Medical treatment
- Cervical orthosis
- Close follow-up with physical examination and radiographic analysis

Operative Treatment

Goals of Surgery

- Operative treatment should prevent or minimize the risk of neurologic deterioration and therefore the risk of paralysis and sudden death.
- Fusion procedures are used in RA patients to decrease motion and to reduce synovial pannus formation and inflammation in the joints.
- Fusion procedures also are used to stabilize the cervical spine to prevent neurologic injury.
  - Once neurologic deficits exist, surgical outcomes less successful.

Potential Indications for Surgery

- In the presence or absence of neurologic signs or symptoms
- Atlantoaxial subluxation with a posterior atlantodental interval of 14 mm
- Subaxial subluxation = 5 mm
- Subaxial subluxation and an SCD of 14 mm or less
- Cervical medullary angle of less than 135 degrees
  - Has a high incidence of progressive myelopathy (Table 14–4, Box 14–1)

Table 14–4: Predictors of Neurologic Recovery and Ranawat Classification*

CLASS	SYMPTOMS	PROGNOSIS
I	Pain but no neurologic deficit	Better postoperative outcomes
II	Subjective weakness	Less recovery and increased morbidity after surgery
IIIa	Ambulatory with weakness and pathologic reflexes	Less recovery and increased morbidity after surgery
IIIb	Nonambulatory with weakness and pathologic reflexes	Less recovery and increased morbidity after surgery

* Paralyzed patients with: Spinal Canal Diameter (SCD) > 14mm had complete recovery post-operatively
  SCD 10–14mm had recovery of one Ranawat class
  SCD < 10mm had no neurologic recovery
* Early decompression in patients with neurologic deficits are associated with improved outcomes.

Seronegative Spondyloarthropathies

- Human leukocyte antigen (HLA) B27 associated with the development of spondyloarthropathies and including the following:
  - AS
  - Reactive arthropathy associated with inflammatory bowel disease
  - Psoriatic arthritis
  - Reiter's syndrome

Ankylosing Spondylitis

- Chronic inflammatory disease affecting the axial skeleton
- Prevalence is 1 in 1,000
- Onset 15-50 years of age

Box 14–1: Surgical Pearls in Treating Rheumatoid Arthritis

- Avoid if possible anterior instrumentation in RA patients with osteoporosis.
- Consider preoperative traction to realign the spine prior to fusion in patients with a multilevel disease.
- Be aware of ending a fusion at an unstable or listhetic segment because this increases the risk of failure.
- Extend fusion levels if there is any uncertainty about the spine stability at the ends of a surgical construct.
- Do not ignore the occiput and the C1-C2 junction
  - If they are significantly involved with disease, fuse them.
- Before fusing just the occipitocervical junction, rule out subaxial instability.
  - Perform a close follow-up to assess for junctional breakdown above and below the fusion level.
  - If a severe deformity exists, consider anterior and posterior stabilization.
  - For example, consider an anterior strut graft with posterior segmental instrumentation.

- Male = female; however, males have a more severe disease expression
- Mostly Caucasian (HLA-B27)
- Propensity toward spinal fractures (rigidity and osteoporosis)
- Development of spinal deformity (related to micro-fractures)
- Usually presenting symptoms of low back pain and morning stiffness
- When spine autofuses, most symptoms resolve
- **Requires the most attention of the seronegative spondyloarthropathies because of the risk of worsening spinal cord or nerve injury from delayed diagnosis of spinal fractures and instability**

Anatomy and Pathophysiology

- HLA-B27 in 88%-96% patients with AS
- Earliest changes are in SI joints followed with cephalad spinal progression
- Pannus formation common
- Initial cartilage destruction and bony erosions
- After a reparative phase, fibrous and bony ankylosis
- Enthesitis at tendon and ligament bony insertions
- In the spine, enthesitis at the insertion of the anulus fibrosus
- Ossification of the anulus producing syndesmophytes and eventually a "bamboo spine"
- Nonskeletal manifestations
  - Aortic insufficiency, cardiac conduction defects, uveitis, uremia, and pulmonary fibrosis (cause of death in 10% patients)
- Spontaneous atlantoaxial subluxation can result from bony erosions

Diagnostic Tools

Plain Radiography

- Squaring the corners of vertebral bodies
- Marginal symmetric syndesmophytes (Fig. 14–2)
  - Syndesmophytes—Vertical paravertebral ossification
  - Osteophytes—More horizontal ossifications
- Bamboo spine (Fig. 14–3)
- Sacroiliitis (Fig. 14–4)
  - Bilateral and symmetric
  - Sequence erosions, sclerosis, and autofusion
  - CT—Test of choice for SI joint involvement
- Arthropathy of large joints resembles RA

Occult Fractures

- Such fractures can occur with minimal trauma or minor motor vehicle collision.
- Plain radiographs can be misleading and hard to interpret.
- CT can be hard to interpret because of the difficulty in obtaining true axial cuts.
- MRI is a more reliable test for occult fractures and hematoma evaluation.

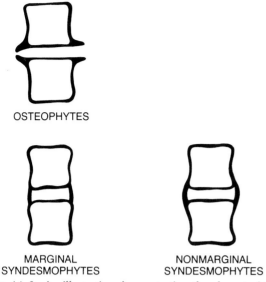

OSTEOPHYTES

MARGINAL
SYNDESMOPHYTES

NONMARGINAL
SYNDESMOPHYTES

Figure 14–2: An illustration demonstrating the characteristic appearance of vertebral osteophytes, marginal syndesmophytes, and nonmarginal syndesmophytes. (Reprinted from Booth et al. 1999.)

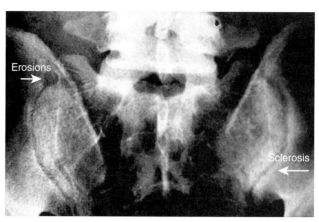

Figure 14–4: An anteroposterior radiograph of the pelvis and sacroiliac joints demonstrating the typical erosions and the sclerosis of sacroiliac joints frequently seen in patients with AS.

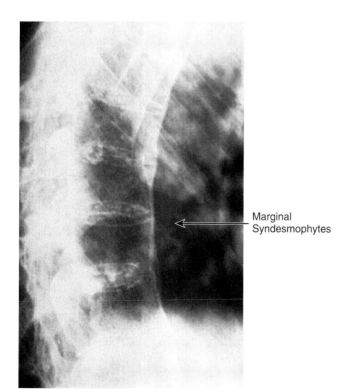

Marginal
Syndesmophytes

Figure 14–3: A lateral plain radiograph of the thoracic spine demonstrating a bamboo spine and marginal syndesmophytes as a result of AS.

- Bone scan can be "hot" because of the disease itself.
- There is a high incidence of neurological compromise if fractures are missed.
- **Always maintain a high index of suspicion for spinal fracture!**

Physical Examination

- Stooped posture
- Rigid kyphotic spine
- Most effective measure of the spinal deformity—Chin-brow to vertical angle
- Compensatory hip flexion contractures common

Nonoperative Treatment

- Radiation therapy
  - Rarely used and predisposes to malignancy
- NSAIDs
  - Control pain and stiffness but do not alter the course of the disease
  - Phenylbutazone and indomethacin most effective
- Steroids
  - Useful for local control but systemically have no proven value
- Disease-modifying agents—Sulfasalazine, cyclophosphamide, and methotrexate may be helpful
- Exercise

Operative Treatment

Indications for Surgery

- Flexion deformity associated with pain and neurologic compromise
- Loss of horizontal gaze
- Stabilize spine fractures (flexion deformity is probably a late consequence of fractures)

- Chin-brow vertical angle to assess the deformity preoperatively

Goals of Surgery

- Restoration of erect posture
- Relief of rib encroachment on abdomen
- Improvement in pulmonary function or diaphragmatic excursion
- Regain horizontal gaze

Surgical Technique

- Fiberoptic intubation
- Spinal cord monitoring (somatosensory-evoked potentials, motor-evoked potentials, electromyogram)
- Consider wakeup test

Surgery of the Cervical Spine in AS

- Extension osteotomy for kyphosis at cervicothoracic junction that limits horizontal gaze
- Postoperative immobilization (halo jacket)

Surgery of the Thoracic Spine in AS

- Costotransverse osteotomies
- Thoracic kyphosis can be corrected by lumbar osteotomy.
- If thoracic osteotomies are indicated, multiple small osteotomies are preferred to a single large osteotomy (to minimize acute angulation of the spinal cord).

Surgery of the Lumbar Spine in AS

- V-shaped posterior osteotomy (Smith-Peterson 1945)
- Osteotomy between L2 and L4
  - Closing wedge osteotomy, decancellation, and pedicle subtraction
  - High neurological complication rate (up to 9%)
- Higher complications seen with unisegmental vs. multisegmental correction
- Closing wedge osteotomy appears to be safer than opening wedge (avoidance of tension forces anteriorly on the aorta)

Inflammatory Bowel Disease

- Shares many musculoskeletal features with AS
- HLA-B27 positive in 5% of cases
- Spondyloarthropathy more prevalent in Crohn's disease than in ulcerative colitis
- Spine involved in 5% of patients (of those, 50%-75% are HLA-B27 positive)
- Spinal involvement usually independent of bowel disease
- Marginal (starting at the endplates) symmetric syndesmophytes
- Sacroiliitis is bilateral and symmetric
- Peripheral arthritis following disease exacerbations

Psoriatic Arthritis

- 7% of patients with psoriasis
- Arthritis precedes skin lesions in 15% of cases
- 20% HLA-B27 positive
- Spine involved in 20% patients
- Shares many musculoskeletal features with Reiter's syndrome
- Nonmarginal asymmetric syndesmophytes (large and bulky) (Fig. 14–5)
- Sacroiliitis is unilateral and asymmetric
- Can involve small joints (e.g., proliferative erosions, soft tissue swelling, periostitis, and ankylosis)
- Arthritis deformans (severe involvement of hands and feet)

Reiter Syndrome

- Triad of urethritis, uveitis, and arthritis
- 90% patients HLA-B27 positive
- Spine involved in 30%-40% patients
- Microbes implicated include Shigella, Salmonella, Yersinia, and Campylobacter
- Disability occurs in 25% (mostly because of calcaneal involvement)
- Unilateral asymmetric sacroiliitis
- Nonmarginal asymmetric syndesmophytes

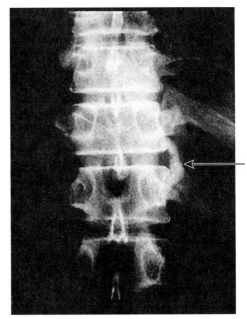

Non-marginal Syndesmophyte

Figure 14–5: An anteroposterior plain radiograph of the thoracolumbar spine demonstrating a nonmarginal syndesmophyte characteristic of psoriatic arthritis and Reiter's syndrome.

Miscellaneous Inflammatory Disorders Affecting The Spine

Calcium Pyrophosphate Dihydrate Deposition Disease

- The common disorder is characterized by calcium pyrophosphate dihydrate deposition disease (CPPD) crystal deposition within soft tissues.
- The incidence of CPPD increases in hyperparathyroidism, hemochromatosis, hemosiderosis, hypomagnesemia, and hypophosphatemia.
- Spinal involvement is common (secondary to knee involvement) but mostly asymptomatic.
- There is a male/female ratio of 1:1 with a typical onset after 50 years of age.

Pathophysiology

- CPPD crystal deposition in hyaline cartilage, fibrocartilage, and periarticular tissues leads to the chondrocalcinosis, the hallmark of the disease. Deposition can lead to secondary arthritis with prominent calcifications, cysts, and erosions, but the clinical significance of this can vary (Box 14–2)
  - Mostly asymptomatic
  - Pain and symptoms similar to those seen in osteoarthritis and RA
  - Compression of neural structures when depositions are located within the spinal canal.
  - Cervical myelopathy rare but reported
  - Spinal stenosis

Diagnostic Tools

- Laboratory test
  - Mildly elevated erythrocyte sedimentation rate
  - Synovial aspiration demonstrating pyrophosphate crystals (gold standard to establish the diagnosis); crystals are rhomboid shaped and positively birefringent
- Plain radiographs
- MRI
  - Indicated if neural compression suspected

Box 14–2:	**Radiographic Features Distinguishing CPPD from Degenerative Joint Disease**

- Prominent calcification
- Involvement of unusual joints and compartments
- Presence of extensive sclerosis, cysts, fragmentation, and osseous debris
- Variable osteophyte formation

Treatment

- Nonoperative treatment
  - NSAIDs
- Operative treatment
  - Surgical decompression is indicated in patients with myelopathic symptoms, symptomatic spinal stenosis, or both nonresponsive to conservative treatment.

References

Akkus S, Tamer MN, Yorgancigil H. (2001) A case of osteomalacia mimicking ankylosing spondylitis. Rheumatology Int 20(6): 239-242.
  A case report of a patient with clinical AS by examination and history with osteomalacia diagnosed through pseudofractures on radiography.

Al Faraj S, Al Mutairi K. (2003) Vitamin D deficiency and chronic low back pain in Saudi Arabia. Spine 28(2): 177-179.
  A clinical study demonstrating that vitamin D deficiency is a major cause of lower back pain in areas of the world where decreased intake is endemic. Screening for vitamin D deficiency and treatment with supplements is recommended in these areas. Measurement of serum 25-OH cholecalciferol is sensitive and specific for detection of vitamin D deficiency and hence for presumed osteomalacia in patients with chronic low back pain.

American Academy of Orthopaedic Surgeons. (2002) Orthopaedic Knowledge Update: Spine 2. North American Spine Society, pp. 393-395.

Barker LR, Burton JR, Zieve PD et al. (1999) Principles of Ambulatory Medicine, 6th edition. Baltimore: Williams and Wilkins.

Booth RE, Simpson JM, Herkowitz HN. (1999) Arthritis of the spine. In: Rothman-Simeone—The Spine (Herkowitz HN et al., eds.), 4th edition. Philadelphia: Saunders.

Bridwell KH, DeWald RL. (1997) The Textbook of Spinal Surgery, 2nd edition. Philadelphia: Lippincott-Raven. pp. 705-706, 1109-1158.

Fardon DF, Garfin SR, Abitol J et al. (2002) Orthopaedic knowledge update: Spine 2. N Am Spine Soc.
  Text distributed by the AAOS that contains core information on all aspects of spinal care.

Freehill, Lenke LG. (1999) Severe kyphosis secondary to glucocorticoid-induced osteoporosis in a young adult with Cushing's Disease: A case report and literative review. Spine, 24: 189-193.
  A case report of a young adult with progressive kyphosis of the thoracic spine managed surgically, demonstrating that unrecognized endogenous production of glucocorticoids in Cushing's disease should be considered in young adult patients with progressive osteoporotic spinal deformities.

Goranov SE, Simeonov SB. (2002) Bone lesions in malignant diseases—I: Current concepts of major pathogenetic mechanisms and forms. Folia Med (Plovdiv) 44(1-2): 7-14.

A review article detailing the metabolic bone sequela of malignant disease. The article describes the natural history of malignant disease and the mechanism causing osteomalacia.

Hadjipavlou AG, Gaitanis LN, Katonis PG et al. (2001) Paget's disease of the spine and its management. Eur Spine J 10(5): 370-384.
This article reviews the literature providing information about the pathomechanics by which Paget's disease alters the spinal structures. It describes spinal entities such as pagetic spinal arthritis, spinal stenosis, and other pathologies. It also assesses the best treatment options and available drugs for treating this disease.

Helms CA. (1995) Fundamentals of Skeletal Radiology, 2nd edition. Philadelphia: Saunders. pp. 122-150.

Hirano T, Hasegawa K, Washio T, Hara T et al. (1998) Fracture risk during pedicle screw insertion in osteoporotic spine. J Spinal Disord 11(6): 493-497.
The structural changes that occur in the pedicles of severely osteoporotic patients were analyzed using quantitative CT scanning. The effect of these structural changes on the risk of pedicle fracture during screw insertion was then assessed. Of the seven fractures that occurred, all were in patients with a DEXA value of less than 0.7 g/cm2 and with screw diameters greater than 70% of the outer diameter of the pedicle. The authors conclude that to avoid fractures in osteoporotic patients, the screw diameter should not exceed 70% of the outer diameter.

Klippel JH, ed. (1997) Primer on the Rheumatic Diseases, 11th edition. Atlanta: Arthritis Foundation. pp. 180-195.

Koval K et al. (2002) Orthopaedic knowledge update 7. AAOS.

Kumar A, Leventhal MR, Freedman EL. (1997) Destructive spondyloarthropathy of the cervical spine in patients with chronic renal failure. Spine 22(5): 573-577.
Eleven patients with chronic renal failure and destructive spondyloarthropathy of the cervical spine were evaluated to determine the results of surgical and nonsurgical treatment. The authors conclude that cervical fusion is an effective method of treating patients with chronic renal failure and destructive spondyloarthropathy: Patients with laminectomy alone had no improvement in pain or neurologic function, one of three patients with anterior fusions had some improvement, and both patients with posterior fusions improved.

Leech JA, Dulberg C, Kellie S et al. (1990) Relationship of lung function to severity of osteoporosis in women. Am Rev Respir Dis 141: 68-71.
In this study, 74 women referred for osteoporosis testing underwent pulmonary function testing. After controlling for age, there was a significant decrease in FVC when hyperkyphosis increases. Regression equations revealed that with each thoracic compression fracture there was a decease in FVC of 9.4%.

Robinson D, Mirosky Y, Halperin N et al. (1998) Changes in proteoglycans of intervertebral disk in diabetic patients: A possible cause of increased back pain. Spine 23: 849-855.
A basic science study demonstrating that disks in patients with diabetes have proteoglycans with lower buoyant density and substantially undersulfated glycosaminoglycan, which—with the specific neurologic damage in these patients—might lead to increased susceptibility to disk prolapse.

Silva MJ, Keaveny TM, Hayes WC. (1997) Load sharing between the shell and centrum in the lumbar vertebral body. Spine 22(2): 140-150.
The authors compared the amount of compressive forces that the cortical shell and the trabecular centrum endure when lumbar vertebral bodies are loaded. They found that the shell accounts for only 10% of vertebral strength in vivo and that the trabecular centrum is the dominant component of the vertebral body in regards to strength.

Smith-Peterson MN, Larson CB, Au Franc OE. (1945) Osteotomy of the spine for correction of flexion deformity in rheumatoid arthritis. J Bone Joint Surgery. 27: 1–11.

Snyder BD, Piazza S, Edwards WT et al. (1993) Role of trabecular morphology in the etiology of age-related vertebral fractures. Calcif Tissue Int Suppl 1: 14-22.
A three-dimensional stereological analysis of trabeculae bone was performed on lumbar vertebral bodies extracted from cadavers between the ages of 27 and 81. The authors found that the number and thickness of trabeculae decreased linearly with density when age increased. They also found that the number of vertically oriented trabeculae changed with density at twice the rate of that seen in the transverse (horizontal) trabeculae.

Velan GJ, Currier BL, Clark BL, Yaszemski MJ. (2001) Ossification of the posterior longitudinal ligament (OPLL) in vitamin D-resistant rickets. Spine 26: 590-593.
A clinical study demonstrating that OPLL in patients with vitamin D-resistant rickets is different from degenerative OPLL and may not be reversible with medical management, leading to surgical treatment of spinal pathology.

Vera CL, Cure JK, Najo WB, Geluen PL. (1997) Paraplegia due to ossification of ligamenta flava in X-linked hypophosphatemia. Spine 22: 710-715.
A case report demonstrating the association between X-linked hypophosphatemia and excessive ossification of the ligamentum flavum. This patient had progressive paraplegia, which was unresponsive to medical management and required surgical intervention. Electromyogram testing and clinical motor strength were regained after surgical laminectomy.

Videman T, Leppavouri J, Kaprio J et al. (1998) Intragenic polymorphisms of the vitamin D receptor gene associated with intervertebral disk degeneration. Spine 23: 2477-2485.
A human study demonstrating that MRI documented disk degeneration and back pain is associated with certain polymorphisms of the vitamin D receptor.

Wittenberg RH, Lee KS, Shea M et al. (1993) Effect of screw diameter, insertion technique, and bone cement augmentation of pedicular screw fixation strength. Clin Orthop (296): 278-287.
The effect screw diameter and different screw insertion techniques on axial pullout force and transverse bending stiffness were compared using a biomechanical model. The axial pullout force of Schanz screws was significantly increased, with a 1-mm increase in screw diameter, but there was no significant increase in transverse bending stiffness. Augmenting pedicle screws with PMMA in the lumbar spine increased both the axial pullout force (approximately twofold) and the transverse bending stiffness.

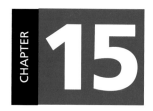

15

The Rheumatoid Spine

Dilip K. Sengupta* and Harry N. Herkowitz §

* M.D., Dr. Med, Assistant Professor, Department of Orthopaedics, Staff Spine Surgeon, Spine Center, Dartmouth-Hitchcock Medical Center, Lebanon, NH
§ M.D., Chairman, Department of Orthopaedic Surgery, William Beaumont Hospital, Royal Oak, MI

Introduction

- Rheumatoid arthritis (RA) most commonly affects the cervical spine.
  - Within 5 years of serologic diagnosis, 30%-50% develop subluxation.
  - Only a few of these (2%-3%) will develop myelopathy 10 years later (12-15 years).
  - Common presenting symptoms are neck pain and neurologic deficit. Patients are at risk for sudden death.
  - Often recognized as asymptomatic radiological instability (Table 15–1).
- The challenges therefore are to identify those who are at risk and to stabilize them to prevent neurological damage.

Pathophysiology

- As in the other joints, RA leads to inflammatory synovitis, which destroys the ligaments and bone, leading to subluxation, pain, and neurological damage.
- Upper cervical spine—Two forms of subluxation may develop:
  - Primarily ligamentous destruction leads to *atlantoaxial subluxation* (AAS).
  - Primarily bony destruction, later in the disease process, leads to *cranial settling,* also known as *superior migration of the odontoid* (SMO) or *basilar invagination.*
- Lower cervical spine—A combination of bony and ligamentous destruction may lead to a "stepladder" pattern

Table 15–1:	Incidence of Cervical Spine Symptoms in RA
SYMPTOM	**PATIENTS WITH SYMPTOM**
Neck pain	40%-80%
Radiological instability	43%-86%
Neurological deficit	7%-34%
Sudden death	10%

of subluxation in multiple segments in the subaxial spine, known as subaxial subluxation (SAS).
- AAS is the most common type of instability (65%) and develops relatively early in the disease process. The subluxation occurs mostly in the anterior, sometimes in the lateral, and rarely in the posterior direction.
- SMO or basilar invagination is the second most common rheumatoid subluxation (20%), develops late in the disease process, and is nearly always associated with AAS. The underlying pathology is predominantly bony destruction. Therefore SMO is rarely reducible and often associated with neurological damage; prognosis is less optimistic.
- SAS is found in approximately 15% of rheumatoid patients. Patients may have a combination of any two or all three types of subluxation (Boden et al. 1998) (Fig. 15–1).

Clinical Presentation

- Most cases are asymptomatic or have minimal pain; most cases also are often recognized at a preoperative checkup

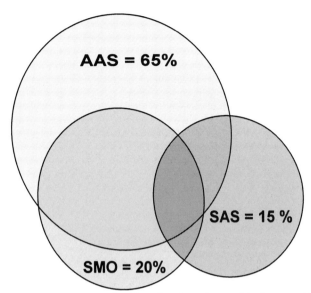

Figure 15–1: Forms of subluxation in patients with rheumatoid arthritis. (*AAS,* atlantoaxial subluxation; *SAS,* subaxial subluxation; *SMO,* superior migration of the odontoid.)

for other joint surgery. Many patients present symptoms of painless myelopathy.

- Common presenting symptoms are the following:
  1. Neck pain and occipital headache
  2. Crepitus in the cervical spine and a palpable "clunk" on movement of the unstable joints of the cervical spine
  3. Neurologic deficit—Myelopathy, radiculopathy, or both
  4. Lhermitte's phenomenon—Electric shock sensation traveling through the body with neck movement
  5. Vertebrobasilar insufficiency (with basilar invagination)—Tinnitus, vertigo, loss of equilibrium, visual disturbances, nystagmus, diplopia, and dysphagia
  6. Urinary dysfunction
  7. Trigeminal nerve tract involvement and facial sensory impairment
  8. Frozen shoulder—If present, often secondary to myelopathy rather than a primary capsulitis
- Neurological assessment is difficult in cases of peripheral joint disease with the involvement of the tendon and muscles.
- Neurological deficit has been classified by Ranawat (Ranawat et al. 1979) (Table 15–2).

Onset and Progression of Cervical Instability

- Instability depends on the severity of the disease process.
- Subluxation appears after the first decade of active disease.
- Radiographic progression of subluxation has been observed in 35%-80% of patients.
- Neurologic progression has been observed in 15%-36% of patients.
- There is a 5-year mortality rate of 17%.

Table 15–2:	Ranawat Classification
TYPE	**CHARACTERISTIC**
Class I	No deficit
Class II	Subjective weakness, hyperreflexia
Class IIIa	Objective weakness, ambulatory
Class IIIb	Objective weakness, nonambulatory

- After the onset of myelopathy, 50% of patients die within 1 year (Crockard et al. 1998).

Risk Factors for the Progression of Cervical Disease (Lipson 1989)

- Male gender
- Severe peripheral disease
- Use of corticosteroids

Radiographic Predictors of Paralysis (Boden et al. 1993)

- Neurological deficits are often irreversible, and surgery only prevents further deterioration. Because cervical instability is common in the rheumatoid population but not all cases progress, it is important to predict neurological deficit to select cases for surgical stabilization before the onset of a neurodeficit.
- Magnetic resonance imaging (MRI) is a superior imaging modality but is impractical for screening cases to predict paralysis. Therefore plain radiographs form the basis of the screening test.

Atlantoaxial Subluxation (Fig. 15–2)

- AAS becomes accentuated in flexion. Lateral flexion–extension plain radiographs are more likely to show instability or dynamic motion.
- The normal anterior atlantodens interval (AADI) is 3 mm in adults and 4 mm in children. AADI greater than 5 mm represents instability.
- Traditionally, AADI has been used clinically to follow RA cervical instability.
- The critical limit of AADI that predicts an impending paralysis and indicates a need for surgery has been desired at 8, 9, or 10 mm by different authors.
- AADI is an unreliable predictor of paralysis because of poor correlation between the AADI and the degree of cord compression as shown by MRI.
- Posterior atlantodens interval (PADI) has been found to be a better predictor of paralysis (Boden et al. 1993): the critical lower limit is 14 mm, which has a 97% sensitivity to predict paralysis.

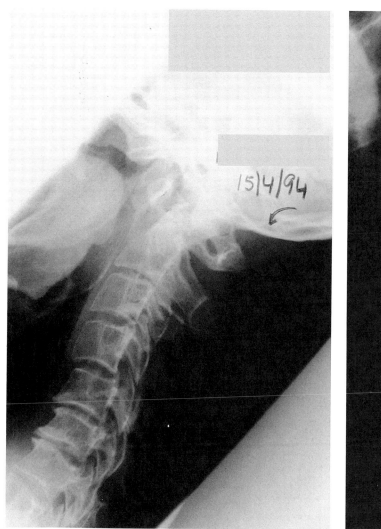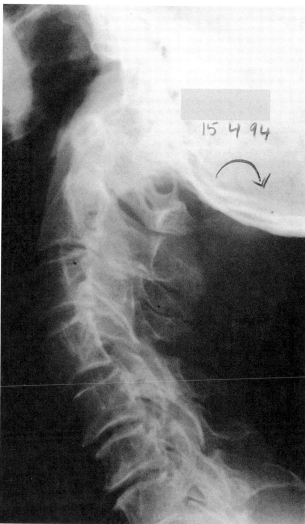

Figure 15–2: Atlantoaxial subluxation may appear as a dynamic instability. The atlantodens interval may become worse in flexion. The presence of dynamic instability may indicate surgical stabilization even when the interval is under the critical limit.

- The negative predictive value of PADI at 14 mm is 94%—that is, when PADI measures ≥14 mm, the chance that the patient will not have paralysis is 94%.
- It is important to recognize that PADI is not the same as space available for the cord; in RA patients, retro-odontoid synovial pannus may occupy as much as 3 mm of space (Fig. 15–3).

Superior Migration of the Odontoid

- SMO is less common than AAS, but it has a higher risk of myelopathy and carries a worse prognosis. It is diagnosed in the lateral radiograph from the station of the tip of the odontoid in relation to the skull base. It is often difficult to recognize the bony reference points in

the lateral radiograph, which has lead to several radiological reference lines to diagnose SMO (Fig. 15–4).

- Clark station is the station of the atlas in relation to the upper, middle, or lower third of the odontoid process in the midsagittal plane. If the anterior arch of the atlas is level with the middle third (station 2) or the caudal third (station 3) of the odontoid process, basilar invagination is diagnosed.
- McRae's line connects the anterior and the posterior margins of the foramen magnum—the tip of the odontoid should lie 1 cm below this line.
- Chamberlain's line is drawn from the margin of the hard palate (easier to recognize on a lateral radiograph) to the posterior margin of the foramen magnum. The odontoid tip should not project beyond 3 mm above this line.
- Both margins of the foramen magnum may be difficult to recognize without a tomogram.

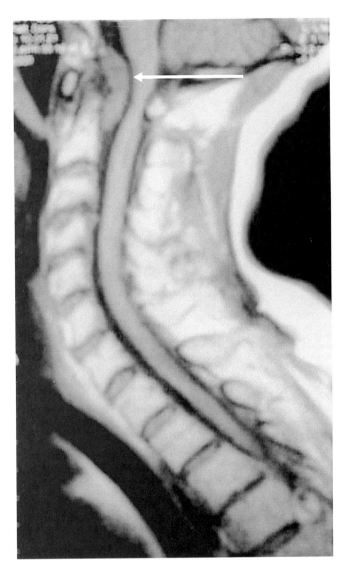

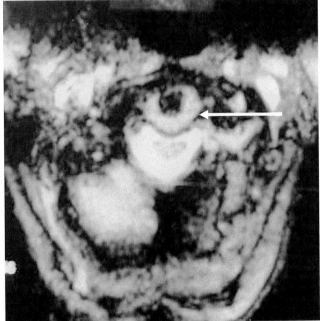

Figure 15–3: The true space available for the cord is not the same as the posterior atlantoaxial distance. The retro-odontoid synovial pannus (arrows) may occupy considerable space, leading to further cord compression. MRI scan is helpful to evaluate the actual space available for the cord, the cord diameter, and the cervicomedullary angle.

McGregor's line connects the posterior margin of the hard palate to the most caudal point of the occiput; the odontoid should not project beyond 4.5 mm above this line (Fig. 15–5).

- The odontoid tip may be difficult to identify in the presence of osteopenia or destruction; in these situations, there are few alternative radiological criteria available to diagnose basilar invagination.
  - Redlund-Johnell criterion is the perpendicular distance from the middle of the lower endplate of the axis to McGregor's line. The normal lower limit is 34 mm in men and 29 mm in women (Redlund-Johnell et al. 1984).
  - Ranawat criterion is an alternative. This is the distance between the center of the pedicle of axis and the transverse axis of the atlas. A measurement of less than 15 mm in males and less than 13 mm in females indicates basilar invagination (Fig. 15–5).

- A study of the different radiological diagnostic criteria by blinded observers on plain radiographs showed that no single screening test had a sensitivity higher than 90%. But when the Clark station, the Redlund-Johnell criterion, and the Ranawat criterion were measured and at least one of the tests was positive, the sensitivity increased to 94% with a negative predictive value of 91%. This means only 6% would have a false-negative diagnosis; however, the specificity was only 56%, meaning that 44% would be falsely diagnosed as having basilar invagination and would undergo unnecessary advanced imaging studies to rule out SMO (Riew et al. 2001).

Subaxial Subluxation (Fig. 15–6)

- SAS tends to occur at multiple levels.
- A characteristic feature is a staircase or stepladder pattern of deformity.

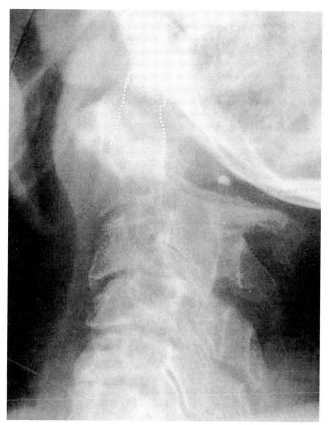

Figure 15–4: SMO may be difficult to quantify on plain radiographs. The anterior and posterior margins of the foramen magnum and the outline of the odontoid process may be obscure.

- SAS is differentiated from degenerative instability by a lack of osteophytes.
- It typically involves C2-C3 and C3-C4 levels—unlike degenerative instability, which tends to occur around the C5-6 level.
- Endplate erosions are evident in 12% to 15% of patients.

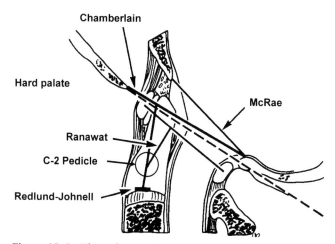

Figure 15–5: The reference lines in the schematic of lateral radiograph of the upper cervical spine for diagnosis of basilar invagination.

- Discovertebral destruction and narrowing may not always accompany SAS.
- Relative translation of the vertebral bodies (>4 mm) is better expressed as a percentage of the anteroposterior diameter of the inferior vertebral body.
- An alternate method is to measure the minimal spinal cord diameter behind the slipped vertebra; this may be a more reliable predictor of cord compression when it is less than 14 mm.
- A flexion–extension view may indicate a dynamic instability.
- An **MRI scan** is indicated whenever there is suspicion of instability on the plain radiographs.
  - Although a PADI greater than 14 mm is generally considered safe, a patient with a PADI of 13 mm could have as much as 12 mm to as little as 8 or 9 mm of space available for the cord, depending on the thickness of the pannus (Boden et al. 1993). MRI scan shows the exact space available for the cord (Fig. 15–3).
  - Space available for the cord may be further reduced in flexion. A flexion–extension MRI scan may show the actual space available for the cord in the presence of dynamic instability (Fig. 15–2).
  - If the spinal cord diameter is 6 mm or less in flexion, paralysis is predicted (Dvorak et al. 1989).
  - The cervicomedullary angle (normally 135 to 175 degrees) can only be measured from an MRI scan. It is reduced in the presence of SMO. Paralysis may be predicted when the cervicomedullary angle is less than 135 degrees (Bundschuh et al. 1988).
- **Tomography** is particularly helpful for quantitating the amount of basilar invagination and should be obtained if there is any suggestion of SMO on plain radiographs. It is important to recognize any degree of basilar invagination when present and to determine whether it is a fixed or a mobile deformity.
- A **computed tomography (CT) scan,** when used with a myelogram, may be particularly helpful in demonstrating cord compression. Measurement from a sagittal reconstruction CT scan may help to more accurately quantify the AAS and basilar invagination, which has shown a much higher correlation with neurologic status than plain radiographic studies.

Predictors of Neurological Recovery

- Ranawat classification—More severe preoperative neurologic deficit tends to have a poorer neurologic recovery. The operative mortality of Ranawat IIIb (nonambulatory) patients is 12.5%, and the survivors have a 61% mortality rate in the first year. This raises the question of justification of surgical intervention in the

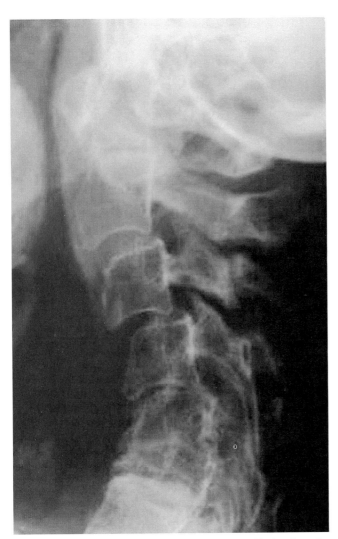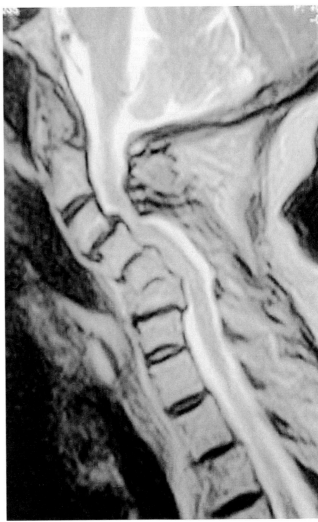

Figure 15–6: SAS in the rheumatoid spine typically involves the upper cervical region around C2 to C4 and often shows a stepladder type of subluxation.

presence of an advanced (IIIb) neurological deficit (Casey et al. 1996).

- Location of disease—SMO has a much worse prognosis than AAS and SAS.
- Preoperative PADI of 14 mm or greater predicts a potentially significant motor recovery after appropriate surgery. In contrast, PADI of less than 10 mm indicates a poor prognosis for neurologic recovery.
- A postoperative subaxial canal diameter less than 14 mm indicates poor prognosis for neurologic recovery.

Goals for Management

- Recognize the problem early (before an irreversible neurologic deficit occurs) by a practical and reliable screening method for serial evaluation.
- Avoid sudden death because of unrecognized spinal cord compression. The reported incidence is 10%.

- Avoid unnecessary surgery because 50% of AAS patients may never develop neurologic symptoms.

Indications for Surgical Stabilization

- *Definite indications* for surgery are the following:
  - Intractable pain
  - Definite neurologic deficit
- *Relative indications* include the group of patients with radiological instability but with minimal symptoms and no neurodeficit.

Atlantoaxial Subluxation

- PADI ≤14 mm indicates further investigation by MRI scan.

- Space available for the cord ≤13 mm, a cervicomedullary angle ≤135 degrees, or a spinal cord diameter ≤6 mm indicates a need for surgery.

Superior Migration of the Odontoid

- Any demonstrable SMO—on plain radiographs, CT scan, or MRI scan—is an indication for surgery because of high morbidity and poor prognosis with surgery in progressive basilar invagination.

Subaxial Subluxation

- SAS exceeding 4 mm in plain radiographs indicates the need for an MRI scan.
- If the residual subaxial canal diameter is less than 14 mm, MRI scan is indicated.
- If MRI shows space available for the cord ≤13 mm or a notable dynamic instability, surgery is indicated.
- A flowchart for the treatment strategy is presented in Fig. 15–7.

Surgical Stabilization

General Considerations

- A posterior atlantoaxial fusion or craniocervical fusion is the preferred method of stabilization. Anterior surgery (transoral decompression, subaxial corpectomy, and stabilization) is infrequently indicated for specific problems.
- A period of preoperative cervical traction using halo is recommended to relieve pain, reduce subluxation, arrest or reverse neurologic deterioration, and correct deformity. If subluxation may be reduced, decompression may be avoided and a less aggressive surgical procedure may be adequate.
- Traction in the recumbent posture in bed may be hazardous, resulting in pressure sores and pneumonia; halo wheelchair traction for 2 or more days is preferable.
- Fiberoptic intubation without neck extension is often indicated.

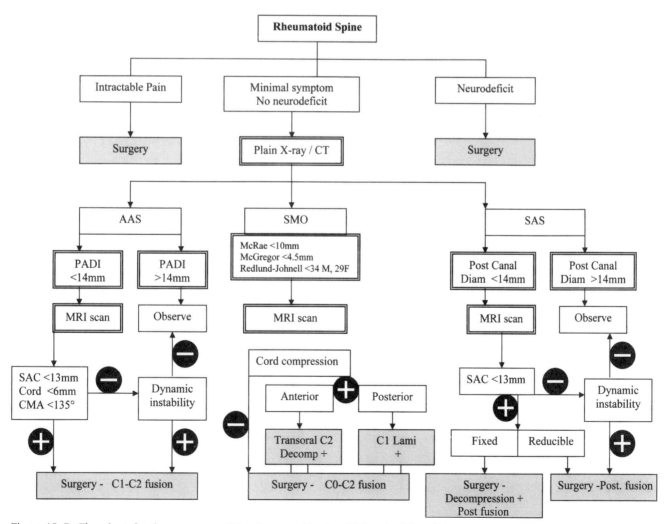

Figure 15–7: Flowchart for the treatment of the rheumatoid spine. (*F*, female; *M*, male.)

- The need for bone grafting is controversial. It is often indicated in young, fit patients. However, many authors question the morbidity of harvesting bone graft in elderly patients with end-stage RA, because studies show little difference in instrumentation failure in the long-term follow-up with or without bone grafting (Crockard et al. 1990).
- It should be emphasized that many of the indications for surgery are essentially preventive, and patients are often debilitated, with fragile skin, poor wound healing secondary to the disease process and steroid medication, osteopenic bone, increased susceptibility to infection, and a high perioperative morbidity and mortality rate.

Types of Surgical Stabilization

Atlantoaxial Subluxation

- AAS can be fixed by a posterior atlantoaxial fusion.
- When the subluxation is small or reducible, C1-C2 fusion may be performed by the Gallie wiring or Brooks wiring technique with an autologous bone graft. C1-C2 transarticular screw fixation, as described by Magerl in 1979, requires the reduction of subluxation but achieves better stabilization and may be performed when the C1 arch is thin or needs to be removed for decompression.
- When the subluxation is irreducible, C1-C2 lateral mass and pedicle screw fixation is an alternative method, but it is technically more difficult (Fig. 15–10).

Superior Migration of the Odontoid

- Posterior occipitocervical fusion is the mainstay of surgery.
- Because of the high morbidity and the poor potential for recovery, a more aggressive surgical approach is necessary.
- Isolated and fixed basilar invagination with no symptoms and no evidence of cord compression may be treated by observation.
- In the presence of cord compression, cervical traction is applied; if reduced, posterior occipitocervical fusion is indicated.
- If cord decompression is not achieved by traction, decompression by C1 laminectomy, in addition to occipitocervical fusion, may be performed.
- Anterior decompression by transoral resection of the odontoid is indicated when there is evidence of significant anterior pannus or marked vertical translocation of the odontoid (>5 mm).

Subaxial Subluxation

- In most cases, posterior cervical fusion with lateral mass instrumentation is needed.
- When evidence of cord compression is present, decompression by laminectomy may be performed with fusion.

- Rarely, when notable subluxation is present and cannot be reduced, anterior decompression with corpectomy and reconstruction with strut bone grafting may be indicated. Graft resorption and progressive collapse is not uncommon. Usually, additional posterior stabilization is advised.

Combined Subluxation

- In patients with combined upper and lower cervical instability, an occipitocervical fusion frequently may be performed, extending the fixation to all the anatomically involved segments in the subaxial cervical spine.
- There is a possibility of an accelerated progression of SAS following an occipitocervical fusion from the occiput to C2 level. Current data in the literature is inadequate to support this view.

Outcome and Complications

- The clinical success rate for cervical fusions in patients with RA ranges from 60% to 90%. It is often difficult to define clinical success in the presence of progressive generalized disease.
- Complications include death (5% to 10%), infection, wound dehiscence, implant breakage or pullout, loss of reduction, nonunion (5% to 20%), and late subluxation below the fused segment.
- Not all nonunions are symptomatic, and their management must be individualized.

Surgical Technique

- The *Gallie wiring technique (1939)* (Fig. 15–8) consists of an autologous bone graft fixed with a wire loop to the posterior arch of the atlas and the spinous process of C2. The advantage is the simplicity of the procedure. The disadvantage is inferior stability against anteroposterior translation of C1 on C2. The technique is not indicated unless the AAS is reduced and should always be supplemented with additional postoperative external support.
- The *Brooks wiring technique (1978)* involves two paramedial, wedge-shaped autologous bone grafts placed posteriorly between the arch of atlas and the lamina of the axis and secured by two wire loops. This technique provides superior rotational stability compared with the Gallie technique. However, it requires the wire loops to be passed under the C1 and C2 lamina in the spinal canal (Brooks et al. 1978).
- *Transarticular fixation of C1-C2 (Magerl 1979)* is a superior technique to wiring and can be performed even after laminectomy of the C1 arch. The fixation is achieved by one posterior screw crossing the atlantoaxial joints on each side; therefore it requires good reduction of the

Figure 15–8: Gallie wiring technique. A wire loop is first passed under the C1 posterior arch upward. A corticocancellous graft from the iliac crest is then placed over the C1 arch and the C2 lamina. The closed end of the loop is then bent down superficial to the graft and hooked around the spinous process of C2, and the free ends are tied together over the graft.

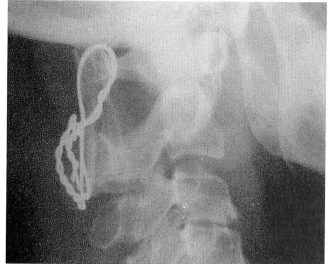

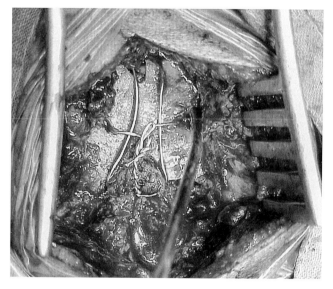

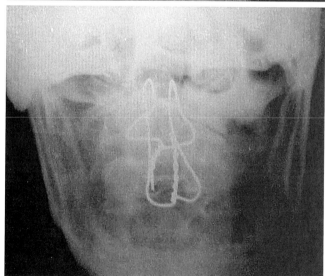

atlantoaxial joint. When performed with wiring, it provides three point fixation and therefore may eliminate the need for postoperative external support (Gebhard et al. 1998). However, the implants are small compared with the weight of the head, and additional external support may still be indicated to prevent implant failure (Fig. 15–9).

- *C1-C2 lateral mass and pedicle screw and rod fixation* provides superior stability (Harms et al. 2001). This is technically more difficult and carries a significant risk of injury to the vertebral artery. A three-dimensional CT reconstruction image using thin-slice CT axial images is an essential prerequisite. Theoretically, it may be performed even in the presence of an unreduced subluxation; however, that makes the procedure even more difficult (Fig. 15–10).

- *Transoral odontoidectomy* (Crockard et al. 1998) has an essential requirement: the ability to open the patient's mouth more than 25 mm. Temporomandibular joint ankylosis or flexion deformity of the neck may prevent

adequate opening of the mouth. An alternative approach is a midline mandibular split retracting the tongue downward. The risk of sepsis is usually overestimated. But poor dental hygiene or sepsis, excessive damage to the pharyngeal mucosa, or dural tear may increase the risk of sepsis and meningitis. Postoperative intraoral swelling is common and may be avoided by application of topical steroid in the oral cavity. Division of palate is not usually required and may be retracted by a suture.

- A midline 4-cm incision is preferred. The important landmark is the anterior tubercle of atlas. The vertebral artery lies 20 mm away from the midline. On either side, 10 mm of the anterior arch may safely be exposed. The arch of atlas and odontoid are removed by a high-speed air drill to decompress the dura. The pannus and the destroyed ligaments should be removed, exposing a clear pulsatile dura, to ensure satisfactory decompression.

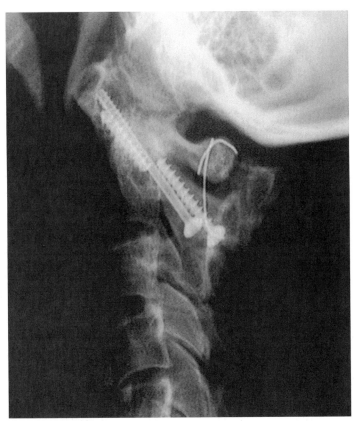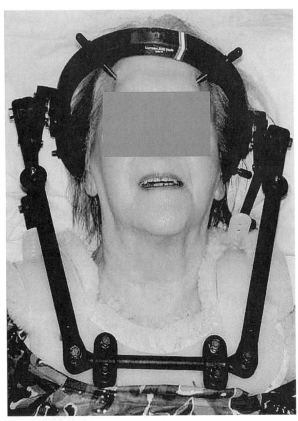

Figure 15–9: Magerl technique of C1-C2 transarticular screw fixation. With wiring, they provide a three-point fixation. Although the technique provides a strong fixation and good rotational stability, the implants are too small and additional external protection with a cervical collar or a halo vest may be recommended to prevent early implant failure.

- Usually anterior fixation is not indicated, and the segment is stabilized by posterior occipitocervical fixation.
- *Occipitocervical fixation* uses rods or plates and screws to connect the occiput to the cervical spine. Solid internal fixation is the aim to avoid cumbersome postoperative external support. In the presence of osteopenic bone, internal fixation may be augmented by metal mesh with or without bone cement.

Summary

- RA affects the cervical spine, causing instability in 50%-80% of subjects, toward the end of the first decade of the disease process.
- Only a small percentage of cases progress to develop a neurological deficit. Once a neurodeficit starts, rapid deterioration is the rule with a mortality rate of nearly 50% within the first year.
- Three types of instability are seen: AAS is the most common (65%) followed by SMO (20%), also known as basilar invagination, and SAS, involving a stepladder pattern of subluxation of multiple segments commonly affecting the C2-C3 and C3-C4 segments.

- Neurological deficit is most common with SMO, which also carries the poorest prognosis.
- Surgical stabilization is always indicated for instability with intractable pain or with any degree of neurological deficit.
- In the absence of significant pain or any neurodeficit, prophylactic surgical stabilization is indicated in cases with impending neurodeficit.
- Impending neurodeficit is predicted when the PADI is less than 14 mm, the space available for the cord is less than 13 mm, the cord diameter is less than 6 mm, the subaxial canal diameter is less than 14 mm, or there is any degree of SMO, as seen in radiographs, CT scans, or MRI scans.
- Posterior stabilization is usually indicated. Anterior decompression by transoral odontoidectomy or cervical corpectomy is rarely indicated for the decompression of anterior cord impingement.
- If the subluxation is reasonably reduced by traction, then AAS is stabilized by atlantoaxial fusion, SMO is stabilized by occipitocervical fusion, and SAS is stabilized by lateral mass instrumentation.
- Decompressive laminectomy of the subaxial cervical spine or removal of the posterior arch of atlas is indicated if persistent subluxation causes cord impingement.

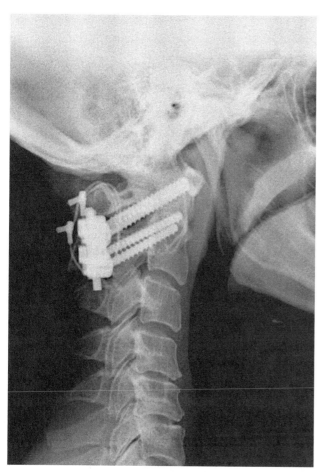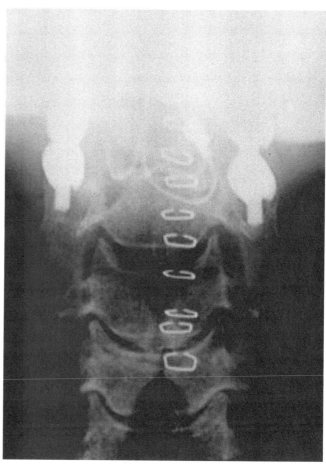

Figure 15–10: C1-C2 lateral mass and pedicle screw–rod instrumentation provides a strong fixation. Theoretically, it may be performed even in the presence of persistent C1-C2 subluxation, unlike Magerl's transarticular screw technique. However, persistent subluxation makes the procedure technically more difficult. In this particular case, additional Brooks wiring was performed to compress a graft between the C1-C2 posterior arch and the lamina.

- Complications are common and include death, infection, wound dehiscence, the loosening of hardware, or implant failure because of osteopenic bone and nonunion.

References

Boden SD, Clark RC, Bohlman HH, Rechtine GR. (1998) Rheumatoid arthritis of the cervical spine. In: The Cervical Spine (Clark RC, ed.). Philadelphia: Lippincott-Raven Publishers, pp. 693-703.

  The authors review the treatment strategy of cervical spine involvement in RA. They describe the radiological predictors of neurologic progression and outcome and outline a flowchart for the management of rheumatoid cervical spine.

Boden SD, Dodge LD, Bohlman HH et al. (1993) Rheumatoid arthritis of the cervical spine: A long-term analysis with predictors of paralysis and recovery. J Bone Joint Surg Am 75(9): 1282-1297.

  For this landmark article, the authors analyzed 73 patients who were managed over 20 years for rheumatoid involvement of the cervical spine and were followed for a minimum of 2 years. The average follow-up was 7 years. The authors found that the most important predictor of the potential for neurological recovery after the operation was the preoperative posterior atlanto-odontoid interval. PADI was a more reliable predictor than AADI.

Brooks AL, Jenkins EB. (1978) Atlantoaxial arthrodesis by the wedge compression method. J Bone Joint Surg Am 60(3): 279-284.

  In this original article, the authors describe a new technique of atlantoaxial stabilization using two sublaminar wires, one on either side, compressing a wedge-shaped graft between the arch of the atlas and the axis. This method is popularly known as Brooks fusion. Although more difficult, this method provides superior rotational stability compared with Gallie fusion.

Bundschuh C, Modic MT, Kearney F et al. (1988) Rheumatoid arthritis of the cervical spine: Surface-coil MR imaging. AJR Am J Roentgenol 151(1): 181-187.

  The authors describe the MRI changes in the rheumatoid cervical spine in 15 patients. They also analyzed the normal range of the cervicomedullary angle (135-175 degrees) in 50 normal subjects. They note that a cervicomedullary angle below 135 degrees indicates a high probability of neurological damage and the need for surgical stabilization.

Casey AT, Crockard HA, Bland JM et al. (1996) Surgery on the rheumatoid cervical spine for the nonambulant myelopathic patient—Too much, too late? Lancet 347(9007): 1004-1007.

In this original article, the authors describe their experience with 134 patients treated surgically for rheumatoid involvement of the cervical spine after the development of objective signs of myelopathy. They found a strong likelihood of surgical complications, poor survival, and limited prospects for functional recovery in nonambulant patients and recommend a strong case for earlier surgical intervention. At a late stage of disease, most patients will have irreversible cord damage.

Crockard A, Grob D. (1998) Rheumatoid arthritis—Upper cervical involvement. In: The Cervical Spine (Clark RC, ed.). Philadelphia: Lippincott-Raven Publishers, pp. 705-713.

The authors review the literature and describe the indications and rationale for surgery and the management principles of upper cervical spine involvement in RA. They also describe the indications, methods, and complications of transoral odontoidectomy.

Crockard HA, Calder I, Ransford AO et al. (1990) One-stage transoral decompression and posterior fixation in rheumatoid atlantoaxial subluxation. J Bone Joint Surg Br 72(4): 682-685.

In this original article, the authors describe their experience with combined anterior transoral decompression with posterior occipitocervical fixation in 68 rheumatoid patients with irreducible anterior neuraxial compression at the craniocervical junction. They found that use of bone graft may be justified in young subjects but question the morbidity of harvesting bone graft in elderly patients with end-stage RA, because studies show little difference in instrumentation failure in the long-term follow-up with or without bone grafting.

Dvorak J, Grob D, Baumgartner H et al. (1989) Functional evaluation of the spinal cord by magnetic resonance imaging in patients with rheumatoid arthritis and instability of upper cervical spine. Spine 14(10): 1057-1064.

In this article, 34 patients with atlantoaxial instability caused by RA were examined with plain x-ray views and functional MRI and were neurologically evaluated. The authors observe that the spinal canal diameter was significantly decreased in the flexed position and emphasize the need for a functional evaluation of the spinal cord by MRI.

Gebhard JS, Schimmer RC, Jeanneret B et al. (1998) Safety and accuracy of transarticular screw fixation C1-C2 using an aiming device: An anatomic study. Spine 23(20): 2185-2189.

In this anatomic study, the safety and accuracy of C1-C2 transarticular screw placement was tested in a normal anatomic situation in cadaver specimens using a specially designed aiming device. Five frozen human cadaveric specimens were thawed and instrumented with 10 C1-C2 transarticular screws according to the technique described by Magerl but using a specially designed aiming device described by the senior author (Jeanneret). The structure at the greatest risk was the atlanto-occipital joint, with one screw found to be damaging the joint.

Vertebral artery or spinal canal penetration was not observed in any of the specimens.

Harms J, Melcher RP. (2001) Posterior C1-C2 fusion with polyaxial screw and rod fixation. Spine 26(22): 2467-2471.

In this article, a novel technique of atlantoaxial stabilization using individual fixation of the C1 lateral mass and the C2 pedicle with minipolyaxial screws and rods is described. In addition, the initial results of this technique on 37 patients are described.

Lipson SJ. (1989) Rheumatoid arthritis in the cervical spine. Clin Orthop (239): 121-127.

In this literature review, the author describes the risk factors for the progression of cervical disease. They found that male gender, severe peripheral disease, and the use of corticosteroids indicate a rapid progression and poor outcome.

Magerl F, Seeman PS. (1986) Stable posterior fusion of the atlas and axis by transarticular screw fixation. In Cervical Spine (Kehr P, Weidner A, eds.). Berlin: Springer-Verlag, pp. 322-327.

The authors described the technique of C_1-C_2 transarticular screw fixation originally developed by Magerl in 1979.

Mikulowski P, Wollheim FA, Rotmil P et al. (1975) Sudden death in rheumatoid arthritis with atlantoaxial dislocation. Acta Med Scand 198(6): 445-451.

In this study, postmortem material of 11 consecutive cases of severe atlantoaxial dislocation with cord compression is reported. The total number of deaths from RA during 5 years was 104, and all were autopsied. They observed sudden death in 7 of the cases. Only 2 cases obtained a correct diagnosis intra vitam.

Pellicci PM, Ranawat CS, Tsairis P et al. (1981) A prospective study of the progression of rheumatoid arthritis of the cervical spine. J Bone Joint Surg Am 63(3): 342-350.

In this prospective study with long-term follow-up, the authors review the incidence of cervical spine involvement in RA and describe the natural history.

Ranawat CS, O'Leary P, Pellicci P et al. (1979) Cervical spine fusion in rheumatoid arthritis. J Bone Joint Surg Am 61(7): 1003-1010.

In this landmark article, the authors describe a new system for the classification of pain and the neural involvement in rheumatoid patients. They also describe a new method of measuring superior odontoid migration.

Redlund-Johnell I, Pettersson H. (1984) Vertical dislocation of the C1 and C2 vertebrae in rheumatoid arthritis. Acta Radiol Diagn (Stockh) 25(2): 133-141.

In a retrospective analysis of 450 patients with RA, the cervical films were reviewed to detect vertical dislocation of the C1 and C2 vertebrae. A frequency of 10% was found among all patients and one of 24% was found among those with cervical arthritis. The authors' method of measuring vertical dislocation using conventional radiography turned out to be superior to the method of McGregor, especially sin cases with severe dislocation. The vertical dislocation was shown to be preceded by a horizontal dislocation, and the appearance of the vertical dislocation diminished or abolished the radiographic appearance of the horizontal dislocation.

Riew KD, Hilibrand AS, Palumbo MA et al. (2001) Diagnosing basilar invagination in the rheumatoid patient: The reliability of radiographic criteria. J Bone Joint Surg Am 83-A(2): 194-200.

The authors studied cervical radiographs of 67 cases of rheumatoid patients (of which 29 had basilar invagination and 38 did not) who had tomograms, MRI, sagittally reconstructed computed tomography scans, or a combination of these to detect the presence of basilar invagination. Three observers, who were blinded to the diagnosis, independently scored each radiograph as positive, negative, or indeterminate according to the criteria for invagination established by various methods. No single diagnostic test had sensitivity above 90%, but a combination of Clark station, Ranawat criterion, and Redlund-Johnell criterion could increase the sensitivity to 94%. However, these combined criteria would result in a 44% false-positive diagnosis.

CHAPTER 16

Vertebral Discitis and Osteomyelitis

Rafael Levin★, Christopher M. Bono §, and Steven R. Garfin †

★M.D., M.Sc., Comprehensive Spine Care, Emerson, NJ
§M.D., Attending Orthopaedic Surgeon, Boston University Medical Center; Assistant Professor of Orthopaedic Surgery, Boston University School of Medicine, Boston, MA
†M.D., Professor and Chair, Department of Orthopaedics, University of California San Diego, San Diego, CA

Introduction

Anatomy

- The vertebral body is composed primarily of cancellous bone, which is highly vascular.
- The posterior arch (lamina, facets, and pedicles) is mostly dense cortical bone.
- The intervertebral disk is made up of the anulus fibrosis (outer with some vascularity) and the nucleus pulposus (inner and avascular).

Classification

- See Table 16–1 for classifications of spinal infections.

Vertebral Pyogenic Osteomyelitis

Epidemiology

- 2%-7% of all cases of osteomyelitis, 1%-2% of osteomyelitis cases in children
- Concomitant involvement of bone and disk (i.e., spondylodiscitis) is the "rule"
- Isolated bone or joint involvement (each represents around 1% of adult cases)
- Isolated discitis more common in younger children but still rare
- Can occur at any age (50% of cases in patients older than 50 years) (Sapico et al. 1979, Emery et al. 1989)
- Incidence increasing, especially in young intravenous (IV) drug abusers
- 2:1 to 3:1 male/female ratio (Currier et al. 1999, Hadjipavlou et al. 2000)
- Cephalad levels more prone to developing secondary epidural abscesses and thus more likely to develop neurologic deficits (Table 16–2)
- Mortality rate below 5% (Sapico et al. 1979)

Etiology (in Order of Frequency)

- Hematogenous spread from any condition causing bacteremia (Perronne et al. 1994)
  - Urinary tract infections and transient bacteremia from genitourinary procedures are the most common sources, followed by soft tissue infections and respiratory tract infections.
  - Frequency increases in association with IV drug abuse.
- Unidentified source (42% in one series—Emery et al. 1989)
- Direct inoculation (e.g., penetrating trauma or invasive spine procedures)

Risk Factors

- Immunocompromised hosts (e.g., diabetes, chronic disease, HIV, malnutrition, or steroids)

Table 16–1: Classification of Spinal Infections

FACTOR	DESCRIPTION
Organism	Bacterial
	Mycobacterial
	Fungal
	Parasitic
Anatomic location	Spondylitis—Confined to bony elements (common with TB)
	Discitis—Confined to disk space
	Spondylodiscitis—Involving bone and disk
	Epidural abscess
	Septic arthritis—Confined to synovial joint (e.g., rare facet joint arthropathy)
	Paraspinal abscess—Outside the vertebral column (e.g., psoas muscle abscess) and may eventually seed or extend to the spine
	Describe by region—Cervical, thoracic, thoracolumbar junction, lumbar, sacral
Route	Hematogenous (most common)
	Direct inoculation (including iatrogenic, e.g., after discography)
	Contiguous spread (e.g., psoas abscess)
Chronicity	Acute (<6 weeks)
	Subacute (6 weeks to 3 months)
	Chronic (>3 months)
Host age	Pediatric or adult

- Elderly males
- IV drug abuse (Currier et al. 1999, Hadjipavlou et al. 2000, Sapico et al. 1979, Perronne et al. 1994)

Causative Bacteria

Gram-positive Aerobic Cocci

- Most common (>80% of all isolates in one series) (Hadjipavlou et al. 2000)
- *Staphylococcus aureus* isolated in more than 50% of all infections (Currier et al. 1999, Hadjipavlou et al. 2000, Sapico et al. 1979)
  - Recent increase in methicillin-resistant *S. aureus* is a growing concern (6.8% of all isolated bacteria in one series) (Hadjipavlou et al. 2000)
- Streptococcus is the second most common followed by coagulase-negative staphylococcus (20% and 15% of

Table 16–2: Location of Vertebral Pyogenic Osteomyelitis and Secondary Epidural Abscesses

REGION	LUMBAR	THORACIC	CERVICAL
Spondylodiscitis	50%	35%	<10%
Secondary epidural abscess (% of total cases)	40%	33%	27%
Secondary epidural abscess (% of cases within a specific spinal region)	24%	33%	90%

isolates in one series, respectively) (Hadjipavlou et al. 2000)

Gram-negative Aerobic Cocci

- 15%-20% of isolates in one series (Hadjipavlou et al. 2000)
- Organisms responsible for urinary tract infections are the most common
  - *Escherichia coli*
  - *Pseudomonas aeruginosa* (also frequent in IV drug abusers)
  - Proteus species

Gastrointestinal Tract Organisms

- Salmonella is rare, but the following is true:
  - Has been reported following acute gastroenteritis or cholecystitis
  - Has a tendency to localize in preexisting diseased tissue
  - Is associated with sickle cell disease

More on Causative Bacteria

- Anaerobic bacteria are rare (e.g., foreign bodies, open fractures, wound infections, diabetes, or human bites).
- Low-virulence organisms such as coagulase-negative staphylococci and diphtheroids require prolonged incubation times. Infection is characterized by the following:
  - Indolent chronic presentations with delayed diagnosis
  - Frequency in elderly patients and those with immunocompromise
- There may be more than one organism (Hadjipavlou et al. 2000).
  - 25% of cultures → No growth
  - 51% of cultures → One bacteria isolated
  - 18% of cultures → Two bacteria isolated
  - 8% of cultures → Polyorganism

Pathology and Pathophysiology

- Mechanisms of **hematogenous** seeding and spread
  - Rich **arterial** anastomosis within the metaphysis of the vertebral body is most likely responsible for initial bacterial seeding of the vertebra.
  - Batson's valveless venous plexus (a presumed mechanism of metastatic spine disease) is not considered to play a significant role in bacterial hematogenous seeding.
  - Initial hematogenous spread into an adult disk is unlikely because of its relative avascularity. In contrast, a pediatric disk has a much richer vascular supply provided by numerous cartilage canals that, however, end in "cul-de-sacs" without an associated venous outflow (Fernandez et al. 2000).

- Once seeded, the vertebral body metaphysis provides bacteria with a low-flow environment that facilitates direct spread into and across the disk into the adjacent vertebral body.
- There is a hypothesized association between osteoporotic compression fractures and osteomyelitis. It may be the result of vascular stasis in the osteoporotic bone.
- Direct inoculation following invasive procedures (such as discography) is rare.
- Mechanisms of **bone and disk destruction** (causing instability and deformity)
  - Disk—Bacterial-produced enzymes that digest disk tissue (not ingested by the bacteria themselves)
  - Bone—Bone resorption by osteoclasts activated by various inflammatory mediators (not bacteria specific)
- **Abscesses** can be formed within the following:
  - Cervical spine—Retropharyngeal abscesses may invade the mediastinum.
  - Thoracic spine—Paraspinous or retromediastinal abscesses may occur.
  - Lumbar spine—Psoas abscesses occasionally distally extend through the sciatic foramen and cause buttock and lower extremity symptoms.
  - Epidural space—Epidural abscesses occur within the spinal canal and outside the dura to compress the spinal cord, cauda equina, nerve roots, or a combination of these.
- Mechanisms of neurologic compromise
  - Direct compression (e.g., epidural abscess, granulation tissue, bone or disk fragments, or deformity)
  - Neural tissue ischemia secondary to inflammation or septic emboli (rare)

Presenting Signs and Symptoms
Clinical History (Sapico et al. 1979, Perronne et al. 1994)

- Back or neck pain is the presenting complaint in more than 90% of adult cases.
- Duration of symptoms
  - More than 3 months before presentation in 50% of cases with a mean of 2 months in one series (Perronne et al. 1994)
  - Acute presentation with septicemia and toxemia extremely rare (in the antibiotic era)
- History of fever with or without chills is found in about 50% of cases.
- Atypical, nonspecific complaints such as chronic chest pain, abdominal pain, and leg pain are present in 15% of cases.
- Patients are often seen by multiple physicians for back or neck pain before accurate diagnosis. A high index of suspicion is important.
- In children, a limp and a refusal to walk are characteristically present. Fever of long duration and ill appearance

are more common in vertebral pyogenic osteomyelitis (VPO) than in discitis in children (Fernandez et al. 2000).

Clinical Signs

- Fever at presentation (>100° F)—About 50% of cases
- Limited range of motion, positive straight leg raise test, or both—15% of cases
- Neurologic deficit on examination—17% of cases

Diagnostic Laboratories and Tissue Analysis

- Erythrocyte sedimentation rate (ESR)—ESR is elevated at presentation in more than 80% of cases (Currier et al. 1999, Hadjipavlou et al. 2000). In treated patients, ESR drops to at least two-thirds of the original value by the completion of antibiotic therapy (Sapico et al. 1979).
- White blood cell (WBC) count—The count is elevated (>10,000/mm^3) in more than 50% of cases. A mean value of 8000/mm^3 was reported in one series (Lifeso 1990). A WBC count has low sensitivity for diagnosis (Currier et al. 1999, Hadjipavlou et al. 2000).
  - ESR and WBC are **higher in the presence of a concomitant epidural abscess.**
- C-reactive protein (CRP)—CRP is sensitive and more specific than ESR for monitoring postoperative spine infections (Thelander et al. 1992).
- Blood cultures—Blood cultures are positive in only 24%-59% of cases and are reliable in detecting the offending organism. They are most useful in children with VPO.
- Urine cultures—These cultures are not reliable.
- Needle biopsy—This is a fluoroscopically (Fig. 16–1) or CT-guided biopsy (74% reliability one series according to Perronne et al. 1994), but the following is true:
  - Nondiagnostic biopsy often occurs if insufficient tissue is obtained.
  - False-negative examinations can occur when the patient is on antibiotics.
- Open biopsy is the gold standard for definitive tissue diagnosis.
  - Lower false-negative rate than closed biopsy but higher risk
  - Indicated if needle biopsy is negative, nondiagnostic, or both despite high clinical suspicion

Imaging
Plain Radiography

- Radiography has a poor ability to differentiate pyogenic from nonpyogenic spine infection.
- Findings lag behind clinical presentation (at least 2 weeks from the onset of infection) (Fig. 16–2).
- Finding include the following:
  - Disk space narrowing with erosive changes in endplates (74% of cases)

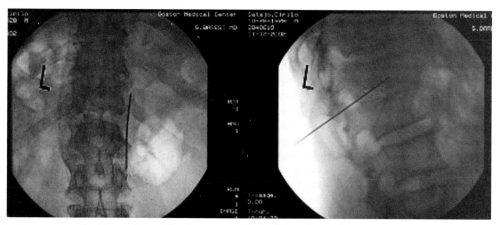

Figure 16–1: Percutaneous needle biopsy is an effective means of obtaining tissue diagnosis or pathogen identification. **It can be performed under CT or fluoroscopic guidance. Tissue from the disk space (shown), vertebral body, or paraspinal abscesses can be obtained. Abscess or soft-tissue masses are better accessed under CT guidance.**

- Lytic changes, diffuse osteopenia, or focal defect (50% trabecular bone destruction before radiographic evidence is noted)
- Bony sclerosis (11%)
- Involvement of transverse, spinous, or both types of processes (7.5%)
- Spontaneous bony fusion in about 50% of cases with a 1- to 5-year follow-up
- Look for fractures and deformity with potential instability.
  - Loss of height as in osteoporotic compression fracture (13%)
  - Kyphosis (acute gibbus at infected segment) or "scoliosis" (i.e., lateral angulation)
  - Translational instability or lateral listhesis
- In children with VPO, plain films were reported diagnostic in only 54% of cases compared with 76% of cases of isolated discitis (Fernandez et al. 2000).
- In infants, findings may be striking.
  - Almost complete dissolution of vertebral body
  - Nearly normal adjacent endplates
  - Late findings possibly mimicking congenital kyphosis

Nuclear Imaging

- Such imaging is useful as an initial screening (earlier detection and localization than plain films).
- The combination of gallium (inflammatory) and technetium (bone) scans provides 94% accuracy in diagnosis. Sensitivity for detection increases with the duration of the infection (Modic et al. 1985).
- Gallium scans normalize before technetium scans; the former is more useful to monitor treatment response (like CRP versus ESR) (Modic et al. 1985).
- Indium—111-labeled leukocyte (WBC) scans are not sensitive in the spine (sensitivity = 17%, accuracy =

31%). The high false-negative rate may be related to leukopenia.

Computerized Tomography

- Best modality for quantifying bone loss (Fig. 16–3)
- Excellent in defining spinal canal compromise.
- Used in computerized tomography (CT)-guided biopsies for tissue diagnosis

Magnetic Resonance Imaging

- Magnetic resonance imaging (MRI) is the imaging modality of choice for spine infections.
- MRI has 96% sensitivity, 93% specificity, and 94% accuracy (Modic et al. 1985). In children, 90%-100% are diagnostic for both VPO and isolated discitis (Fernandez et al. 2000).
- Such imaging can detect both epidural and paravertebral abscesses.
- It is best to differentiate infection from malignancy, benign tumors, degenerative disk disease, and osteoporotic compression fractures.
- Changes in MRI occur about the same time as gallium scans (Modic et al. 1985).
- MRI can be used as a screening study of the entire spine without ionizing radiation.

Magnetic Resonance Imaging Findings

- T1-weighted images—Decreased signal around adjacent endplates and disk space
- T2-weighted images—High signal intensity in bodies near adjacent endplates and disk space
- Loss of definition of endplate—Disk interface with irregular disk margins
- Disk and involved portions of vertebral bodies enhance with gadolinium contrast

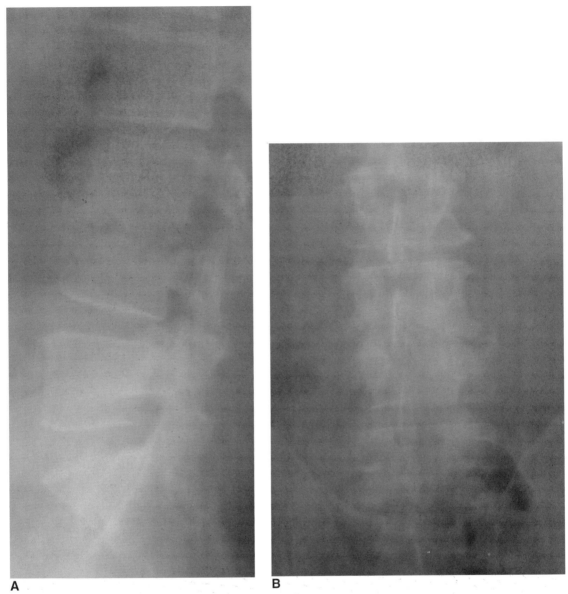

A **B**

Figure 16–2: Radiographs of a 47-year-old diabetic man with a 10-week history of back pain attributed to "arthritis." At the time of presentation, he was being treated for an open, nonhealing ulcer of the foot. Findings on plain radiographs (A and B) include disk space narrowing, fluffy endplate changes, diffuse osteopenia, and— with more longstanding disease—sclerosis.

- Absence of intranuclear cleft in the involved disk (Table 16–3 and 16–4)

Magnetic Resonance Imaging Limitations

- Claustrophobic, motion-dependent patients
- Cost and availability (though this is becoming less of an issue)
- Cannot readily screen the entire skeleton (versus a bone or gallium scan)
- Changes persist longer after clinical resolution than after a bone or gallium scan
- Difficult to discern normal increased disk signal in children from infection

Treatment Goals

- Establish tissue diagnosis and identify the organism
- Prevent bacteremia and sepsis
- Provide long-term pain relief
- Prevent or relieve neurologic deficits
- Restore spinal stability and near-anatomic alignment

Treatment Principles

- Perform medical optimization (i.e., improve nutrition and immune response).
- Treat extraspinous infection sources (e.g., urinary tract, respiratory tract, and gastrointestinal tract).

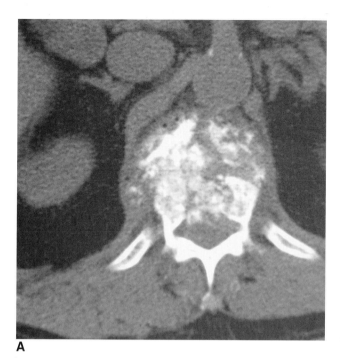
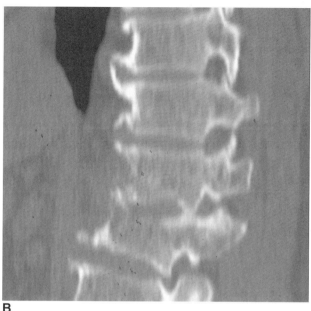

A   **B**

Figure 16–3: CT is useful in characterizing the extent of bony destruction. A, Axial images enable quantification of canal compromise. B, Sagittal reformation can also be helpful in visualizing bone loss.

- Avoid antimicrobial chemotherapy prior to the identification of an organism if possible.
- If biopsy is not possible, nondiagnostic, or negative (but clinical suspicion is high), a full course of broad-spectrum antimicrobial treatment may be initiated.

- In septic patients, broad-spectrum antimicrobial coverage should be administered immediately following biopsy and until a definitive diagnosis is made.
- Antimicrobial therapy is tailored according to cultures to minimize toxicity and resistance.

Table 16–3: Magnetic Resonance Imaging Differentiation of Infection, Fracture, and Tumor

DIAGNOSIS	T1	T2	DIFFERENTIATING CHARACTERISTICS
Pyogenic vertebral osteomyelitis	Decreased signal within disk and adjacent endplates Loss of endplate definition	Increased signal within disk and adjacent endplates with loss of endplate definition	Disk and endplate involvement > vertebral body involvement Hyperintense abscesses on T2 (more common in pyogenic than in tuberculous) Tuberculous spondylitis usually does not involve contiguous vertebral bodies (exception—advanced cases extend through anterior expansion) Soft tissue mass is poorly defined
Osteoporotic compression fracture	Decreased signal in the involved vertebral body Usually incomplete marrow replacement along the vector of compressive force in nontraumatic cases	Increased signal in the involved vertebral body Usually incomplete marrow replacement along the vector of compressive force in nontraumatic cases	Return to isointensity on T1 and T2 with fracture resolution Marrow preservation in the posterior third of the body and decreased anterior signal intensity on T1 Disk disruption and body fragmentation can be seen in traumatic benign compression fractures
Metastatic or neoplastic disease	Decreased signal, relatively well-defined area of mottled, infiltrative edema Pedicle often involved	Increased signal, relatively well-defined area of mottled, infiltrative edema Pedicle often involved	No disk or cartilaginous endplate involvement (i.e., does not cross disk space) Noncontiguous segment involvement is frequent No restoration of normal signal intensity (versus fracture); changes tend to progress Pathologic compression fractures—Diffuse, complete replacement of vertebral body marrow by tumor is noted, less so in multiple myeloma Soft tissue masses are eccentric, large, well defined (versus infection)

Table 16–4: Differential Diagnosis	
BENIGN	**MALIGNANT**
Infection	Metastatic carcinoma
Scheuermann's disease	Lymphoproliferative disease
Trauma	Lymphoma
Degenerative disease	Myeloma
Osteoporotic compression fracture	Primary mesenchymal sarcoma
Neuropathic spinal arthropathy	Radiation-induced sarcoma
Sarcoidosis	Chondrosarcoma
Paget's disease	Malignant fibrous histiocytoma
Hyperparathyroidism	
Benign tumor	

- Apply IV antibiotics for 6 weeks followed by oral antibiotics until resolution (clinically in laboratories).
- ESR and CRP levels are useful indicators of response to treatment.
- Immobilization is continued for at least 3 months if surgical stabilization is not performed.
- Nonoperative management can generally control infection, but surgery may be more effective in preventing neurologic deficit, instability, kyphosis, and chronic pain (26% versus 64% with residual back pain for operative and nonoperative treatment, respectively) (Hadjipavlou et al. 2000).

Operative Treatment
Indications

- To obtain tissue diagnosis when closed biopsy is nondiagnostic or negative (with high clinical suspicion of infection)
- To decompress a clinically significant abscess or granuloma
- Cases that have failed nonoperative management
- Neurologic deficit attributable to the infection
- Evidence of progressive deformity or instability
- Intractable pain not responsive to conservative measures

Operative Principles

- An anterior approach is the most useful for vertebral body debridement (corpectomy) and reconstruction of anterior column support (Lifeso 1990, Emery et al. 1989).
- An anterior approach is effective for decompression of the spinal canal if offending elements are anterior (most cases).
- Autogenous bone grafting (e.g., iliac crest, rib, or fibula) follows debridement or corpectomy to reconstruct the anterior column (Lifeso 1990, Emery et al. 1989). Despite concerns about implanting metal or allograft in the presence of infection, both autograft-filled titanium cages and cortical strut allografts have demonstrated good clinical results in children and adults in the setting of vertebral discitis and osteomyelitis (Govender et al. 1999, Dietze et al. 1997).

- Posterior fusion and instrumentation following anterior surgery (staged, 1 to 2 weeks) is indicated for cases with significant kyphotic deformity, for cases with multilevel debridement or corpectomy, or when postoperative orthoses cannot be used (Hadjipavlou et al. 2000, Dietze et al. 1997).
- Thoracic and lumbar VPO have been successfully treated by combined debridement and internal fixation using only a posterior approach (either staged or as a single procedure). Simultaneous use of autogenous interbody bone grafting had no increased permanent complications and allowed early mobilization in one series (Rath et al. 1996).
- Laminectomy alone for decompression is generally contraindicated because it further destabilizes the spine (Currier et al. 1999, Hadjipavlou et al. 2000, Lifeso 1990). It may be indicated for posterior epidural abscess with minimal to no bone involvement.

Prognosis and Outcomes

- Higher failure rates have been associated with nonoperative treatment in immunocompromised patients.
- The death rate is significantly higher in the elderly and patients with underlying immunoincompetence.
- There is a higher chance for permanent neurologic deficit with the following:
  - Advanced age
  - Immunocompromise
  - More cephalic level
  - Diabetes mellitus
  - Rheumatoid arthritis
- Neurologic recovery rates are higher with anterior than with posterior decompression (Currier et al. 1999, Lifeso 1990).
- Fusion rates with operative treatment are 90%-100% (Currier et al. 1999, Hadjipavlou et al. 2000, Lifeso 1990).
- Spontaneous fusion, either bony or fibrous, approaches 100% at 2 years for nonoperatively treated patients.
- Residual deformity or instability is more common in the thoracic spine, in the thoracolumbar junction, and in cases with more than 50% destruction of the vertebral body (Fig. 16–4).
- Vertebral osteomyelitis in the infant has the following:
  - A poor prognosis and high recurrence rate
  - Late radiographic appearance virtually identical to that of congenital kyphosis
- Vertebral osteomyelitis in IV drug abusers has an excellent prognosis.

Epidural Abscess
Epidemiology

- Most cases are in adults (and rarely in children).
- Incidence is 0.2-1.2 per 10,000 hospital admissions.

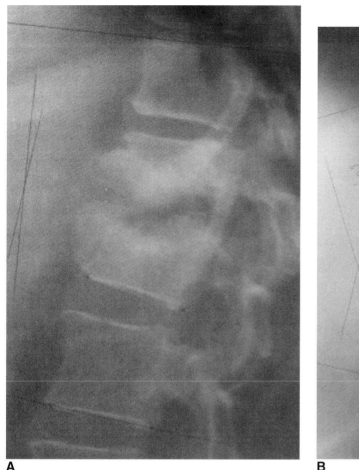
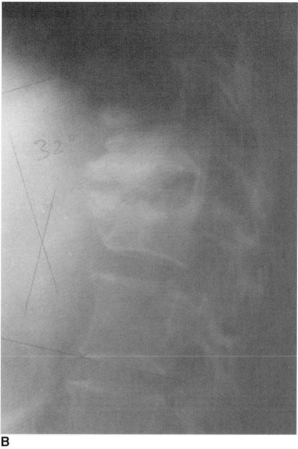

A   **B**

Figure 16–4: Radiographs of the spine of a morbidly obese woman "successfully" treated with a 6-week course of antibiotics. **Despite a normalized ESR and CRP at 2 years, she remained bedridden with intractable pain.** Supine (A) and standing (B) radiographs demonstrate an approximate 20 degrees of increase in kyphosis.

- Postoperative epidural abscesses represent 16% of all epidural abscesses.

Etiology

- Source identified in 60% of cases
- Can be hematogenous, contiguous (from VPO), or direct inoculation (usually iatrogenic)
- Associated with VPO in 28% of cases
- Skin and soft tissue infections the source in 21%
- The organism—*S. aureus* in about 60% of cases, gram-negative rods in 18% of cases (increasing in frequency and more common in IV drug abusers)
- Regional or location frequencies
  - Thoracic in 51%
  - Lumbar in 35%
  - Cervical in 14%
  - Posterior in 79%
  - Anterior in 21% (more common in lumbar spine and following vertebral osteomyelitis)
- Neurologic deficits most common in the thoracic region

Natural History

- Four chronologic stages (with variable and unpredictable transition time between each stage)
  - Local spine pain → Radicular pain → Weakness → Paralysis
- *Exception*—Patients with preceding VPO will have a predictable delay between the phases of spine pain and radicular pain followed by rapid progression. In these patients, neurologic deficits are reported in 82% of cases with an abscess located in the thoracic spine (Hadjipavlou et al. 2000).

Clinical Presentation

- Highly variable, leading to misdiagnosis and delayed treatment in about 50% of cases
- Complaints depend on acuity of presentation and stage of disease
- Localized spine tenderness often present
- Nuchal rigidity and other meningeal-type signs possible
- Neurologic deficit

Diagnosis

- Acute cases—More signs and symptoms of systemic illness
- Laboratory evaluation
  - ESR—Elevated in 100% of cases in one series (Hadjipavlou et al. 2000)
  - WBC—Variably and unreliably elevated
  - CRP
  - Abscess fluid—Diagnostic in more than 90% of cases
  - Blood cultures—Positive and diagnostic in 60% of cases
  - Cerebrospinal fluid analysis—Not routine, only if there are meningeal signs, and with positive cultures in around 17% of cases

Imaging

- Plain radiography and nuclear studies are generally negative unless there is VPO or discitis.
- CT is useful if MRI is contraindicated.
- MRI is the imaging modality of choice.
  - MRI findings include an intense focal signal on T2 (this may sometimes lead to false-negative scans in cases of long abscesses and concomitant epidural abscess and meningitis because of the limited contrast between bright cerebrospinal fluid and abscess).
  - *Warning*—Do not mistake abundant epidural fat or venous lakes for abscesses.
  - Epidural metastasis and subdural abscesses should be considered in the differential.

Treatment

- Epidural abscess = **surgical urgency**
- In general, surgical decompression and debridement with chemotherapy should be considered in every case involving the cervical and thoracic spine.
- An epidural abscess in the presence of a worsening neurologic deficit is a **surgical emergency.**
- Use fusion if the spine is unstable (iatrogenic or from VPO).
- *Exception*—One may consider nonoperative treatment consisting of antimicrobial therapy with close monitoring if the following are true:
  - Surgery would endanger the patient's life (comorbidites).
  - There is an absence of any neurologic deficits or signs when an epidural abscess is present in the lumbar spine.

Antibiotic Management

- Broad-spectrum IV antibiotic therapy should be started immediately after a culture specimen is obtained. With a progressive neurologic deficit **in a patient who cannot undergo surgery**, broad-spectrum antibiosis is initiated without culture.
- Gram-negative coverage is important in IV drug abuse.

- Duration should be 2-4 weeks after operating if complete debridement and wound closure is achieved; there should be 6 weeks with concomitant VPO or discitis followed by 6 weeks of oral antibiotics.

Operative Procedure

- Approach determined by the location of the abscess
  - Laminectomy for a posterior abscess
  - Anterior decompression for an anterior abscess (usually with VPO as described previously)

Prognosis

- After surgery, 78% of patients with either acute or chronic epidural abscesses have full or near full recovery.
- There is a poor prognosis for neurologic recovery if one of the following are true:
  - Complete paralysis for more than 48 hours
  - Complete paraplegia within the first 12 hours
  - Complete sensory loss
  - Diabetes
  - Advanced age
  - Female
  - HIV
  - Associated VPO
- The presence of granulation tissue instead of a frank abscess is a positive prognostic factor.

Granulomatous Spine Infections

- Epidemiology—Worldwide, tuberculosis (TB) is the most common granulomatous spine infection.
- Of patients infected with TB, only 10% develop bone or joint involvement. Of those patients, 50% develop spinal TB, making the spine the most common site of skeletal involvement. In addition, 10%-47% have a neurologic deficit.
- Age at presentation and incidence is influenced by public health availability.
  - Infants or children—In *under*developed regions (because of malnutrition and overcrowding)
  - Any age (adults and children)—In develop*ing* countries
  - Elderly or immunocompromised—In develop*ed* countries

Etiology

- Hematogenous spread is the most common route (pulmonary or genitourinary infections).
- Direct extension from visceral lesions has also been described.

Pathogenesis and Pathology (Table 16–5)

- Most involve the anterior spine.
- Vertebral body is initially seeded.

Table 16–5: Pathologic Findings in Tuberculosis Spondylitis versus Pyogenic Spine Infections				
	DISK INVOLVEMENT	**TIME COURSE**	**DEFORMITY**	**PARASPINAL ABSCESSES**
TB spondylitis	Rare	Slow progression	Frequent, significant	Larger, common
Pyogenic spondylitis	Always	Relatively fast progression	Less frequent, usually not as significant	Small, not common

- Involvement of adjacent levels—From expansion of an anterior granuloma that eventually bridges a disk space to involve an adjacent vertebral body
- Less common—Primary involvement of posterior elements (i.e., laminae)
- Secondary pyogenic infections—Through sinus tracts or iatrogenically after debridement procedures
- Neurologic deficits may develop acutely or by chronic progression.
- Mechanisms of neurologic deficits are as follows:
  - Cord compression (e.g., granuloma or abscess, sequestered bone or disk fragment, and instability)
- About half of infections are widespread at presentation. Focal TB infections represent the other half and can be further divided into three types:
  - Peridiscal (most common)—Starts in metaphysis and spreads under the anterior longitudinal ligament to adjacent vertebral bodies, skipping intervening disks
  - Central (rare)—Starts within a single vertebral body and may be mistaken for a tumor
  - Anterior (rare)—Starts under the anterior longitudinal ligament and can involve multiple segments

Clinical Presentation

- Pain comes with evidence of systemic illness—fever, malaise, and weight loss. The duration of symptoms before presentation is typically long (a mean of 5 months versus 2 months for VPO).
- Thoracic spine is most commonly involved followed by lumbar and, rarely, cervical or sacral involvement.
- Examination demonstrates local tenderness, muscle spasm, and limited range of motion.
- Paraplegia is more likely with thoracic or cervical involvement; it is more common in adults than in children.
- IV drug abusers can have a more disseminated disease that is more acutely toxic and rapidly progressive.

Diagnosis

- Definitive diagnosis is by tissue biopsy of spinal or extraspinal lesions, whichever is more accessible. Culturing mycobacterium can be difficult, may require a long time, and may have up to a 50% false-negative rate.
- Differential diagnosis includes other infections, neoplasms, sarcoidosis, and Charcot spine.
- Indicators of exposure to TB include a positive response to purified protein derivative skin testing (can be positive

in those inoculated with the bacillus Calmette-Guérin vaccine)
- ESR, CRP, and urine and sputum cultures are helpful but do not supplant tissue diagnosis.

Imaging

- Plain radiographs—Findings depend on infection type
  - Peridiscal type—Most common in the lumbar spine; similar to VPO with disk narrowing followed by bone destruction (Fig. 16–5)
  - Central type—Most common in the thoracic spine; resembles tumor bone destruction or collapse
  - Anterior type—Scalloping of the anterior aspect of adjacent vertebrae
- Nuclear imaging—Not sensitive for diagnosing and monitoring TB spine infections
- CT—Best for bony detail; may show some soft tissue changes in the paraspinal area

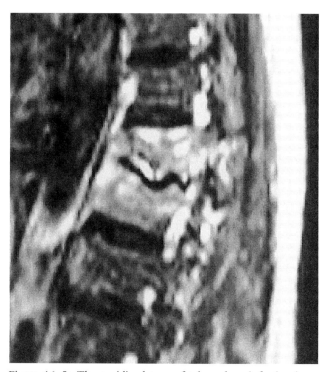

Figure 16–5: The peridiscal type of tuberculous infection is the most common. The vertebral bodies are primarily affected, with relative preservation of the disk space. Eventually, it can become collapsed. Spread to contiguous levels occurs by way of an anterior soft tissue mass.

- MRI—Modality of choice; unique characteristics of TB versus pyogenic infections are as follows:
  - Disk space often spared
  - Involvement of anterior bodies over contiguous segments
  - Paraspinal abscesses and granulomas distinguished with the use of gadolinium (abscesses in TB spondylitis are usually longer than in pyogenic infections) (Fig. 16–6)
- Disadvantage—Centrally located TB in the vertebral body and an isolated epidural TB granuloma can be indistinguishable from metastatic lesions

Treatment

- Prescribe antibiotics for a longer duration than for pyogenic infections.
- A 6-month, 3-drug regimen including isoniazid, rifampin, and pyrazinamide is the standard first line treatment for drug-sensitive TB in most Western countries. Compliance is key to avoid drug resistance, particularly in high-risk patients such as those with HIV.
- Primary or secondary drug resistance requires aggressive individualized, high-dose, multiagent chemotherapy. Infectious disease consultation is recommended.
- Immobilization—Bracing and short periods of bed rest immobilization are best in cases in which surgery is too risky or not indicated.

Operative Treatment Indications

- Similar to those for pyogenic infection **except** for the failure of response after 3-6 months of nonoperative treatment

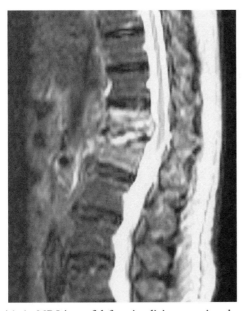

Figure 16–6: MRI is useful for visualizing anterior abscesses and soft-tissue granuloma. In this case, a large granuloma can be noted anterior to the T12 and L1 vertebral bodies.

Operative Treatment Goals

- Abscess drainage, debridement, neural decompression, stabilization, and deformity correction
- The Hong Kong procedure
  - Anterior approach for anterior pathology (Fig. 16–7)
  - Radical debridement (i.e., corpectomy) and removal of all necrotic tissue
  - Strut grafting or fusion using autograft or allograft, which restores the anterior column and maintains sagittal balance; fusion rates >95% (Dietze et al. 1997, Govender et al. 1999)
  - Better results when the infection is active (versus "burnt out")
- **Laminectomy alone is contraindicated** except in rare cases of isolated posterior involvement. If done, the surgeon **must** consider instrumentation and fusion.
- Posterior instrumented fusion to supplement anterior corpectomy and fusion involving more than two segments are possible (Guven et al. 1994).
- Costotransversectomy (for thoracic disease)—This posterior-only approach allows anterior debridement, limited anterior column reconstruction, and the use of posterior instrumentation and fusion.
- Cervical cord compression requires aggressive early intervention, anterior decompression and strut grafting, and staged supplemental posterior instrumented fusion as needed. Cervical **laminectomy alone is contraindicated** because of the high risk of kyphosis and instability.

Outcomes and Prognosis

- Overall prognosis with early diagnosis, compliance to chemotherapeutic regimen, and surgical intervention, when indicated, produces excellent results in the following areas:
  - Eradication of infection (close to 100%)
  - Neurologic recovery
  - Correction of deformity and instability
- The overall mortality rate should be less than 5% but may be as high as 11% with severe neurologic deficit.
- Negative prognostic factors include the following:
  - Advanced age
  - Immunocompromised host
  - Severe neurologic deficit
  - Extensive involvement of vertebral bodies
  - Severe deformity
  - Children—At risk for progressive deformity after anterior debridement and fusion (continued posterior growth)
- Neurologic recovery is best with aggressive surgical debridement and fusion, even in patients with paraplegia of long duration. Negative predictors of neurologic recovery include the following:
  - Involvement of meninges

Figure 16–7: This 74-year-old man had a 3- to 4-month history of intractable back pain. Cultures from a CT-guided biopsy were negative until 3 weeks, after which mycobacterium tuberculosis was identified. The patient was started on a three-drug regimen and placed in a form-fitting brace. However, upon ambulation with the brace in place, the patient complained of an inability to move his right foot normally. Neurologic examination demonstrated a new onset weakness of ankle dorsiflexion and plantar flexion. A, Plain radiographs demonstrated 35 degrees of segmental kyphosis at the T12-L1 junction. B and C, An MRI displayed anterior spinal cord compression from disk and bone fragments. The patient underwent emergent anterior decompression by corpectomy of T12 and L1 and anterior column reconstruction with structural allograft. D, This was followed by a staged posterior procedure that included posterior pedicle screw instrumentation and fusion with autograft from T10 to L3. Excellent correction of kyphosis was achieved. At a 3-month follow-up, ankle dorsiflexion was nearly normal and plantar flexion remained slightly weak (grade 4/5).

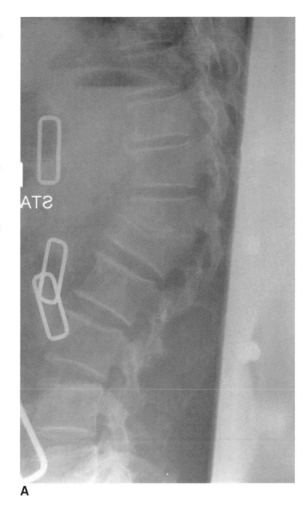

A

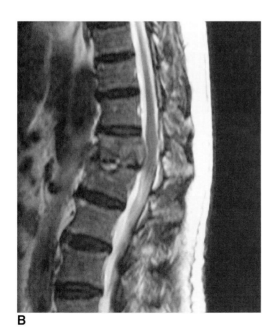

B

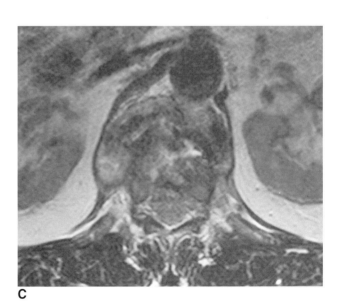

C

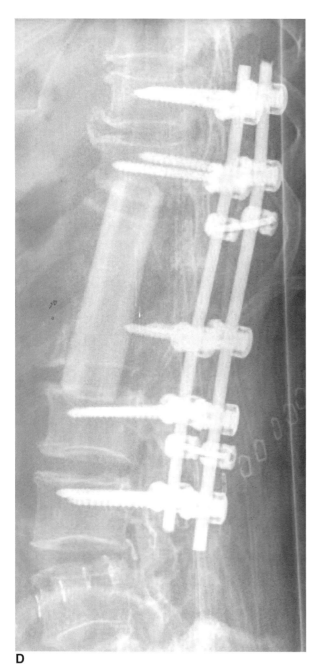

D

Figure 16–7: cont'd

- Atrophic cord
- Deficit of long duration
- Severe deficit
- Late onset of deficit in patients with resolved (inactive) disease

References

An HS, Vaccaro AR, Dolinskas CA et al. (1991) Differentiation between spinal tumors and infections with magnetic resonance imaging. Spine 16: S334-S338.

Thirty cases of biopsy-proven spinal tumors or infections were studied by MRI. Key distinguishing findings included the following: 1. Disk and vertebral body involvement was the most consistent finding with pyogenic infection on both T1- and T2-weighted images versus tumors in which the disk was consistently spared. 2. Loss of definition of the vertebral endplate was more common with infection versus tumor. 3. Contiguous vertebral body involvement was more common in infection than tumor. 4. Fat planes were frequently obscured in infection but are usually intact with tumor. The authors conclude that MRI is the imaging modality of choice for early detection and differentiation of spine infection from tumor.

Currier BL, Eismont FJ. (1999) Infections of the spine. In: The Spine—Rothman-Simeone (Herkowitz HN et al., eds.). Philadelphia: WB Saunders, pp. 1207-1258.

This chapter offers a detailed comprehensive literature review the history, epidemiology, pathology, clinical presentation, diagnostic workup, and treatment of all spine infections. Resources used in this review include articles taken from the infectious disease, radiology, pediatric, neurosurgery, and orthopedic surgery literature.

Dietze DD, Fessler RG, Jacob RP. (1997) Primary reconstruction for spinal infections. J Neurosurg 86: 981-989.

This article details a retrospective study of 18 cases of VPO and 2 cases of TB spondylitis treated surgically by debridement and fusion. Interbody fusion was performed in 18 of the procedures (10 used autologous and 8 used allogeneous bone) and posterolateral fusion (with autograft) was performed in 14 cases. Spinal instrumentation was used in 15 cases (4 anterior and 11 posterior). The authors conclude that primary arthrodesis with autograft or allograft with or without instrumentation can be performed in acute spinal infections with good results.

Emery SE, Chan DPK, Woodward HR. (1989) Treatment of hematogenous pyogenic vertebral osteomyelitis with anterior debridement and primary bone grafting. Spine 14: 284-291.

A retrospective review of 21 adult cases of VPO from a single center. All cases were treated with anterior debridement and 19 of 21 with autogenous strut grafting using iliac crest or rib grafts. Mean follow-up was 4 years with a minimum of 2 years. All cases with preoperative neurologic deficit (6 patients, most Frankel grade D) had complete motor recovery. Of the 19 attempted fusions, 18 were successful. The average increase in kyphosis was only 3 degrees. The authors conclude that single-stage anterior debridement and autologous bone fusion combined with IV antibiotics is a safe and efficacious method for eradication of infection, improved neurologic recovery, and spinal stabilization.

Fernandez M, Carrol CL, Baker CJ. (2000) Discitis and vertebral osteomyelitis in children: An 18-year review. Pediatrics 105: 1299-1304.

This paper reports the results from a retrospective review of 36 children with discitis and 14 with VPO. The mean age at presentation was 2.8 years for discitis and 7.5 years for VPO. Duration of symptoms was 33 and 22 days for discitis and VPO, respectively. VPO patients were more febrile (79% versus 28%) and appeared more systemically ill. The authors conclude that age and clinical presentation can help to distinguish discitis from VPO. Although radiographs were generally helpful for diagnosing discitis, MRI was the diagnostic modality of choice for diagnosing VPO in children.

Govender S, Parbhoo AH. (1999) Support of the anterior column with allografts in tuberculosis of the spine. J Bone Joint Surg Br 81B: 106-109.

The authors describe a retrospective review of 47 cases of pediatric TB spondylitis (mean age was 4.2 years). The preoperative gibbus deformity averaged 53 degrees. All patients were treated by anterior decompression and fusion using fresh frozen humerus allograft. At a 2-year follow-up, kyphosis averaged 15 degrees. Cross trabeculation between the allograft and the vertebral body was observed, on average, 6 months postoperatively, with remodeling evident by about 30 months.

Guven O, Kumano K, Yalcin S et al. (1994) A single-stage posterior approach and rigid fixation for preventing kyphosis in the treatment of spinal tuberculosis. Spine 19: 1039-1043.

Guven and associates document the results of their retrospective review of 10 cases of TB spondylitis treated by single-stage posterior instrumented fusion without anterior debridement or fusion. Minimum follow-up was 17 months. The authors conclude that in select patients, posterior rigid fixation and antibiotic chemotherapy can provide satisfactory stabilization and prevention of late kyphosis but avoid the morbidity of anterior surgery.

Hadjipavlou AG, Mader JT, Necessary JT, Muffoletto AJ. (2000) Hematogenous pyogenic spinal infections and their surgical management. Spine 25: 1668-1679.

In this retrospective study of 101 cases of pyogenic spinal infections (excluding postoperative infections), all patients underwent tissue biopsy, plain radiographs, gadolinium-enhanced MRI scans, and bone or gallium radionuclide scans to aid in diagnosis. Of the patients, 58 were treated surgically. Spondylodiscitis was by far the most common form of pyogenic spinal infection, with hematogenous seeding from a distant site the most common source. Epidural abscess complicated spondylodiscitis most often in the cervical region. This was followed by the thoracic and lumbar areas.

Lifeso RM. (1990) Pyogenic spinal sepsis in adults. Spine 15: 1265-1271.

Twenty adults with VPO and neurologic deficit were treated surgically with posterior spinal decompression. Anterior autogenous tricortical iliac crest grafting was also performed in 11 of these cases. Better neurologic recovery and a return to ambulatory status was found in the patients who underwent the anterior procedure at a minimum 2-year follow-up. The author concludes that anterior decompression and fusion is the optimal treatment for achieving pain relief, stabilization, and neural decompression. His experience demonstrates that autogenous iliac crest grafts incorporate well even in the presence of infection.

Modic MT, Feiglin DH, Piraino DW et al. (1985) Vertebral osteomyelitis: Assessment using MR. Radiology 157: 157-166.

Modic et al. performed a prospective evaluation using MRI, radiography, and nuclear studies of 37 patients clinically suspected of having VPO. Their findings were as follows: 1. MRI had a sensitivity of 96%, a specificity of 92%, and an accuracy of 94%. 2. Combined gallium and bone scan had a sensitivity of 90%, a specificity of 100%, and an accuracy of 86%. 3. Plain

radiography had a sensitivity of 82%, a specificity of 78%, and an accuracy of 73%.

Perronne CJ, Saba J, Behloul Z et al. (1994) Pyogenic and tuberculous spondylodiscitis (vertebral osteomyelitis) in 80 adult patients. Clin Infect Dis 19: 746-750.

The article details the results of a retrospective review of 31 cases of TB and 49 cases pyogenic spondylodiscitis from a single hospital in France. Blood cultures were positive in 56% of cases of pyogenic spondylodiscitis. Needle biopsy provided bacteriologic diagnosis in 74% of cases. Staphylococcus and tuberculous infections had high rates of neurological deficits (32% and 33%, respectively) compared with other pathogens.

Rath SA, Neff U, Schneider O et al. (1996) Neurosurgical management of thoracic and lumbar vertebral osteomyelitis and discitis in adults: A review of 43 consecutive surgically treated patients. Neurosurg 38: 926-933.

In this study, the 40 patients underwent combined posterior debridement and internal fixation with transpedicular screw–rod systems. Autologous interbody bone grafting was performed simultaneously in 18 patients and in a second, staged procedure in 21 patients. Most cases were VPO, though 6 patients had TB infection. Of patients with neurological deficit, 88% had improvement of at least one Frankel grade. The authors conclude that most patients with thoracic and lumbar osteomyelitis can be successfully treated by debridement and internal fixation using a posterior approach.

Sapico FL, Montgomerie JZ. (1979) Pyogenic vertebral osteomyelitis: Report of nine cases and review of the literature. Rev Infect Dis 1: 754-776.

A comprehensive literature review of 318 cases with VPO definitively diagnosed by tissue biopsy. Based on these studies, the authors calculated epidemiologic incidence, estimated the natural history, and reported the results of various types of treatment.

Thelander U, Larsson S. (1992) Quantification of C-reactive protein levels and erythrocyte sedimentation rate after spinal surgery. Spine 17: 400-404.

In this prospective study, the CRP level and ESR were measured before and after operation in patients undergoing four types of spine surgery (microdiscectomy, standard discectomy, anterior interbody fusion, and posterior interbody fusion). The CRP increased in all patients from normal preoperative levels to a peak of 46+/−21 on postoperative day two after microdiscectomy and anterior fusion, 92 +/−47 on day three after conventional discectomy, and 173 +/−39 on day three after poster interbody fusion. In all cases, the CRP normalized between 5 and 14 days postoperatively. The ESR peaked after about 5 days and remained elevated between 21 and 42 days after surgery. The authors conclude that the CRP is a better test than ESR for early detection of postoperative infection.

Vaccaro AR, Shah SH, Schweitzer ME et al. (1999) MRI description of vertebral osteomyelitis, neoplasm, and compression fracture. Orthopedics 22: 67-73.

This excellent review article compares the MRI characteristics of spine infection, malignancy, and compression fractures. Distinct MRI criteria are presented to aid accurate diagnosis. The authors also highlight the limitations of MRI in particular cases.

Primary and Metastatic Spinal Tumors

Luke S. Austin★, Jonathan N. Grauer §, John M. Beiner †, Brian K. Kwon ‡, and Alan S. Hilibrand ‖

★ Medical Student, Thomas Jefferson University, Philadelphia, PA
§M.D., Assistant Professor, Co-Director Orthopaedic Spine Surgery, Yale–New Haven Hospital; Assistant Professor, Department of Orthopaedics, Yale University School of Medicine, New Haven, CT
†M.D., B.S., Attending Surgeon, Connecticut Orthopaedic Specialists, Hospital of Saint Raphael; Clinical Instructor, Department of Orthopaedics, Yale University School of Medicine, New Haven, CT.
‡ Orthopaedic Spine Fellow, Department of Orthopaedic Surgery, Thomas Jefferson University and the Rothman Institute, Philadelphia, PA; Clinical Instructor, Combined Neurosurgical and Orthopaedic Spine Program, University of British Columbia; and Gowan and Michele Guest Neuroscience Canada Foundation/CIHR Research Fellow, International Collaboration on Repair Discoveries, University of British Columbia, Vancouver, Canada
‖ M.D. Associate Professor of Orthopaedic Surgery, Director of Education, Thomas Jefferson University, the Rothman Institute, Philadelphia, PA

Introduction

- The most common bony site for musculoskeletal tumors is the spine.
- The overwhelming majority of these tumors are metastatic in nature. However, a small number are primary benign or malignant lesions.
- Spinal tumors can be difficult to differentiate from other common diseases such as osteoarthritis, osteoporosis, and infection.
- Early diagnosis is associated with improved outcomes. Thus a thorough understanding of the common presenting signs and symptoms is imperative.
- This chapter reviews the different tumors found in each of three categories: primary benign, primary malignant, and metastatic. This chapter also reviews the basic pathogenesis, presentation, diagnostic workup, treatment, and complications of spinal neoplasms.

Pathogenesis and Pathophysiology

Primary Tumors

- Primary tumors of the spine develop from the transformation of any tissue of the spinal column.
- Primary bone tumors are uncommon and represent less than 5% of all spinal neoplasms.
- The cellular mechanisms of transformation are the same as those found elsewhere in the body. In other words, cells acquire certain capabilities, which include the following (Hahn et al. 2002):
  - Self-sufficiency in growth factors
  - Resistance to exogenous growth-inhibitory signals
  - Resistance to apoptosis
  - Immortalization (the ability to proliferate ad infinitum)

- Sustained angiogenesis
- Mutation in protooncogenes, tumor suppressor genes, and genes that govern cellular proliferation are responsible for endowing cells with these acquired attributes (Fig. 17–1).
- Benign lesions remain local, whereas malignant lesions possess the capability of metastasizing. Of note, lesions may be locally quiescent or aggressive regardless of whether they are benign or malignant.

Metastatic Tumors

- Metastatic tumors spread from distant parts of the body. In the musculoskeletal system, common metastatic sources include (in descending order) breast and prostate, thyroid, lung, and kidney.
- Metastatic spread to the spine is thought to occur according to the "seed and soil" theory. Tumor emboli seed the blood stream and embed in natural filters such as the highly vascularized red marrow of the vertebrae (Harrington 1986).
- Thoracic spinal metastases often originate from the lungs and breast. Seeding to the spine is thought to occur

through the valveless paravertebral venous plexus first described by Batson (1942).
- Lumbar metastases commonly originate from the prostate, which drains to the pelvic plexus and then to the capillaries of the local vertebrae by way of the lumbar Batson's plexus.

Presentation and Diagnostic Tools

History

- A careful history of anyone with a suspected spinal tumor is essential.
- In this patient population, pain (localized or radicular) is the most common chief complaint noted in 85% of cases. Other common presenting symptoms are motor weakness in 41%, mass in 16%, and other symptoms in 2% of patients (Weinstein, McLain 1987).
- **Pain secondary to a spinal tumor is classically localized, progressive, unrelenting, nonmechanical,**

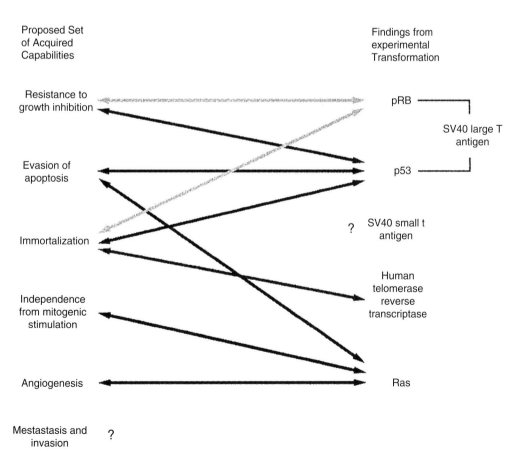

Figure 17–1: Transformation associated with cellular proliferation becoming deregulated. **On the left are the five acquired capabilities theorized to be needed in the transformation of cells. On the right are some of the known mutations in biochemical pathways that bestow these capabilities on cells. (Hahn et al. 2002.)**

and worse at night. **This is in contrast to pain from muscle spasm, degenerative arthritis, or other causes, which often relents with rest.**

- A patient's age, symptoms, and localizing complaints may help to narrow a differential diagnosis.
- A history of a primary tumor elsewhere in the body raises the concern of metastases.
- With primary tumors, certain characteristics help to predict the lesion type (Table 17–1).
  - Younger patients are more likely to have benign lesions.
  - The presence of a neurologic deficit, especially if rapid in onset, is associated with malignant lesions.
  - Primary tumors in the vertebral body are more likely to be malignant than those in the posterior elements.
  - Primary tumors found in the cervical spine are nearly always benign (Weinstein, McLain 1987).
- A careful history of neurologic symptoms should be ascertained. This helps to assess the aggressiveness of the lesion.
- Furthermore, the patient should be questioned about systemic signs and symptoms of malignancy, such as fevers, chills, night sweats, lethargy, unexplained weight loss, or changes in appetite.
- Especially in older patients, a targeted review of any potential metastatic source should be performed.
  - Risk factors for **breast cancer** include a first-degree relative with breast cancer, known mutations (such as BRCA-1, BRCA-2, Li-Fraumeni, and HNPCC mutations), any history of increased estrogen exposure (such as early menarche, late menopause, nulliparity, and prolonged hormone replacement therapy), and radiation exposure.
  - The main risk factor for **prostate cancer** is increased age (the disease is rarely found before the age of 45). Patients often complain of bladder outlet obstruction

in the form of hesitancy, decreased stream, and nocturia.

- There are several types of **thyroid cancer,** and they appear in different ways. Risk factors include iodine excess (papillary), iodine deficiency (follicular), radiation exposure, and genetic factors. Common presenting situations are an asymptomatic thyroid nodule, bone fractures from metastasis, and endocrine abnormalities.
- The most common risk factor for **lung cancer** is a history of smoking. Patients often have a cough or a change from a baseline cough. Hemoptysis and dyspnea are also common.
- **Renal cell carcinoma** has been linked to tobacco use and analgesic abuse. These patients have a classic triad of hematuria, flank pain, and palpable abdominal mass.

Physical Examination

- Physical examination, similar to history, should focus on two areas:
  - The spine and any resultant neurologic sequelae
  - Potential metastatic sources
- Examination of the spine includes palpation, range of motion, and neurologic function.
- A baseline neurological examination is imperative. Multiple studies have shown that the pretreatment neurological examination correlates with the post-treatment outcomes. The neurological examination should include the following:
  - Detailed motor examination, which may be compromised because of anterior spinal cord compression
  - Sensation examination, including light touch, pain, and vibration
  - Assessment of long tract findings such as reflexes, which may be abnormal secondary to cord compression
- As with the history, an examination targeted at potential metastatic foci should be performed.
  - Patients with **breast cancer** often have a hard, fixed, nontender breast mass; nipple retraction; skin erythema; or edema.
  - **Prostate cancer** may be associated with a large, hard, nodular prostate on digital rectal examination.
  - In **thyroid cancer,** a painless, palpable thyroid nodule and cervical lymphadenopathy may be found.
  - With **lung cancer,** distant or tubule breath sounds indicating pleural effusion or areas of hyperresonance indicative of atelectasis may be identified.
  - The most common finding on physical examination in **renal cell carcinoma** is a palpable abdominal mass.

Imaging Studies

- Several imaging modalities may be used in the evaluation of a potential spinal tumor (Table 17–2).

Table 17–1:	Clinical Features of Patients with Spinal Neoplasms*	
	BENIGN PRIMARY	**MALIGNANT PRIMARY**
Age at diagnosis	<21 years	>21 years
Neurological deficit	<33% of time	>50% of time
Sudden onset of neurological deficit	–	+
Vertebral location	More common in posterior elements	More common in the vertebral body
Spinal location	Of 31 cases	Of 51 cases
Cervical	6 (19.4%)	0 (0%)
Thoracic	12 (38.7%)	21 (41.2%)
Lumbar	6 (19.4%)	12 (23.5%)
Sacrococcygeal	7 (22.5%)	18 (35.3%)

* (Weinstein, McLain 1987.)

Table 17–2:   Imaging Modalities

IMAGING MODALITY	ADVANTAGES	DISADVANTAGES
Plain radiography	Simple and inexpensive Differentiates many pathologies and is satisfactory for diagnosing a majority of spinal tumors Helpful in the diagnosis of benign versus malignant neoplasms	Low sensitivity for small lesions—30%-50% of cancellous bone loss is needed for radiographic evidence of bone destruction Not sufficient for the development of a treatment plan
Bone scan	High sensitivity for spinal lesions that show osteoblastic activity The most sensitive tool for detecting metastases	Low specificity (cannot differentiate degeneration, fracture, infection, and neoplasm) Uptake does not correlate with the extent of tumor involvement
CT	Demonstrates bone better than other modalities Often important in preoperative planning	Impractical as a screening tool; the lesion must first be localized with radiography, bone scan, or MRI
MRI	High sensitivity, particularly when performed with intravenous gadolinium Excellent, noninvasive way of evaluating soft tissues Provides information on vascularity, presence of hemorrhage, and edema	High cost Extent and level of cord compression does not consistently correlate with symptoms or outcome
Myelography	Good visualization of epidural metastasis and cord compression	Invasive Extent and level of cord compression does not consistently correlate with symptoms or outcome
Angiography	Effective in assessing highly vascular tumors such as metastatic renal cell and thyroid carcinomas, aneurysmal bone cysts, and hemangiosarcomas Selective embolization of the neoplasm may decrease bleeding during surgery	Invasive

- **Plain radiography** should be the initial imaging modality in working up any spinal pathology (Fig. 17–2, *A*). This can help to identify spinal pathology. In particular, plain radiography has been shown to identify some abnormalities suggestive of tumor more than 90% of the time (Weinstein 1989).

- However, plain films have a low sensitivity for small lesions and lesions of the thoracic spine. In fact, 30%-50% of cancellous bone loss is required for a lesion to be noted on plain radiographs (Shimizu et al. 1992). For this reason it is often not until cortical bone destruction, such as that of the pedicle, occurs that a lesion will be noted with plain radiography (Fig. 17–3, *B*).

- **Bone scans** (technetium-99m) have high sensitivity but low specificity for metastatic and spinal lesions and may show uptake secondary to any fracture or degenerative disease (Fig. 17–2, *B*). Also, certain nonosteoblastic tumors, such as multiple myeloma, may not be detected.

- **Computed tomography** (CT) is excellent for visualization of bone and is often useful in surgical planning.

- **Magnetic resonance imaging** (MRI) provides exceptional definition of soft tissues and edema and has widely replaced myelography as the gold standard for the evaluation of epidural metastases and cord compression (Fig. 17–2, *C*).

- **Angiography** is effective in the assessment of highly vascularized tumors that may compromise surgery by excessive bleeding. Some such tumors are aneurysmal bone cysts, hemangiosarcomas, and thyroid and renal cell carcinomas. Angiography may also be used with selective **embolization** as a way to manage these lesions. This must be done close to the time of surgery or there is the risk of recanalization or collateral compensation.

- **Positron emission tomography** (PET) scans using F-18-fluorodeoxyglucose, a radiolabeled glucose molecule, measure local glucose metabolism. They can be used to detect and stage neoplastic lesions, characterize benign versus malignant lesions, and evaluate recurrent disease. Furthermore, PET scans are proving to be an excellent tool in the detection of spinal metastases with a greater specificity than bone scans.

- See the diagnostic and treatment flowchart in Fig. 17–4.

Laboratory Studies

- Laboratory studies can be used to help differentiate tumor from infection, which are often in the same differential. White blood cell count, sedimentation rate, and C-reactive protein should all be elevated with infection and normal or only slightly elevated with tumor.

- Multiple myeloma is associated with protein spikes on serum or urine analysis.

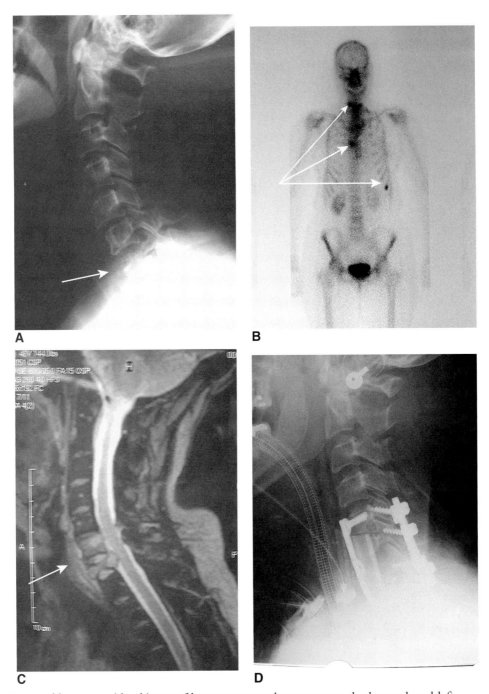

Figure 17–2: A 48-year-old woman with a history of breast cancer and mastectomy who has neck and left upper extremity pain. **A,** Plain radiograph shows C7 collapse. **B,** Bone scan reveals cervical, thoracic, and rib lesions. **C,** MRI shows the involvement of C6 and C7 with anterior soft tissue mass. The patient underwent anterior C6 and C7 corpectomies with allograft fibula and plate reconstruction and posterior supplemental stabilization.

- Lymphoma is associated with elevated white blood cell counts.

Biopsy

- Imaging studies, coupled with a thorough history and physical examination, are often adequate for determining the diagnosis and stage of a spinal lesion. However, when these fail to produce a definitive diagnosis, a biopsy may be required.
- The three-biopsy techniques are **needle biopsy, incisional biopsy,** and **excisional biopsy** (Table 17–3).
- All specimens should be sent for pathology, Gram stain, and culture.

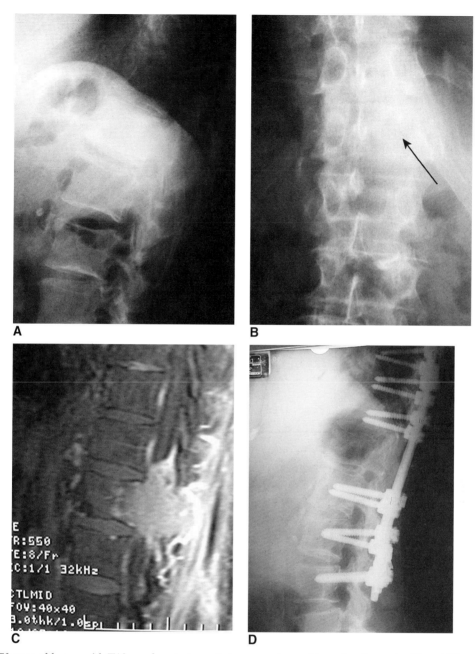

Figure 17–3: A 73-year-old man with T12 renal metastases. Anteroposterior and lateral radiographs (**A** and **B**) reveal the missing pedicle as shown by the arrow (often know as a blinking owl sign). This is further defined by MRI (**C**). The patient underwent posterior decompression and instrumented fusion after embolization (**D**).

Staging

- Staging of tumors serves several important functions:
  - Provides a common language for description
  - Allows the development of treatment protocols
  - Allows critical analysis of outcome results with different treatment modalities
- The **Enneking system** is a commonly used staging system of musculoskeletal tumors. This has three stages for benign lesions and three grades for malignant lesions (Fig. 17–5).

1. Benign stage 1 lesions are latent.
   - They grow slowly and typically are asymptomatic.
   - They have a true capsule with well-defined margins on plain radiographs.
   - Hemangioma is a typical example.
2. Benign stage 2 lesions are active.
   - They produce mild symptoms secondary to slow growth.
   - They elicit positive findings on bone scan.
   - They have a slender true capsule and do not extend out of their bony vertebral compartment.

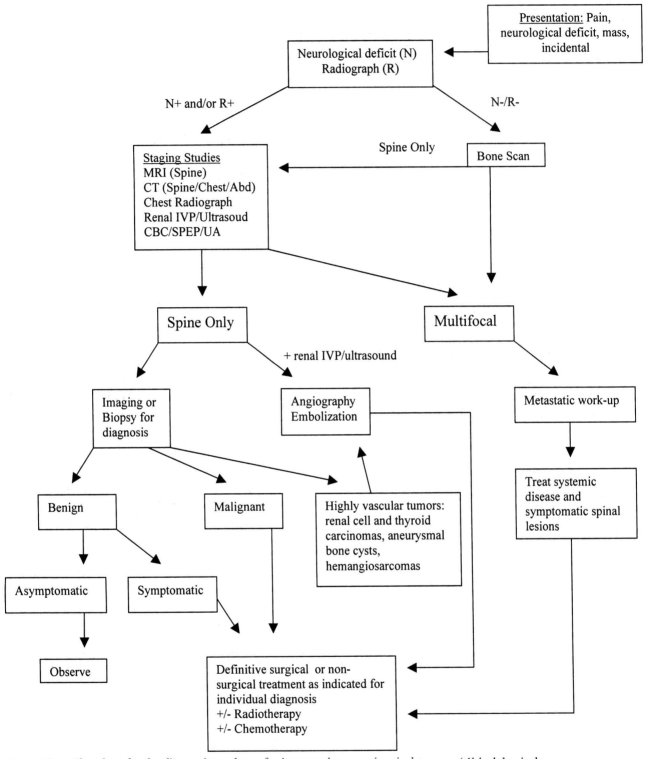

Figure 17–4: Flowchart for the diagnostic workup of primary and metastatic spinal tumors. (*Abd*, abdominal; *CBC*, complete blood count; *IVP*, intravenous pyelography; *N*, neurological deficit; *R*, radiograph; *SPEP*, serum protein electrophoresis; *UA*, urinalysis).

Table 17–3:	Methods of Biopsy*		
METHOD OF BIOPSY	**INDICATIONS**	**POSITIVE RESULTS**	**NOTES**
Needle biopsy	Ideal for differentiating possible diagnoses	65% of lytic lesions 25% of blastic lesions	Most spinal lesions can be safely accessed with CT guidance
Incisional biopsy	Useful when diagnosis cannot be determined by needle biopsy	>85%	A small longitudinal, midline, or paravertebral incision should be used
			Tissue contamination from biopsy or subsequent hematoma must be excised if definitive surgical resection is required
Excisional biopsy	Occasionally suitable for posterior lesions Generally used when a presumptive diagnosis has been made and biopsy is planned as the definitive intervention, such as in benign lesions	>85%	Uncommonly used for staging and diagnosis

* (Statistics from Boland et al. 1982.)

- Osteoid osteoma is a typical example.
3. Benign stage 3 lesions are aggressive.
   - They do not have a true capsule and often protrude through their pseudocapsule into surrounding tissue.
   - They are not confined to the vertebral compartment.
   - They are usually positive on bone scan with fuzzy borders.
   - Giant cell tumor is a typical example.
- The Enneking system grades malignant tumors as low grade (1), high grade (2), and tumors with distant metastases (3).
   - Malignant grade 1 and 2 tumors are further subdivided into intracompartmental (confined to the vertebrae) (A) or extracompartmental (extending out of the vertebrae) (B).
- The Enneking classification system has limitations when applied to spinal lesions.

- The extent of the lesions is not truly defined.
- The outcome is not directly related to the stage or grade.
- The **Weinstein-Boriani-Biagini (WBB) System** has been developed to describe spinal lesions. The system provides a three-dimensional description of tumor invasion by using anatomical zones, layers, and vertebral segments (Fig. 17–6).
- The vertebrae are divided into 12 pie-like anatomical zones starting at the spinous process and rotating clockwise.
- The tumor is also described by its involvement in different vertebral layers designated A through E: A is extraosseous soft tissue, B is intraosseous (superficial), C is intraosseous (deep), D is extraosseous (extradural), and E designates extraosseous (intradural).
- Further included in the WBB staging system is the spinal segment or segments involved.

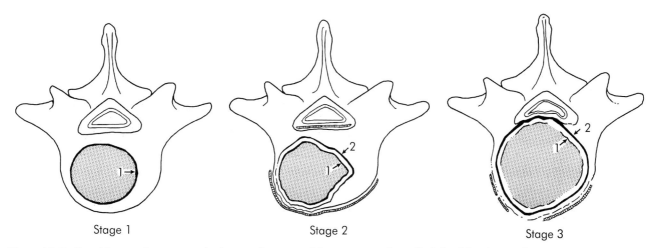

Stage 1   Stage 2   Stage 3

Figure 17–5: Enneking staging system. **A,** A stage 1 tumor with a true capsule, well-defined borders, and no reactive zone *(a)*. **B,** A stage 2 tumor with a slender true capsule that does not extent outside the bony vertebrae and a small reactive zone *(b)*. **C,** A stage 3 tumor with a pseudocapsule, with a large reactive zone, and not confined to the vertebral compartment.

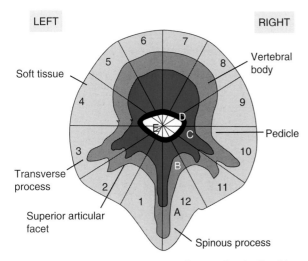

Figure 17–6: WBB staging system. The vertebra is sliced into 12 sections in a clockwise fashion starting at the spinous process. There are also five tissue layers designated A through E.

- A study performed by Hart et al. in 1997 on the clinical outcomes of giant cell tumors of the spine demonstrated the effectiveness of preoperative planning using the combination of the WWB and Enneking staging systems. Patients treated with complete resection at the referral treatment center had an 18% recurrence rate, whereas patients treated outside the referral center had an 83% recurrence rate.

Review of Specific Tumors

Primary Benign Tumors

- Primary benign tumors of the spine occur most commonly before the age of 21 and are seen more frequently in males.
- The most commonly occurring tumors are osteoid osteoma, osteoblastoma, aneurysmal bone cyst, eosinophilic granuloma, osteochondroma, giant cell tumor, and hemangioma. Table 17–4 lists their common characteristics.

Table 17–4:	Primary Benign Spinal Tumors*					
TUMOR TYPE	**GENDER**	**MOST COMMON SYMPTOM**	**VERTEBRAL LOCATION**	**RADIOGRAPHIC APPEARANCE**	**AGE**	**NOTE**
Osteoid osteoma	Male > female	Pain at night, relieved by salicylates	Posterior elements	Isolated radiolucency with surrounding sclerosis <2 cm in diameter	<30 years	Associated with scoliosis
Osteoblastoma	Male > female	Pain Night pain not as frequent as in osteoid osteomas	Posterior elements	Destructive, expansile lesions, some with sclerosis or calcification >2 cm in diameter	<20 years	Associated with scoliosis
Osteochondroma	Male > female	Pain or neurological symptoms during appositional bone growth	Posterior elements	Difficult to visualize on plain films because of the radiolucent cartilaginous cap	<30 years	Most commonly found in the cervical spine
Giant cell tumor	Female > male	Pain Neurological symptoms in 33% of cases	Vertebral body	Lytic, expansile lesion with matrix calcification and sclerosis	<30 years	Marginal resection necessary for a cure 10% incidence of sarcomatous change with radiotherapy
Hemangioma	Female > male	Rarely symptomatic	Vertebral body	Variable striations and honeycomb appearance	Variable	Radiotherapy effective if symptomatic Angiography and embolization useful
Aneurysmal bone cyst	Female > male	Pain	Posterior elements	Lytic, expansile lesion and fluid Fluid levels on MRI and CT[AU3]	<20 years	
Eosinophilic granuloma	Male > female	Rarely symptomatic	Vertebral body	Vertebral plana	<20 years	Self-limiting Radiological appearance similar to Ewing's sarcoma and infection

* (Abdu et al. 1998, Sanjay et al. 1993, Weinstein, McLain 1987.)

- The description of these tumors as benign is a misnomer because of their association with the spine. This association can lead to significant morbidity and mortality.
- However, a study performed by Weinstein and McLain demonstrated the 5-year survival rate to be quite favorable—at 86% (Weinstein, McLain 1987). They found no correlation between the method of treatment used and the survival or recurrence rates, except in the case of giant cell tumors.
- **Osteoid osteoma** and **osteoblastoma** are histologically identical lesions differentiated based on size. Lesions less than 2 cm in diameter are classified as osteoid osteomas, and lesions greater than 2 cm are classified as osteoblastomas. Both of these tumors have a propensity to cause scoliosis secondary to pain; however, this is more common with osteoid osteomas. The classic presentation of the osteoid osteoma is a young patient with back pain worse at night and ameliorated by salicylates.
- **Osteochondromas** are theorized to be an aberration in bone formation rather than a true neoplasm. They typically arise in long bones and rarely in the spinal column, with a propensity for the cervical spine. They are usually solitary but may appear at multiple sites. The latter is associated with a genetic disorder known as hereditary multiple exostoses.
- **Giant cell tumors** are more aggressive than other benign tumors of the spine.
  - They are generally Enneking stage 3 tumors.
  - They are responsible for 75% of all deaths from primary benign tumors (Weinstein, McLain 1987).
  - They tend to recur (Fig. 17–7) and case reports have demonstrated histologically benign primary giant cell tumor with metastases to the lungs.
  - They have a 10% incidence of malignant transformation following irradiation (Sanjay et al. 1993).
- **Hemangiomas** are highly vascularized tumors. They are rarely symptomatic but when symptoms occur, they are generally in the older population. The true incidence of this lesion is difficult to estimate because these lesions are generally only noted incidentally.
  - There are some atypical hemangiomas, which can have a soft tissue extension beyond the confines of the vertebral body.
- **Aneurysmal bone cysts** are uncommon lesions in the spine that occur most often in the lumbar spine. Among benign neoplasms, aneurysmal bone cysts are unique in their propensity to affect adjacent vertebrae.
- **Eosinophilic granulomas** are self-limiting. However, care must be taken to ensure the proper diagnosis because these neoplasms are difficult to distinguish radiographically from more malignant lesions, such as Ewing's sarcoma and infection. Open biopsy to obtain an adequate specimen is recommended.
- Overall, benign spinal tumors have been found to have a 21% recurrence rate irrespective of the extent of the

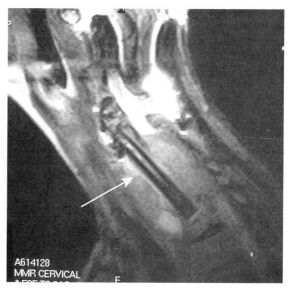

Figure 17–7: Example of an aggressive giant cell tumor (arrow) at the cervicothoracic junction. It recurred only 5 weeks after resection and allograft fibula reconstruction.

initial excision; half of the recurrences were giant cell tumors (Weinstein, McLain 1987). The 5-year survival rate for the group is 86% (Weinstein, McLain 1987).

Primary Malignant Tumors

- Primary malignant tumors of the spine generally occur in the older population and are more common in males.
- Overall, survival rates of patients with primary malignant tumors vary considerably with tumor type (Table 17–5).
- The most commonly occurring primary malignant tumors of the spine in descending order are solitary plasmacytoma, chordoma, chondrosarcoma, lymphoma, Ewing's sarcoma, and osteosarcoma. Table 17–6 lists some of their common characteristics.
- **Solitary plasmacytomas** are B-cell lymphoproliferative tumors and are thought to be a mild, unifocal form of multiple myeloma.
  - Solitary plasmacytomas have a better prognosis than multiple myeloma.

Table 17–5:	Incidence and Survival Rates of Patients with Primary Malignant Spinal Tumors*	
TUMOR TYPE	**N**	**MEAN SURVIVAL (MONTHS)§**
Solitary plasmacytoma	15	38
Chondrosarcoma	4	28
Chordoma	11	28
Ewing's sarcoma	4	28
Osteogenic sarcoma	3	18
Lymphoma	5	13
Others	4	36

* (Weinstein, McLain 1987.)
§ Survival scores truncated to 60 months.
† N, Number of subjects.

- Most lesions will eventually progress into multiple myeloma over time.
- MRI and serum M-protein levels should be followed indefinitely because of the likelihood of progression.
- **Chordomas** arise from the transformation of notochordal remnants.
  - Most tumors are seen in the sacrococcygeal and suboccipital regions.
  - Sacrococcygeal tumors can often be palpated through digital rectal examination.
  - Local recurrence is a poor prognostic indicator.
- **Chondrosarcomas** are slow-growing tumors that metastasize late in the course of disease (Fig. 17–8).
  - They often present symptoms of pain and a palpable mass.
  - These tumors are resistant to both radiotherapy and chemotherapy.
- **Lymphomas** are malignant disorders of lymphoid cells. Included in this category are Hodgkin's lymphoma,

lymphosarcoma, and reticulum cell sarcoma. It is important to elucidate the type of lymphoma because they are treated differently and carry different prognoses.
- **Ewing's sarcomas** are malignant round cell tumors that carry a worse prognosis when they arise in the spinal column. In the spine, the neoplasms have a predilection for the sacrum. Establishing a diagnosis using imaging modalities is difficult, and biopsy is often necessary.
- **Osteosarcomas** arise form the malignant transformation of mesenchymal cells. The diagnosis of osteosarcoma carries a poor prognosis.

Metastatic Tumors

- The most common tumors seen by orthopedists are metastatic tumors of the spine.
- Metastatic disease of the spine arises most commonly from adenocarcinomas of the breast and prostate, thyroid, lungs, and kidney in order of decreasing frequency.

Table 17–6: Primary Malignant Spinal Tumors*

TUMOR TYPE	AGE	PRESENTING SYMPTOMS	5-YEAR SURVIVAL RATE	RADIOGRAPHIC APPEARANCE	TREATMENT
Solitary plasmacytoma	Fifth or sixth decade	Back or lower limb pain	60%	Solitary punched-out lesion similar to that seen in multiple myeloma	Radiotherapy (highly radiosensitive) Surgical treatment indicated for stabilization and palliation Treatment correlates with the level of M light chain component on SPEP §
Chordoma	Fifth or sixth decade	Constipation, urinary frequency, or nerve root compression secondary to mass effect	86%	MRI is the study of choice and will give off a high intensity on T2-weighted images	Surgical extirpation with wide margins Sparing bilateral, midsacral nerve roots preserves some bladder and bowel function Adjuvant radiation for incomplete resection
Chondrosarcoma	>35 years	Pain and palpable mass	21% to 55%	Extensive bony destruction and a soft tissue mass with matrix calcification	Surgical extirpation with wide margins Resistant to radiotherapy and chemotherapy
Lymphoma	Variable with mean of 46 years	Local pain	58% for isolated lesion (reticulum cell sarcoma) 42% for diffuse lymphoma	Osteolytic lesions, ivory vertebra, and paravertebral soft tissue masses	For isolated lesion, treat with radiotherapy Treat diffuse lymphoma with radiotherapy and adjuvant chemotherapy
Ewing's sarcoma	Second decade	Pain and neurological deficit	33%	Sclerotic lesion with spiculated bone growth and often with a soft tissue mass	Combined radiotherapy and chemotherapy Surgery reserved for instability and neurological deficit
Osteosarcoma	<20 years	Pain and neurological deficit	Poor with median survival of 6-10 months	Mixed lytic and sclerotic lesion with cortical destruction and soft tissue calcification	Surgical extirpation with wide margins Combined chemotherapy and radiotherapy

* (Barwick et al. 1980, Camins et al. 1978, Cheng et al. 1999, Grubb et al. 1994, McLain et al. 1989, Ostrowski et al. 1986, Shives et al. 1986, Shives et al. 1989.)
§ *SPEP,* serum protein electrophoresis.

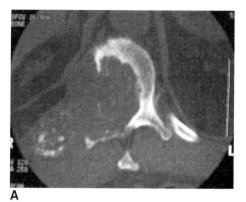
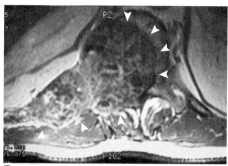

Figure 17–8: A 54-year-old man with a chondrosarcoma arising from the right T11 costovertebral junction. **Involvement can be seen by CT (A), and MRI (B).**

- Of patients with carcinomas, 50% to 70% will go on to develop skeletal metastases of which the spine is the most common site (Harrington 1986). Of patents with breast cancer, 85% will develop skeletal metastases (Weinstein 1988).
- Within the spine, metastases are more common in the vertebral body than in the posterior elements. This is thought to be because of the rich vascular supply to the vertebral bodies.
- Because the spine is the first source of symptoms of metastatic disease in 20% of patients (Schiff et al. 1997), a metastatic workup is often justified (see the preceding section covering presentation and diagnostic tools).
- Table 17–7 lists the best studies for the localization of the primary tumor when the initial manifestation is spinal metastasis.
- Surgical management of spinal tumors for specific indications has become more common as a result of patients living longer with metastatic disease.

Treatment
General Considerations

- The goals of treatment for a patient with a spinal tumor are as follows:
  - Establishment of a definitive diagnosis
  - Conservation or restoration of neurological function
  - Maintenance of spinal stability
  - Pain relief
  - Control of local and systemic spread
- Nonoperative treatment modalities include observation, radiotherapy, chemotherapy, brace wear, and pain management. In certain instances, surgical intervention may be warranted.
- Observation alone may be considered for patients with benign lesions that have self-limited natural histories (e.g., osteoid osteoma). Alternatively, observation may be considered for patients with end-stage lesions for which supportive measures are chosen.
- Radiation therapy is indicated in patients with the following (Tomita et al. 1983):
  - Cord compression caused by soft tissue tumor elements without compromise of the surrounding bony support architecture
  - Tumors responsive to radiation such as hematopoietic, prostatic, and breast cancers
- Chemotherapy is generally used for patients with systemic disease.
- Surgical indications include the following (Tomita et al. 1983, Harrington 1986):
  - Cord compression secondary to fracture or deformity
  - Instability
  - Progressive pain despite nonoperative treatment modalities
  - Isolated spinal lesions unresponsive to nonoperative treatment
- **Several variables must be defined prior to the development of a treatment plan:**
  - Specific tumor diagnosis—Primary benign, primary malignant, and metastatic tumors are treated

Table 17–7:	**Usefulness of Localizing the Primary Site of Neoplasm* §**		
STUDY	**N**	**POSITIVE STUDIES**	**STUDIES POSITIVE FOR MALIGNANCY (%)**
Chest radiograph	67	21	31
Chest CT	40	26	65
Abdominal or pelvic CT	31	24	77
Bone marrow biopsy	22	12	55
Serum immunoelectrophoresis	17	11	65
Abdominal ultrasound	11	4	36
Mammography	8	0	0
Barium enema	8	0	0
Upper gastrointestinal series	5	1	20

* (Schiff et al. 1997.)
§ Patients had spinal epidural metastasis as the initial manifestation of malignancy.
† N, Number of subjects.

differently; therefore diagnosis is the first step in management.

- Stage—The degree of spinal involvement and the potential involvement of distant sites will affect the treatment plan.
- Neurological status—This is the primary indicator of the post-treatment outcome. Patients with severe neurological deficits such as the inability to walk, paraplegia, and the loss of bowel and bladder function are less likely to regain significant function after treatment. Furthermore, rapid onset of neurological symptoms in less than 1 week is a poor prognostic indicator and suggestive of an aggressive neoplasm.
- Prognosis—Historically, radiation therapy has been encouraged for patients with poor prognoses, and surgery has been used more frequently for patients with longer predicted survival. However, with the decrease of surgical morbidity with more advanced surgical treatment methods, more cases are being considered for surgical intervention.
- Structural stability—Instability can only be addressed using operative techniques. Radiation therapy can increase instability.
- Pain status—Pain is the most common presenting complaint and indication for treatment.
- Prior to surgical intervention, patients must be evaluated and treated for the metabolic consequences of their tumor. For example, hematocrit, clotting factors, and immune status may all be affected by a malignancy.
- **There are two main surgical approaches to the spine—anterior and posterior.** The decision of which to use directly affects outcome.
  - Historically, decompressive laminectomy was the procedure of choice, but it did not address anterior pathology and predisposed patients to postoperative instability.
  - Currently, anterior approaches are more commonly selected.
  - To address the area of greatest pathology, reconstruction may be anterior, posterior, or both.
- Weinstein found that in patients with neurological deficits because of cord compression from primary or metastatic tumors, a satisfactory outcome was achieved in 80% of patients treated with anterior decompression and in only 37% of those treated with posterior decompression (Weinstein 1991).
- Posterior stabilization is generally necessary after laminectomy.
- Anterior column reconstruction can be performed with autograft, allograft, methyl methacrylate cement, or synthetic or metallic materials.
  - Autograft and allograft allow potential incorporation and biological fusion.
  - Patients who receive postoperative irradiation have decreased chances of achieving biological fusion.

- Methyl methacrylate offers instantaneous stability but may fail over time and should not be used in patients with a projected survival of 1 year or more.

Primary Benign Tumors

- By definition, benign tumors pose only a local problem. As such, these lesions have an excellent prognosis, irrespective of treatment. Management can be observation or local resection with or without reconstruction, depending on the effect of the lesion on the structural integrity of the spinal column and the effect on neural elements.
- The one notable exception to the relatively good prognosis of benign spinal lesions is giant cell tumors because of their local aggressiveness and high incidence of recurrence.
- When benign tumors are symptomatic, they often manifest themselves through back pain, neurological deterioration, or scoliotic deformities. These generally improve with surgical intervention.
- If surgery is needed, **osteoid osteomas** and **osteoblastomas** are treated with marginal excision. When margins are unobtainable, adjuvant radiotherapy can help to decrease recurrence rates with rare malignant degeneration.
- **Osteochondromas** are treated with excision only if a neurological deficit is present.
- **Giant cell tumors** are locally aggressive and have a propensity to recur; therefore they do not have the same favorable prognosis as other tumors in this class.
  - To achieve a cure, marginal resection in necessary (Fig. 17–7). If marginal resection is impossible, curettage, cryotherapy, and methyl methacrylate packing can decrease the rate of recurrence.
  - Irradiation is not indicated because of the 10% incidence of sarcomatous change (Sanjay et al. 1993).
- **Hemangiomas** are often incidental findings that require no intervention. Rarely, atypical hemangiomas may have a soft tissue component, which leads to compression of the neural elements. Once this diagnosis is established, such lesions may be treated with radiotherapy. If operative treatment is preferred, preoperative angiography and embolization can be used to reduce the perioperative bleeding and postoperative complications.
- **Aneurysmal bone cysts** are treated with excision.
  - Preoperative angiography with embolization has been associated with superior clinical results.
  - The injection of a fibrosing agent with or without surgery has been shown to give good outcomes.
- Biopsy of **eosinophilic granulomas** is often definitive treatment with most lesions resolving completely after the procedure. Symptomatic lesions can be treated with radiotherapy and immobilization with excellent results.

Primary Malignant Tumors

- All primary malignant spinal tumors have poor overall survival rates, meaning most patients will eventually succumb to the disease. However, short-term survival correlates with tumor type (Table 17–5).
- The one exception is solitary plasmacytoma, which has a greater long-term survival secondary to its radiosensitivity.
- Complete excision at initial surgery is the mainstay of treatment for primary malignant tumors. Surgical extirpation improves quality of life, and the ability to obtain surgical margins is the number one factor in determining survival.
- For tailored treatment suggestions of individual tumor types, see Table 17–6.

Malignant Disease

- Treatment of metastatic disease to the spine is controversial. Generally, metastatic disease is treated with chemotherapy. Spinal lesions require specific intervention on a symptomatic basis.
- Patients with evidence of spinal metastases without neurological impingement or vertebral collapse should be treated with chemotherapy and hormonal manipulation. This treatment provides excellent pain relief in most patients.
- The decision to use irradiation or surgery depends on the presence or absence of structural compromise and the extent of neurological impingement.
  - Patients with neurological compromise without structural instability or major bony destruction often receive adequate results from radiotherapy alone. If neurological deficits occur rapidly in a matter of days, adjuvant high-dose steroids are recommended.
  - Patients with intractable pain, neurological deficits, or both secondary to vertebral collapse with objective cord compression because of nontumorous elements may benefit from surgical intervention.

Complications

Radiotherapy

- Localized radiotherapy is relatively safe; most complications are secondary to irradiation and subsequent cellular mutation and death in the field being treated.
  - Cellular death can lead to local immunological incompetence, bone marrow suppression, radiation myelopathy, and osteonecrosis or osteitis, leading to further instability of the spinal column.
  - Radiation-induced cellular mutagenesis leading to future neoplasm is a concern in patients with a significant life expectancy.

- Multiple studies have demonstrated that radiotherapy increases the likelihood of surgical complications and therefore is not recommended preoperatively. Preoperative irradiation increases the incidences of postoperative wound infection and wound dehiscence, and it has been reported to negatively affect neurological recovery.

Surgery

- In a study of 80 patients performed by Wise et al. in 1999, 25% had either major or minor complications.
- The best predictive factors of postoperative complications are poor neurological status, insidious onset of neurological deficits, prior radiotherapy, and malnutrition.
- The most common surgical complications are as follows (in descending order): wound infections, urinary tract infection, hardware failure, pulmonary embolism, death, disseminated intravascular coagulation, paraplegia, and osteomyelitis.

References

Abdu WA, Provencher M. (1998) Primary bone and metastatic tumors of the cervical spine. Spine 23(24): 2767-2777.
> The authors review 73 articles about tumors of the cervical spine, focusing on presentation, workup, staging, and treatment.

Barwick KW, Huvos AG, Smith J. (1980) Primary osteogenic sarcoma of the vertebral column: A clinicopathologic correlation of ten patients. Cancer 46(3): 595-604.
> The article provides survival rates of patients with osteosarcoma.

Batson OV. (1942) The role of the vertebral veins in metastatic processes. Ann Intern Med 16: 38-45.
> Batson describes the anatomical pathway for metastases of tumor emboli to the vertebral column.

Boland PJ, Lane JM, Sundaresan N. (1982) Metastatic disease of the spine. Clin Orthop Rel Res (169): 95-102.
> This article provides a statistical analysis of the diagnostic efficacy of needle, incisional, and excisional biopsy.

Camins MB, Duncan AW, Smith J et al. (1978) Chondrosarcoma of the spine. Spine 3(3): 202-209.
> The authors describe the value of radiological studies, the effectiveness of treatment, and the survival figures of chondrosarcoma of the spine.

Cheng EY, Ozerdemoglu RA, Transfeldt EE et al. (1999) Lumbosacral chordoma: Prognostic factors and treatment. Spine 24(16): 1639-1645.
> A retrospective study of the prognostic factors and treatment of patients with chordoma.

Grubb MR, Currier BL, Pritchard DJ et al. (1994) Primary Ewing's sarcoma of the spine. Spine 19(3): 309-313.
> A retrospective study of 36 patients with primary Ewing's sarcoma of the spine. They found the 5-year survival rate to be 33%, and there was no correlation between prognosis and location of the tumor.

Hahn WC, Weinberg RA. (2002) Rules for making human tumor cells. New Engl J Med 347(20): 1593-1603.

> The authors review 121 articles on the pathogenesis of cancer. They conclude that a cell must ascertain specific acquired capabilities to transform into a malignant cell.

Harrington KD. (1986) Metastatic disease of the spine. J Bone Joint Surg Am 68(7): 1110-1115.

> A review article using 31 references on the pathophysiology, clinical coarse, diagnostic studies, and treatment of metastatic disease of the spine.

Hart RA, Boriani S, Biagini R et al. (1997) A system for surgical staging and management of spine tumors: A clinical outcome study of giant cell tumors of the spine. Spine 22(15): 1773-1782; discussion 1783.

> This study designed the Weinstein-Boriani-Biagini system and applied it to the staging of giant cell tumors of the spine. The study looked at the recurrence rate of giant cell tumors.

McLain RF, Weinstein JN. (1989) Solitary plasmacytomas of the spine: A review of 84 cases. Journal of Spinal Disord 2(2): 69-74.

> This study looked at 84 cases of solitary plasmacytoma of the spine. Survival rates, progression to multiple myeloma, and treatment modalities are described.

Ostrowski ML, Unni KK, Banks PM et al. (1986) Malignant lymphoma of bone. Cancer 58(12): 2646-2655.

> The study assessed 422 patients with malignant lymphoma of the bone. The authors looked at prognostic factors, survival rates, and treatment modalities.

Sanjay BKS, Sim FH, Ummi KK et al. (1993) Giant cell tumors of the spine. J Bone Joint Surg Br 75B: 148-154.

> This is a study of 24 patients with giant cell tumors of the spine. They found that giant cell tumors should be excised with wide margins secondary to high recurrence rates and that radiotherapy should not be used because of the 10% rate of sarcomatous change.

Schiff D, O'Neill BP, Suman VJ. (1997) Spinal epidural metastasis as the initial manifestation of malignancy: Clinical features and diagnostic approach. Neurology 49(2): 452-456.

> The authors performed a retrospective review of 322 patients with spinal epidural metastasis. They accessed patient presentation, the site of the primary tumor, and the diagnostic workup of spinal epidural metastasis.

Shimizu K, Shikata J, Iida H et al. (1992) Posterior decompression and stabilization for multiple metastatic tumors of the spine. Spine 17(11): 1400-1404.

> The study assessed surgical indications, procedures, complication of posterior decompression, and stabilization for multiple metastatic tumors of the spine. The authors conclude that the surgery is cautiously indicated considering the nature of the primary tumor.

Shives TC, Dahlin DC, Sim FH et al. (1986) Osteosarcoma of the spine. J Bone Joint Surg Am 68(5): 660–668.

Shives TC, McLeod RA, Unni KK et al. (1989) Chondrosarcoma of the spine. J Bone Joint Surg Am 71(8): 1158-1165.

> The article assesses the initial presentation, diagnostic workup, survival rates, and treatment of patient with chondrosarcoma. The authors conclude that surgical extirpation with wide margins is the preferred method of treatment.

Tomita T, Galicich JH, Sundaresan N. (1983) Radiation therapy for spinal epidural metastases with complete block. Acta Radiolog Oncol 22(2): 135-143.

> A series of 533 patients with spinal epidural metastases and complete block were studied. The authors describe the management and outcomes of these patients

Weinstein JN. (1991) Differential diagnosis and surgical treatment of primary benign and malignant neoplasms. In: The Adult Spin—Principles and Practices (Frymoyer JW, ed.). New York: Raven Press, pp. 829-860.

> The author explains the differential diagnosis and treatment of primary and malignant neoplasms. He concludes that the anterior surgical approach is superior to the posterior approach when the pathology originates in the vertebral body.

Weinstein JN. (1989) Surgical approach to spine tumors. Orthopedics 12(6): 897-905.

> This is a review of 25 articles on the surgical approach to spine tumors. The article focuses on treatment goals, diagnostic workup, surgical and nonsurgical treatment, and outcomes.

Weinstein JN, Collalto P, Lehmann TR. (1987) Long-term follow-up of nonoperatively treated thoracolumbar spine fractures. J Orthop Trauma 1(2): 152-159.

> This article was used as a statistic reference. The author concludes that 85% of patients with breast cancer will develop skeletal metastases, most of them in the spine.

Weinstein JN, McLain RF. (1987) Primary tumors of the spine. Spine 12(9): 843-851.

> The authors studied the primary benign and malignant tumors of the spine. Particular focus was given to statistical analysis of presenting symptoms, location, treatment, and outcomes.

Wise JJ, Fischgrund JS, Herkowitz HN et al. (1999) Complication, survival rates, and risk factors of surgery for metastatic disease of the spine. Spine 24(18): 1943-1951.

> This was a retrospective study of the complication, survival rates, and risk factors of surgery for metastatic disease of the spine. The authors conclude that complications were related to preoperative neurological deficit and preoperative radiotherapy.

CHAPTER 18

Intradural Spinal Neoplasms

James S. Harrop

M.D., Assistant Professor, Department of Neurosurgery, Division of Spinal Disorders, Jefferson Medical College, Philadelphia, PA

Introduction

- The central nervous system or neuraxis consists of the brain, the brainstem, and the spinal cord.
- Neoplasms affecting the spinal cord and its coverings are uncommon and affect only a minority of the population.
- Primary spinal cord neoplasms are infrequent and comprise approximately 0.5% of newly diagnosed tumors with an overall incidence of 1 per 100,000 patients per year.
- Spinal cord and spinal nerve root neoplasms are similar in histopathology to intracranial lesions and account for approximately 15% of central nervous system tumors.
- Primary spinal cord tumors originate from normal spinal parenchyma; secondary neoplasms are metastatic to the spinal cord and canal.
- Spinal cord neoplasms are generally classified as follows:
  1. Extradural (50%-60%) (Fig. 18–1)
  - Outside the spinal cord
  - Most commonly metastatic disease
  2. Intradural extramedullary (35%-45%) (Fig. 18–2)
  3. Intradural intramedullary (2%-7%) (Fig. 18–3)
- The following are imaging modalities for diagnosis and evaluation:
  - Plain film radiographs
  - Magnetic resonance imaging (MRI)
  - Computerized tomography (CT)
  - Myelogram
  - Angiography
  - Bone scan

Anatomy

- The spinal cord is an extension of the brainstem and connects the cerebrum to the peripheral nervous system.
- The spinal cord is proximally defined by the occipital condyles and skull base and extends distally to the thoracolumbar junction.
- The spinal cord is enclosed in the dural sac and is encased in cerebrospinal fluid (CSF) within the spinal canal (Fig. 18–4).
- The terminal end of the spinal cord, or conus medullaris, has a variable anatomic position because of axial growth and development (Malas et al. 2001).
  - The neonatal spinal cord terminates between the first and third lumbar vertebrae.
  - The adult spinal cord terminates between the twelfth thoracic and the second lumbar vertebrae.
  - The spinal cord terminates into a fine fibrous structure called the filum terminale (Williams 1995).
  - The filum terminale continues distally and attaches to the dorsum of the first coccygeal vertebrae.
- The spinal cord is a cylindrical structure and in the adult male measures approximately 45 cm in length and weighs 30 grams (Williams 1995).
- There are 31 pairs of spinal nerves that arise from the spinal cord:
  - 8 cervical
  - 12 thoracic
  - 5 lumbar

■ **Extradural Lesion**

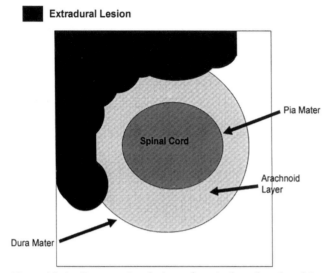

Figure 18–1: Cross-sectional view of a spinal cord enclosed in a dural sac. Note the extradural lesion causing mass effect and encasing the dural sac.

- 5 sacral
- 1 coccygeal
- The spinal cord is a highly organized, somatotopically arranged tissue composed of two functionally and anatomic distinct regions (Fig. 18–5).
  - The central portion consists of the **gray matter** made up of the neuronal cell bodies and supporting structures. Ventral gray matter contains large alpha motor neuron cell bodies, also referred to as anterior horn cells. Dorsal gray matter predominately receives input through afferent sensory neurons.
  - **White matter** encircles the gray matter and is composed of both myelinated and unmyelinated axonal tracts.

■ **Intradural Extramedullary Lesion**

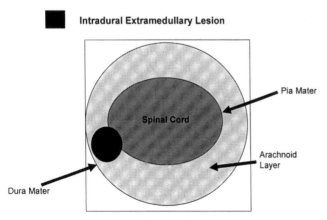

Figure 18–2: Cross-sectional view of a spinal cord enclosed in a dural sac. Note the intradural lesion causing mass effect on the spinal cord and located within the dural sac but outside the spinal cord parenchyma.

■ **Intradural Intramedullary Lesion**

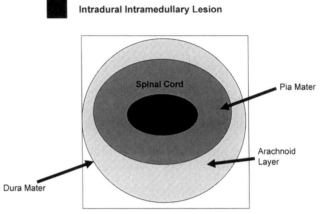

Figure 18–3: Cross-sectional view of a spinal cord enclosed in a dural sac. Note the intraparenchymal or intramedullary lesion causing mass effect on the spinal cord and enlarging the spinal cord.

- The ventral motor and dorsal sensory neurons unite outside of the spinal cord to form the spinal nerves, which exit the spinal canal through the neural foramen.
- The central canal is a continuum of the fourth ventricle from the brainstem (Fig. 18–5).
- The meninges cover the brain and spinal cord and consists of multiple layers (Fig. 18–4).
  1. Dura mater
  2. Arachnoid
  - Located between the pia and the dura mater
  - Consists of a web-like tissue space
  - CSF accumulates and circulates in this space
  3. Pia mater
  - In direct contact with the spinal cord
  - Adherent to blood vessels entering the spinal cord
  - Directly attaches the spinal cord to the dura mater through 18-24 sets of dentate ligaments
- The epidural venous vessels, termed Batson's plexus, are unique because the veins do not contain valves to prevent retrograde flow.
- The spinal cord receives blood through the anterior and posterior spinal arteries.
- The vascular supply of the spinal cord is variable and has an inconsistent distribution of vertebral or radicular arteries.
- The aorta contributes the greatest arterial supply through numerous segmental arteries, which further branch into medullary and radicular arteries.
  - The number of radicular arteries can range from 2 to 17. Most commonly, there are between 6 and 10 (Williams 1995).
  - Although the radicular arteries provide extramedullary blood supply to the nerve root and dura mater, the medullary artery bifurcates into ventral and dorsal divisions to form the spinal arteries.

Spinal Cord Anatomy

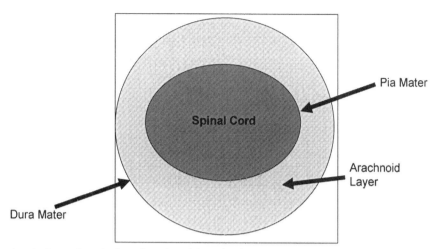

Figure 18–4: Cross-sectional view of a spinal cord enclosed in a dural sac.
Note that the dural sac consists of the three layers of the meninges: a thick outer layer of dura mater and two thinner and looser layers (arachnoid and pia layers).

Spinal Cord Anatomy

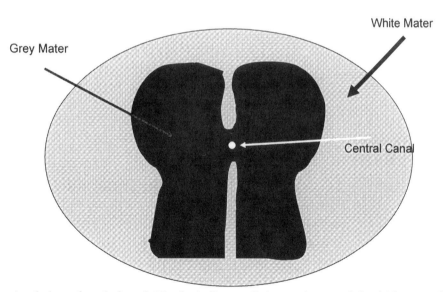

Figure 18–5: Cross-sectional view of a spinal cord. Histologically, two distinct regions are defined. The central gray matter composed of the neuronal cell bodies and the white matter composed of myelinated neuronal axons and nerve fiber tracts. The central canal in located centrally and is an extension of the fourth ventricle.

- The largest radicular artery, the artery of Adamkiewicz (arteria radicularis anterior magna), arises from between T9-T12 and is typically on the left-hand side (Williams 1995).
- The vessels that supply the spinal cord are end arteries; therefore there are no anastomoses between capillary beds (Williams 1995).

Classification

- There are multiple classification systems for the organization and categorization of spine and spinal cord neoplasms.
- The most common classification systems used by surgeons are based on anatomic location (Box 18–1).

Box 18–1:	Classification Systems for Spinal Cord Neoplasms

Anatomic Location

Intradural

- Intramedullary
  - Ependymoma
  - Astrocytomas
  - Hemangioblastomas
  - Other
- Extramedullary
  - Schwannoma
  - Neurofibroma
  - Meningioma
  - Subarachnoid metastasis
  - Other

Extradural

- Metastatic disease
- Primary osseous neoplasms

- Limited because they do not provide for neoplasms involved in or invading multiple anatomic planes
- The second major classification system is based histopathology (Box 18–2).
  - Limited in that it requires biopsy to confirm histopathologic diagnosis

Intradural Extramedullary Neoplasms

- Intradural extramedullary neoplasms are located in the subarachnoid space, which consists of the arachnoid tissue, circulating CSF, nerve rootlets, dentate ligament, filum terminale, and vascular structures (Fig. 18–2).
- Lesions that arise in this space are typically benign overgrowths of normal anatomic structures.
- More than 90% of the lesions are either nerve sheath tumors or meningiomas.
- Lesions may also appear in this location because of leptomeningeal seeding from systemic oncological disease or drop metastasis from supratentorial intracranial neoplasms.

Box 18–2:	Classification Systems for Spinal Cord Neoplasms

Histopathology Criteria

- Intraparenchymal neoplasms
  - Glial origin
  - Nonglial origin
- Nerve sheath neoplasms
- Other

Nerve Sheath Tumors

- Nerve sheath tumors are the most common spinal cord neoplasm and are located in the intradural extramedullary space (Fig. 18–2).
  - Schwannomas
  - Neurofibromas
- There is a prevalence of 0.001% in the general population.
- They appear in approximately 4% of patients with neurofibromatosis.
  - Neurofibromatosis patients with spinal deformity account for approximately 50% of the cases.
- There is equal incidence in male and female patients.
- Typical presenting symptoms are as follows:
  - Axial back pain
  - Painful radiculopathy
  - Often in the soft tissues of the cervical spine, the ventral extension of these neoplasms can be palpated in the anterior neck
- Benign peripheral nerve tumors contain Schwann cells, collagen, and reticulin fibers.
  - Both neurofibromas and schwannomas consist predominately of Schwann cells.
  - Neurofibromas are composed of a significant proportion of fibrous tissue.
- These nerve sheath lesions are usually solitary, encapsulated, and well circumscribed, having a globular configuration (Fig. 18–6).
- As neoplasms grow or enlarge, the following occur:
  - Uninvolved nerves are displaced.
  - Neoplasms may not only extend and expand in the spinal canal but also follow the tracts along the exiting nerve roots through the neural foramina.
  - A globular intracanicular component connects through thin waist to the foramina followed by a second globular component located in the extra-axial compartment (i.e., a dumbbell lesion) (Fig. 18–7).

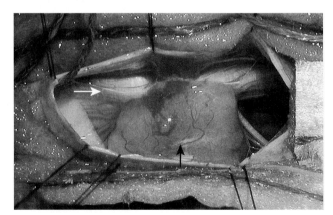

Figure 18–6: Intraoperative photograph of surgically exposed nerve sheath neoplasm (black arrow). **Note the nerve rootlets run parallel to the neoplasm (white arrow).**

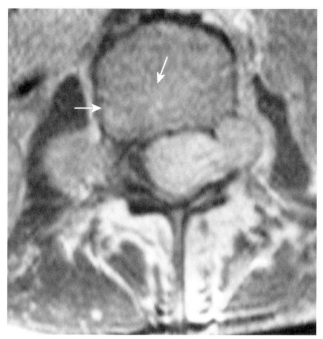

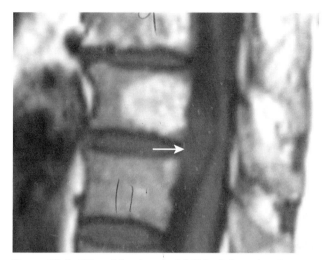

Figure 18–8: T1-weighted sagittal MRI of thoracic spine illustrates the schwannomas (arrow) that compress the spinal cord centrally. The neoplasm exits the neural foramina with the nerve root.

Figure 18–7: T1-weighted axial MRI with contrast of lumbar spine illustrates brightly enhancing schwannomas that have bilobed configuration. The neoplasm exits the neural foramina with the nerve root and has a significant extraspinal component (large arrow). Also note the large intracanicular component (little arrow).

Radiology Characteristics

- Plain radiographs may demonstrate osseous structures with bone remodeling and reabsorption because of chronic increased pressure.
  - Widening of the neural foramina
  - Increase in the interpedicular distance
  - Scalloping of the vertebral bodies
- CT provides greater details of the spinal anatomy compared with plain radiographs.
  - CT of a nerve sheath tumor appears as either a paraspinal or an intraspinal mass of decreased signal attenuation (Modic et al. 1994).
- MRI has the highest definition of all imaging modalities available.
  - Nerve sheath tumors have an increased T1 signal intensity compared with paraspinal muscles (Fig. 18–8), and the T2 signal is markedly intense because of increased water content (Fig. 18–9).
  - The central portions of a nerve sheath tumor can be hypointense on T2 signal images (Modic et al. 1994).
  - These tumors may have the appearance of a "target," based on a bright T1 signal after contrast administration with a central hypodense region.
  - Infusion of a contrast material, gadolinium, clearly defines the tumors relationship to the surrounding

neural structures. Nerve sheath tumors enhance homogenously and brightly (Fig. 18–10).

Neurofibromatosis

- Neurofibromatosis is one of the most common genetic disorders in the United States.
- There is an incidence of approximately 1 in every 3000 to 4000 children.

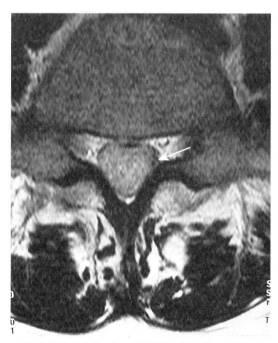

Figure 18–9: T2-weighted axial MRI of lumbar spine illustrates the signal characteristics of brightly homogenous schwannomas (arrow). The neoplasm is centrally located in the canal and displaces the nerve roots laterally.

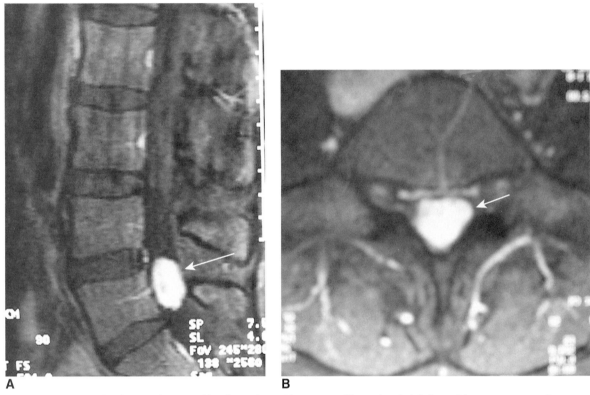

A **B**

Figure 18–10: A, T1-weighted sagittal MRI of lumbar spine with contrast illustrating brightly and homogeneous enhancement of lumbar schwannoma (arrow). B, T1-weighted axial MRI of lumbar spine with contrast illustrating brightly and homogeneous enhancement of lumbar schwannoma (arrow).

- Patients with these genetic mutations, such as neuro-fibromatosis, are at a much greater risk for nerve sheath neoplasms.
- Neurofibromatosis type II patients have bilateral acoustic neuromas (vestibular schwannomas) commonly with intracranial meningiomas and schwannomas (Fig. 18–11).

Schwannomas

- Schwannomas are the most common spinal nerve or cord tumor.
- Schwannomas were previously referred to as neuril-emomas or neurinomas.
- They are slow growing nerve sheath tumors (benign).
- Most are solitary but can occasionally occur as multiple lesions.
- Age of presentation is 20-50 years.
- Schwannomas have a predilection for the following:
  - Flexor surfaces
  - Main nerve trunks
- They arise eccentrically from within the nerve, and nerve bundles are stretched over the surface of the tumor.
- Characteristic diagnostic features are shooting pain and paresthesia induced by palpation of the nerve.

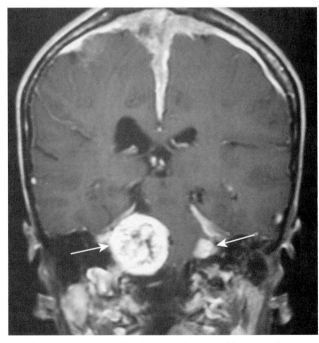

Figure 18–11: T1-weighted coronal MRI of brain with contrast in neurofibromatosis type II patient. Demonstrates bilateral acoustic neuromas (vestibular schwannomas) (arrows) along with thickening of the dura mater.

- Two-thirds of patients with neurofibromatosis develop schwannomas.
  - May precede the development of vestibular tumors (brain)
- Spinal nerve roots giving origin to schwannoma are frequently nonfunctional.

Neurofibromas

- Neurofibromas are slowly growing nerve sheath tumors (benign).
- Most are solitary (90%) but can occasionally occur as multiple lesions.
  - Multiple tumors are seen in neurofibromatosis type 1 (Fig. 18–12).
- Age of presentation is 20-30 years.
- Clinical features
  - Solitary tumors are located primarily on cutaneous nerves.
  - Patients complain of painful swelling, but palpation does not produce pain and paresthesia characteristic of schwannomas.
  - Neurofibromas more often cause weakness and sensory symptoms when noncutaneous sites are involved.

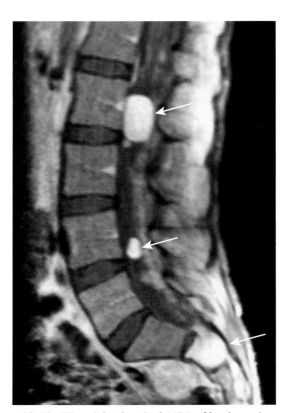

Figure 18–12: T1-weighted sagittal MRI of lumbar spine with contrast in neurofibromatosis type 2 patient. **Demonstrates multiple homogenously enhancing nerve sheath tumors (arrows).**

- Neurofibromas, unlike schwannomas, involve and entangle multiple nerve fascicles and travel parallel to the nerve.

Malignant Nerve Sheath Neoplasms

- Such neoplasms usually arise from transformed solitary or plexiform neurofibromas.
- Irradiation of neurofibromas has also been implicated.
- Benign intradural extraparenchymal lesions have been reported to have a malignant transformation rate between 1% and 12% of cases.
- A higher percentage of malignant nerve sheath tumor degeneration has been reported with patients with underlying chromosomal alterations, such as neurofibromatosis.
- In the minority of the patients affected with a secondary malignant nerve sheath neoplasm, there appears to be a 1- to 2-decade latency period from the time of initial diagnosis to the time of malignant degeneration of these lesions.

Meningiomas

- Meningiomas comprise approximately 25% of intradural extramedullary neoplasms and are second only to nerve sheath neoplasms in frequency in this tumor subtype.
- Meningiomas are believed to arise from an arachnoid cap of meningothelial cells.
- Meningiomas are more common in the intracranial compartment than in the spinal region.
- Spinal meningiomas are very slow-growing lesions and typically appear in a delayed manner because of compression of the spinal cord parenchyma.
- The incidence per region of spinal meningiomas reflects the length of the spinal cord segment with the thoracic spinal cord having the highest incidence, followed by the cervical cord and rarely the lumbar region (Solero et al. 1989).
  1. Frequency per spinal column region
     - Cervical—10%–20%
     - Thoracic—80%–90%
     - Lumbar—1%–5%
  2. Spinal classification
     - Intradural—90%
     - Extradural—5%
     - Both—5%
- Patients present symptoms between the fifth and seventh decade of life because of difficulty in ambulating, gait abnormalities, or pain (Levy et al. 1982, Solero et al. 1989).
  - Pain is the most frequent initial symptom and occurs in between 50% and 70% of patients (Levy et al. 1982, Solero et al. 1989).
  - Pain is typically diffuse and localized over the spinal region affected by the lesion.
  - In approximately 20% of patients, the pain can be of a radicular nature because of nerve root compression or local irritation (Levy et al. 1982, Solero et al. 1989).

- The obscurity of these presenting symptoms can causes confusion for the examining physician, resulting in a delay of the correct diagnosis.
- Pediatric cases are extremely uncommon and occur in the setting of underlying genetic alterations, such as neurofibromatosis or previous irradiation to the spinal canal.
- Women have a greater predilection for spinal meningiomas and comprise 75%-85% of the cases believed to be related to hormonal influences (Levy et al. 1982).
  - Thoracic meningiomas predominate in females (87%).
  - Cervical meningiomas have a slight female predilection (61%).
  - In the lumbar spine, there is an equal incidence between the sexes (Solero et al. 1989).
- Cervical region meningiomas are commonly ventrally located (Levy et al. 1982, Solero et al. 1989).
- The physical examination findings of spinal cord compression include the following:
  - Hyperreflexia of the limbs
  - Motor weakness
  - Other long-tract signs

Radiology

- Plain radiographs unfortunately provide little data and are diagnostically of minimal value.
- CT imaging of meningiomas appear as well-circumscribed intradural lesions with a higher density than the spinal cord tissue and homogeneously enhance after contrast administration (Modic et al. 1994).
- MRI is the imaging modality of choice because of excellent soft tissue definition.
  - The T1- and T2-weighted images signal the intensity of meningiomas and are isointense to the spinal cord parenchyma.
  - Although the T1 signal intensity is consistent, there is a degree of variability in the T2 signal intensity, with the T2-weighted image being somewhat more hyperintense (Fig. 18–13).
  - The infusion of contrast or gadolinium causes the well-circumscribed tumors to brightly enhance homogeneously (Sze et al. 1988).

Surgical Excision

- Spinal cord meningiomas are benign. Many surgeons believe most of these lesions should be completely excised (Fig. 18–14).
- The tumors are located lateral or dorsal to the spinal cord, which facilitates surgical resection and gross total removal (more than 95% of the tumor volume) (Figs. 18–13 and 18–14).
- Neurologic recovery and function with good to excellent results have been reported in 80%-90% of cases (Levy et al. 1982, Solero et al. 1989).
- The recurrence rate is 6%.

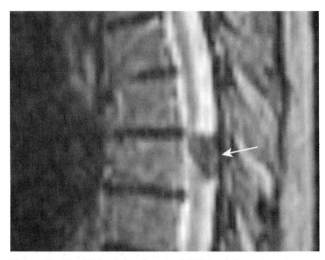

Figure 18–13: T2-weighted sagittal MRI of thoracic spine. Demonstrates the posterior location of the spinal meningioma (arrow) in relationship to the spinal cord. This is a calcified meningioma that presented with weakness in the lower extremities of numerous years.

- Calcified meningiomas have a worse prognosis and in 75% of cases result in neurologic decline because of manipulation of the spinal cord during resection (Levy et al. 1982).

Leptomeningeal Seeding

- The subarachnoid space or intradural extramedullary location provides for CSF to circulate around the spinal cord and nerve roots.
- Primary or metastatic spinal or intracranial neoplasms can breach the pia and arachnoid planes and invade the subarachnoid space.

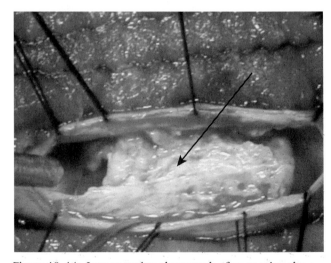

Figure 18–14: Intraoperative photograph after opening the dura mater in the midline and encountering a calcified meningioma (arrow). Note the dura mater is sutured upward and the spinal cord is deep to the meningioma.

- Although central nervous system neoplasms have direct access to the spinal fluid pathways, metastatic disease has a greater propensity for symptomatic CSF dissemination.
- These are not amendable to surgical resection because of diffuse and invasive pathology.
- MRI with contrast has the greatest sensitivity for visualization of intradural extramedullary lesions (Sze et al. 1988).

Intramedullary Neoplasms

- Intramedullary or primary spinal cord neoplasms account for approximately 2%-4% of adult central nervous system neoplasms (Fig. 18–3).
- In the pediatric population, the incidence of primary spinal cord neoplasms for unknown reasons is much greater and approximately 10%.
- The histologic diagnosis of these primary spinal cord neoplasms include the following:
  - Astrocytomas
  - Ependymomas
  - Hemangioblastomas

Adult Population

- In adults, 85% to 90% consist of either astrocytomas or ependymomas.
  - Ependymomas have the highest incidence of 60% to 70%.
  - Hemangioblastomas account for an additional 5% of spinal cord tumors.
  - Paragangliomas, oligodendrogliomas, and gangliogliomas account for the remaining lesions.
  - It is exceedingly rare to have intraparenchymal manifestation of metastatic disease in the spinal cord.

Pediatric Population

- Astrocytomas consist of between 55% and 65% of intramedullary neoplasms.

Radiology

- Plain radiographic abnormalities are seen in less than 20% of patients with intrinsic spinal cord neoplasms.
  1. A structural spinal abnormality, such as scoliosis, may be the presenting symptom of a spinal cord neoplasm.
  2. Remodeling of the osseous structure often involves expansion of the spinal canal.
  - Scalloping of the vertebral bodies
  - Increased interpedicular distance
- Spinal myelography is an invasive radiological procedure.
  - It may reveal nonspecific widening of the spinal canal and spinal cord or possibly a block of the contrast agent.
- CT may show nonspecific findings such as cord enlargement and osseous erosion.

- MRI with and without gadolinium is the imaging modality of choice.
  - MRI clearly defines the anatomic boundaries of the lesions with associated syringomyelia and intraparenchymal cavitations (Fig. 18–15).
  - It demonstrates enlargement of the spinal cord.
  - Varying the signal intensity, T1 versus T2 signals, can further define the suspected lesions histology. T1 images provide detailed anatomic images. Widening of the spinal cord or cystic cavitations may be appreciated. T2 images detail pathologic processes and higher water content. Edema from the neoplasm may be visualized with more detail.
- The natural history of a spinal cord neoplasm is defined by the histology of the tumor.
- The overall 5-year survival rate for patients with an intrinsic spinal cord neoplasm is greater than 90%.
- The greatest predictor of a patient's neurologic function after surgical intervention is his or her preoperative neurological condition.
- The McCormick grading or classification system provides a means of classifying patients' preoperative clinical and functional status (Box 18–3).
  - Unfortunately there are limited nonsurgical treatment alternatives for these lesions, and pharmacologic treatment is of limited clinical benefit.

Corticosteroid Therapy

- Therapy decreases vasogenic edema but does not treat the underlying pathology of the disorder.
- Prolonged steroid use is associated with gastric ulceration, steroid induced psychosis, myopathy, hyperglycemia, and immunosuppression.

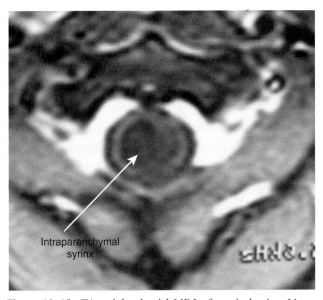

Intraparenchymal
syrinx

Figure 18–15: T1-weighted axial MRI of cervical spine. Note the large intraparenchymal cyst or syrinx (arrow) that displaces the spinal cord to a thin ribbon of tissue.

Box 18–3:	McCormick Classification for Clinical or Functional Outcome

- Grade I
  - Neurologic examinations normal, mild deficit, gait normal
- Grade II
  - Sensorimotor deficit, mild to moderate gait difficulty, severe dysesthetic syndrome, independent ambulation
- Grade III
  - Severe neurologic deficit, brace or cane needed for ambulation, bilateral upper extremity impairment
- Grade IV
  - Severe deficit; wheelchair, cane, or brace required; usually not independent

Chemotherapeutic Agents

- Chemotherapeutic agents are of limited success in the treatment of spinal cord neoplasms because they are unable to penetrate the central nervous system's blood–brain barrier to perfuse and inhibit the growth of these lesions.

Radiosurgery

- Radiosurgery has been used in the treatment of these lesions.
  - Although symptomatic control may be achieved short term, when compared with surgical resection, tumor recurrence and malignant transformation has been observed with a higher frequency after radiotherapy.
  - Postsurgical radiation is not recommended for intramedullary spinal cord neoplasms because this has not been shown to improve quality of life or increase length of survival.
  - Radiation therapy may be most effective in treating malignant lesions only or applied for lesions not surgically approachable.
  - Radiosurgery techniques are being redefined such that radiation beams are directed over a large field and converge as a highly focused beam onto the spinal tumor.

Goal of Surgery

- The goal of surgery is to prevent further neurologic deterioration through aggressive resection (Brotchi et al. 1999, Cooper 1989, Cristante et al. 1994, Epstein et al. 1993, Epstein et al.1992, Greenwood 1954).
  - There is a less than 5% risk of recurrence for low-grade tumors. Approximately 10% of patients will have progression of residual tumor (Brotchi et al. 1999).
  - Neurologic outcome is again related to preoperative neurologic status.
  - It is common to see immediate postoperative neurologic worsening, such as posterior column dysfunction or worsening motor deficit.

- After any intervention or change in clinical status, these patients should be reevaluated clinically and with appropriate imaging studies.

Ependymomas

- Ependymomas are a histologic subtype of intramedullary spinal cord tumors and arise from the cuboidal ependymal cells that surround the ventricular system and center canal of the spinal cord (Fig. 18–5).
  - Cauda equina or filum terminale ependymomas are histologically of the myxopapillary subtype.
- Ependymomas are the most common adult primary spinal parenchymal neoplasm but are twice as likely to occur in the neuraxis outside the spinal cord.
  - Primary brain and brainstem ependymomas may disseminate to the spinal cord as a result of metastatic seeding through the cerebrospinal pathways.
- Mean age of presentation is 43 years, and there is a slightly greater predilection for females to be affected than males.
- Pain is the most common presenting symptom and is often only localized to the spine (65%).
- Clinical signs of spinal cord tumors most commonly are weakness of the limbs caudal to the spinal levels of involvement and gait abnormalities such as a spastic paraparesis or ataxia.
- Physical examination may reveal the following:
  - Reflex abnormalities
  - Sensory changes
  - Sphincter dysfunction
  - Paraspinal muscle spasms
- Lesions are located in the center of the spinal cord parenchyma. Enlargement and compression of the central canal may result in obstruction and accumulation of CSF at the proximal and distal ends of the lesion.
- Hemorrhage in the neoplasms at the rostral and caudal poles of the neoplasm is more common in ependymomas than in astrocytomas.
- MRI signal characteristics of ependymomas
  - T1-weighted MRI has either an isointense or hypointense signal relative to the spinal cord signal and enhances brightly with contrast (Fig. 18–16).
  - T2-weighted images reveal a hyperintense signal (Fig. 18–17).
  - Signal hyperintensity may also be secondary to associated spinal cord edema.
  - Contrast administration results in a strong homogeneous enhancement of the neoplasm, and there is a clear margin between the parenchyma and the ependymoma of the spinal cord (Fig. 18–16).
  - Axial imaging the spinal cord retains its symmetric appearance with a centrally located circular lesion.
- Spinal ependymomas have a much better life expectancy compared with their brain or brain-stem ependymoma counterparts.

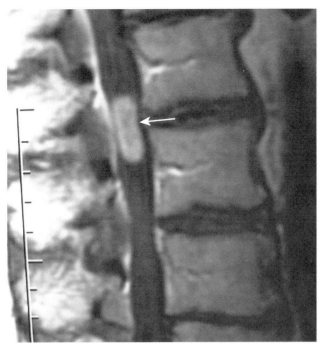

Figure 18–16: T1-weighted sagittal MRI with contrast of lumbar spine. This ependymoma (arrow) enhances uniformly with heterogenous signal characteristics.

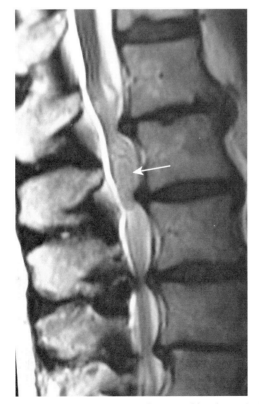

Figure 18–17: T2-weighted sagittal MRI of lumbar spinal ependymoma (arrow).

- Patients typically deteriorate because of the progression of local disease or the recurrence of a previously excised neoplasm.

Surgical Treatment

- Gross total resection of intraparenchymal spinal cord ependymomas results in long-term disease free control of the lesion (McCormick et al. 1990).
- The presence of a capsule aids surgical resection (Fig. 18–18).
- Patients in whom a gross total resection has been performed must be followed for local recurrence.
- There is no need for adjuvant therapy (Brotchi et al. 1999, Epstein et al. 1993).
- If subtotal resection is performed, additional therapy is often advocated because radiotherapy can decrease the incidence of recurrences by controlling the growth of macroscopic tumor cells.

Astrocytomas

- Astrocyte cells function as support cells and provide nutritional support to the neurons and axons.
- Neoplastic transformation of these supporting glial cells results in the formation of astrocytomas.
- Spinal cord astrocytomas may occur during any period of life but are most common during the first 3 decades of life.
- Spinal astrocytomas are four to five times more common than ependymomas during the first 2 decades of life.
- Most spinal cord astrocytomas are low-grade tumors; 10% of pediatric and 20% of adult tumors are more aggressive and infiltrating, categorizing them as a higher grade or "malignant."
- Equal incidence is found in males and females.
- Spinal cord astrocytomas have a similar clinical presentation as spinal cord ependymomas.
  - The tumor enlarges and causes compression of the neuronal structures, resulting in motor and sensory disturbances,
  - Patients have the following symptoms:
  1. Pain either along the spinal axis or radicular in nature

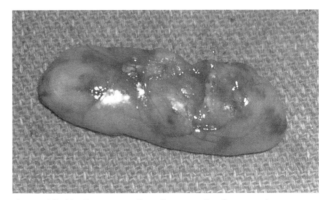

Figure 18–18: Intraoperative photograph of resected encapsulated ependymomas imaged in Figs. 18–16 and 18–17.

2. Bowel and bladder disturbances
3. Gait difficulties
- Patients present in a delayed manner because of the tumors' relatively slow growth (most are of a low histologic grade).
- Initial symptoms are often ill defined and nonspecific, resulting in a delay in the diagnosis.
1. Low-grade astrocytomas have a mean symptom duration prior to diagnosis of 41 months.
2. Malignant astrocytomas have a mean symptom duration prior to diagnosis of only 4 to 7 months.

Radiology or Magnetic Resonance Imaging

- T1 images have an isointense or hypointense signal.
- T2 images display a hyperintense signal characteristic of the associated edema in the spinal cord parenchyma.
- Contrast creates a heterogeneous enhancement, which is nearly always present in astrocytomas, but the intensity varies (Fig. 18–19).
- Astrocytomas are infiltrative in nature; therefore the neoplasm border is less defined than that seen with ependymomas.
- Cystic cavitations may be present but are less frequent than those seen with spinal ependymomas.

- Astrocytomas are eccentrically located in the spinal parenchyma on axial MRI (Fig. 18–19, B).

Surgical Therapy

- Radical surgical excision of low-grade astrocytomas (Epstein et al. 1992) is associated with an excellent long-term prognosis and minimal morbidity.
- Higher grade neoplasms, such as anaplastic astrocytomas, do not usually benefit from surgery.
  - These neoplasms enlarge in a fusiform manner and displace the spinal cord parenchyma.
  - More aggressive or higher grade neoplasms have an ill-defined plane and are infiltrative into the spinal parenchyma, thus preventing surgical excision. Lower grade lesions tend to have a more defined dissection plane.

Hemangioblastomas

- Spinal cord hemangioblastomas are the third most frequent intramedullary spinal cord neoplasm.
- They are present in approximately 5% of patients with a primary spinal cord tumor and are the most common intraparenchymal neoplasm of nonglial origin.
- Location
  - Cervical—50%-60%
  - Thoracic—35%-45%
  - Conus medullaris—2%-6%

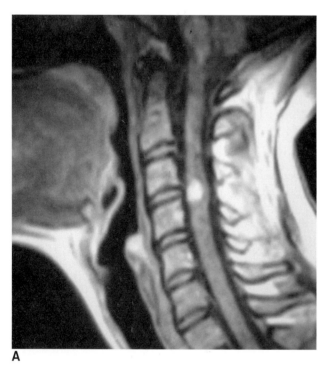

A

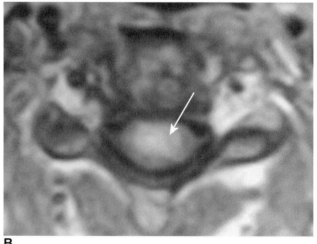

B

Figure 18–19: Cervical spinal card astrocytoma. A, T1-weighted sagittal MRI with contrast of cervical spine of astrocytomas. Note the absence of discrete borders between the neoplasm and the normal spinal parenchyma. These neoplasms tend to enlarge, have more associated edema, and have more heterogenous signal characteristics as they become more aggressive and form a higher grade malignancy. B, T1-weighted axial MRI with contrast of cervical spine of astrocytomas. Note the absence of discrete borders between the neoplasm and the normal spinal parenchyma (arrow) after contrast administration.

- Predilection for a younger patient population
  - Onset of symptoms is typically by the fourth decade.
  - In younger patients, 80% are symptomatic by the fifth decade.
- Patients have the following symptoms with most intramedullary neoplasms:
  - Pain
  - Decreased posterior column sensation
  - Rarely, a sudden neurological deterioration because of acute hemorrhage
- Associated with von Hippel-Lindau syndrome, an inherited disease
  - The syndrome is an autosomal dominant disorder with an almost 100% penetrance rate.
  - It affects the small arterioles in the body and predisposes these patients to malignancies.
  - The spinal cord is affected in approximately a third of the patients with this syndrome.
- Other associated lesions
  - Cerebellar hemangioblastomas
  - Renal carcinomas
  - Retinal angiomas
  - Pheochromocytoma
- Although spinal cord hemangioblastomas may be associated with significant morbidity, mortality is related to urologic disorders, kidney failure, malignancies, and cerebellar hemangioblastomas.
- MRI is essential in the evaluation of a patient with von Hippel-Lindau syndrome or any patient with a suspected spinal hemangioblastoma.

Spinal Imaging

- MRI
  - T1 images are isointense compared with the spinal cord.
  - T2 images are hyperintense compared with the spinal cord.
  - Cystic tumor nodules are apparent in approximately 80% of patients.
  - Heterogeneous nodules found within the cystic cavities enhance strongly with contrast administration. In 15% of patients, the nodule has an extramedullary extension.
- Spinal angiograms may help to define the hemangioblastomas anatomy, demonstrating a vascular blush and identifying a prominent draining vein.
  - These tumors are connected to the pia-arachnoid tissue and receive a prominent vascular supply through an arteriole network.
  - Newer angiography and microcatheterization techniques provide a greater visualization of the blood flow through these lesions.

Other Lesions

- Numerous other lesions may become evident because of their mass effect or compression on the spinal cord.

They may initially be interpreted as a spinal cord neoplasm.

Vascular Disorders

- Cavernomas
- Arteriovenous fistulas

Miscellaneous Neurologic Diseases

- Multiple sclerosis
- Transverse myelitis
- Sarcoidosis
- These neurologic diseases differ from neoplasms in that there is typically no associated mass effect. A careful analysis of the clinical evaluation and imaging modalities can differentiate these processes. A spinal arteriogram may be beneficial to further define the disorder in a limited number of vascular cases.

Intramedullary Spinal Cord Metastasis

- Exceedingly uncommon
- Dissemination through hematogenous routes—that is, arterial or venous—and possibly through the nerve root sheath
- Clinical presentation similar to intrinsic spinal tumors

References

Brotchi J, Lefranc F. (1999) Current management of spinal cord tumors. Contemp Neurosurg 21(26): 1-8.
  Large retrospective series of 239 patients with low-grade spinal tumors treated with operative treatment. After treatment, 5% worsened, 50% stabilized, and 40% improved with surgical excision.

Cooper PR. (1989) Outcome after operative treatment of intramedullary spinal cord tumors in adults: Intermediate and long-term results in 51 patients. Neurosurgery 25(6): 855-859.
  Retrospective review of 51 patients treated with microsurgical resection of intrinsic spinal cord neoplasms. Postoperatively, the neurological conditions of 21 patients were improved or stabilized and those of 16 patients were worse. Patients with ependymomas who had gross total resection fared the best.

Cristante L, Herrmann HD. (1994) Surgical management of intramedullary spinal cord tumors: Functional outcome and sources of morbidity. Neurosurgery 35(1): 69-74.
  Retrospective review of a postoperative functional assessment reported deterioration in 65.4% of patients by the Cooper scale. Surgery on tumors of the cervicothoracic and upper thoracic region had a relatively higher morbidity in this series.

Epstein FJ, Farmer JP, Freed D. (1993) Adult intramedullary spinal cord ependymomas: The result of surgery in 38 patients. J Neurosurg 79(2): 204-209.
  Review of 38 patients that underwent surgery for an intramedullary spinal cord ependymoma. The patients' postoperative neurologic examinations were proportional to preoperative status. There were no tumor recurrences at 2 years without radiation therapy.

Epstein FJ, Farmer JP, Freed D. (1992) Adult intramedullary astrocytomas of the spinal cord. J Neurosurg 77(3): 355-359.

Review of 25 adult patients with intramedullary astrocytomas treated by radical excision alone. Low-grade tumors treated with radical excision were associated with minimal morbidity and an excellent long-term prognosis. However, surgery was not beneficial for anaplastic spinal astrocytomas.

Greenwood J Jr. (1954) Total removal of intramedullary tumors. J Neurosurg 11: 116-121.

Classic article detailing the surgical approach and resection of intraspinal tumors.

Levy WJ, Bay J, Dohn D. (1982) Spinal cord meningioma. J Neurosurg 57: 804-812.

Retrospective review of 97 cases of spinal meningiomas, which demonstrated poor results among those with calcified or recurrent tumors. The cervical tumors were almost all anterior to the spinal cord.

Malas MA, Salbacak A, Buyukmumcu M et al. (2001) An investigation of the conus medullaris termination level during the period of fetal development to adulthood. Anat Sci Int 76(5): 453-459.

Radiographic analysis of the termination level of the conus medullaris from fetus to adulthood in a total of 285 individuals. The tip of the conus medullaris of prematures and neonates ranged from the L1 to L3 vertebrae. The tip of the conus medullaris in children resided between the T12 and L3 vertebrae, and in the adults it resided between the T12 and L2 vertebrae.

McCormick PC, Torres R, Post KD. (1990) Intramedullary ependymoma of the spinal cord. J Neurosurg 72(4): 523-532.

Retrospective review of 23 patients who had operative excision of intramedullary spinal cord ependymomas. Patients were followed from 8 months to 10 years postoperatively, and no patient exhibited clinical or radiological evidence of tumor recurrence.

Modic MT, Masaryk TJ, Ross JS. (1994) Spinal tumors. In: Magnetic Resonance Imaging of the Brain and Spine (Modic MT et al., eds.). St. Louis: Mosby, pp. 946-953.

Radiographic textbook that details the imaging characteristics of spinal cord neoplasms on plain radiographs, CT, and MRI.

Solero CL, Fornari M, Giombini S et al. (1989) Spinal meningiomas: Review of 174 operated cases. Neurosurgery 25(2): 153-160.

Retrospective review of 174 spinal meningiomas in which complete tumor excision was achieved in 96.5% of the patients. Surgical mortality was about 1%. A microsurgical technique, which was used in the last 29 cases, was reported to be highly effective.

Sze G, Abramson A, Krol G. (1988) Gadolinium-DPTA in the evaluation of intradural extramedullary spinal disease. AJNR 9: 153-163.

The authors evaluated the use of gadolinium contrast agent administration in intradural extramedullary lesions. The study showed that MRI with contrast was able to visualize the intradural lesions with greater efficiency than CT myelogram.

Williams PL, ed. (1995) Gray's Anatomy, 38th edition. New York: Churchill Livingstone, pp. 974-1018.

Detailed anatomic textbook that characterizes the relationship of the spine, spinal cord, and blood supply.

CHAPTER 19

Pathophysiology and Pharmacologic Treatment of Acute Spinal Cord Injury

Brian K. Kwon★, Jonathan N. Grauer §, and Alexander R. Vaccaro †

★ M.D., Orthopaedic Spine Fellow, Department of Orthopaedic Surgery, Thomas Jefferson University and the Rothman Institute, Philadelphia, PA; Clinical Instructor, Combined Neurosurgical and Orthopaedic Spine Program, University of British Columbia; and Gowan and Michele Guest Neuroscience Canada Foundation/CIHR Research Fellow, International Collaboration on Repair Discoveries, University of British Columbia, Vancouver, Canada
§M.D., Assistant Professor, Co-Director Orthopaedic Spine Surgery, Yale-New Haven Hospital; Assistant Professor, Department of Orthopaedics, Yale University School of Medicine, New Haven, CT
† M.D., Professor of Orthopaedic Surgery, Thomas Jefferson University and the Rothman Institute, Philadelphia, PA

Introduction

- Approximately 12,000 new spinal cord injuries occur each year in North America, adding to an estimated 200,000 people who live with chronic spinal cord paralysis.
- Of the new injuries, 55% occur in individuals under the age of 30; 80%-85% of the new injuries are sustained by males.
- Motor vehicle accidents and acts of violence account for more than half of the new injuries (Fig. 19–1).
- More than half of spinal cord injuries occur at the cervical level.
- An intensive search is under way to develop pharmacologic strategies that will provide neuroprotection for the acutely injured spinal cord. The development of such interventions requires an understanding of the pathophysiological processes triggered at the time of injury.

Concepts of Primary and Secondary Damage After Spinal Cord Injury

- **Primary damage** to the spinal cord is caused by the mechanical forces imparted to the spinal column at the time of trauma. In the setting of nonpenetrating trauma, the osteoligamentous spinal column can fail under a combination of flexion and extension, lateral bending, axial compression, and rotational or distractive forces.
- **Secondary damage** refers to injury of the adjacent neural tissue that escapes the initial mechanical forces but subsequently succumbs to the pathophysiological processes triggered by the primary injury (Fig. 19–2).
- The extent of both the primary and the secondary damage is directly related to the energy delivered to the spinal cord at the time of impact.

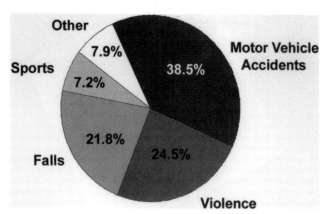

Figure 19–1: Etiology of SCI since 1990. From the National Spinal Cord Injury Statistical Center, Birmingham, AL, May 2001.

Acute Pathophysiological Processes

- Several acute processes have been identified that are thought to contribute to secondary damage after spinal cord injury. These include vascular abnormalities and ischemia, free radical generation and lipid peroxidation, excitotoxicity and loss of ionic homeostasis, and an inflammatory or immune response.

- These processes are interrelated, often feeding back on one another to lead to the necrotic or apoptotic death of cells within the spinal cord—neurons, oligodendrocytes, astrocytes, and microglia (Fig. 19–3).

- Almost everything that is understood about these acute pathophysiological processes comes from animal models of spinal cord injury (Box 19–1). Very little comes from human studies.

Alterations in Vascular Perfusion

- Spinal cord injury provokes significant cord hypoperfusion and ischemia as the result of mechanical disruption of the microvasculature, which causes hemorrhage, intravascular thrombosis, vasospasm, and edema (Tator et al. 1991). The microvasculature is primarily affected; the larger caliber vessels, such as the anterior spinal artery, normally are spared.

- Unfortunately, the hypoperfusion and ischemia appear to be worst in the gray matter, where neurons have high metabolic demands and are extremely sensitive to ischemia.

- Spinal cord blood flow is normally autoregulated, which maintains a fairly constant perfusion within the microvasculature of the cord during systolic blood pressure fluctuations between approximately 50 and 130 mm mercury (Hg).

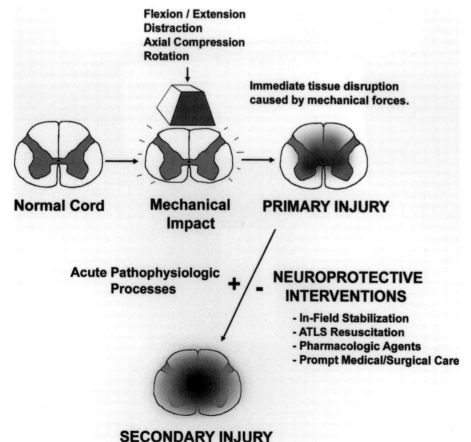

Figure 19–2: Primary and secondary damage after spinal cord injury. A variety of mechanical forces cause immediate tissue disruption, thus imparting the primary injury. This rarely transects the spinal cord. Adjacent tissue that survives the primary injury is vulnerable to acute pathophysiological processes that quickly follow. Neuroprotective interventions aim to minimize the destructive effects of these processes (*ATLS*, advanced trauma life support).

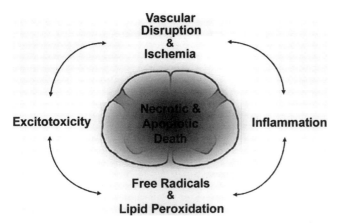

Figure 19–3: Acute pathophysiological processes after spinal cord injury.
The initial trauma initiates several processes that contribute to the necrotic and apoptotic death of cells within the spinal cord. These are interrelated processes that often have positive feedback on one another to worsen injury.

- This autoregulation is lost after spinal cord injury, leaving the cord vulnerable to fluctuations in systemic arterial pressure. Systemic hypotension secondary to hypovolemic shock, neurogenic shock, or both can therefore exacerbate spinal cord hypoperfusion and ischemia and worsen the secondary injury.
- Every effort should be made to maintain the systolic blood pressure in these patients—a mean arterial pressure of 90 mm Hg has been recommended.

Box 19–1: Animal Models of Spinal Cord Injury

- **Blunt injury models**—Impactor or weight drop and clip or balloon compression
  - The New York University and Ohio State University spinal cord impactors are widely used "weight drop" rodent models of spinal cord injury. They produce consistent injuries of varying severities by precisely striking the dorsal aspect of the spinal cord.
  - The contusion initiates many pathophysiological processes thought to mimic the human condition. Over time, the cord develops cystic changes similar to those seen in chronically injured humans.
  - Because the injury is, by nature, anatomically incomplete, an unpredictable number of axons are spared at the periphery. The evaluation of strategies to promote axonal regeneration requires knowledge of which axons are cut—therefore, these blunt injury models are difficult to use in studies of axonal regeneration.
- **Sharp injury models**—Complete or partial transection
  - Because the injury can reliably disrupt all the axons of the spinal cord, or all the axons in part of the spinal cord, these are more useful models for studying axonal regeneration.
  - These models poorly represent the typical human injury and are therefore less appropriate to use for studies of acute pathophysiology.

Free Radicals and Lipid Peroxidation

- Free radicals are molecules that possess unpaired electrons, making them highly reactive to lipids, proteins, and deoxyribonucleic acid (DNA). Molecular oxygen itself (O_2) possesses two such unpaired electrons.
- Oxygen-derived free radicals include superoxide (O_2^-), hydrogen peroxide (H_2O_2), and highly reactive hydroxyl radical (OH^-). Another highly reactive free radical, peroxynitrite ($ONOO^-$), is formed by the interaction of superoxide with nitric oxide (NO).
- Free radicals can cause a progressive oxidation of fatty acids in cellular membranes (lipid peroxidation), whereby the oxidation process geometrically generates more free radicals that can propagate the reaction across the membrane surface (Fig. 19–4).
- Oxidation by free radicals can injure key mitochondrial respiratory chain enzymes, alter DNA and DNA-associated proteins, and inhibit sodium-potassium adenosine triphosphatase (ATPase)—all of which can contribute to the death of the cell.
- The inhibition of lipid peroxidation is thought to be a major neuroprotective property of several pharmacologic agents that have been evaluated for spinal cord injury, including methylprednisolone, tirilazad mesylate (an antioxidant), and GM1 ganglioside.

Excitotoxicity and Electrolyte Imbalances

Glutamate and Calcium Homeostasis

- Glutamate release and accumulation occurs rapidly after spinal cord injury in response to ischemia and membrane depolarization (Box 19–2).
- N-methyl D-aspartate (NMDA) receptors allow calcium into the cell when activated by glutamate, which may also trigger the release of calcium from intracellular stores into the cytoplasmic compartment.

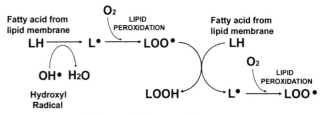

Figure 19–4: Lipid peroxidation reaction.
Notice that there is a geometric "chain reaction" to the lipid peroxidation process. The free radical OH^- generates a lipid radical L• from fatty acids in the lipid membrane. After oxidation of L•, another lipid molecule from the membrane is claimed in an oxidation reaction that generates yet another lipid radical, which can propagate the reaction further. If this process goes unchecked, we can envision how the cell membranes would be disrupted.

- The pharmacologic blockade of NMDA receptors has been extensively evaluated as a potential treatment of spinal cord and other central nervous system (CNS) injuries and neurodegenerative disorders.
- The cytosolic concentration of calcium is normally extremely low and tightly controlled; elevated intracellular calcium concentrations can activate many calcium-dependent processes that can lethally alter cellular metabolism (Box 19–3).

Sodium Homeostasis

- Sodium homeostasis across membranes significantly influences osmotic pressure and, thus, water distribution. Like calcium, sodium concentrations are normally high in the extracellular compartment and low in the intracellular compartment.
- Loss of sodium homeostasis is particularly important in the pathophysiology of axons and glial cells within spinal cord white matter after injury.
- Sodium can enter the intracellular compartment through several channels (Box 19–4). (Restoration of sodium homeostasis depends heavily on ATP-dependent pumps (e.g., $Na^+K^+ATPase$)
- Blocking sodium influx with pharmacologic antagonists of voltage-gated sodium channels and alpha-amino-3-hydroxy-5-methyl-4-isoxazole propionic acid (AMPA) or kainate receptors has been shown to be neuroprotective, particularly of axons and glial cells within white matter (Rosenberg et al. 1999). This confirms the importance of sodium homeostasis in secondary injury.

Inflammatory and Immunologic Response

Cellular and Noncellular Components

- Inflammatory and immunologic responses are highly interrelated processes that represent a universal defense and reparative reaction to tissue injury (Fig. 19–5).
- Cellular components are either blood-borne and invade the area (neutrophils, macrophages, and lymphocytes) or reside within the CNS and are activated by injury (microglia and astrocytes). The cellular response to CNS injury can cause further injury by phagocytosing tissue and by expressing noncellular elements such as cytokines and arachidonic acid metabolites (Popovich et al. 1997).

Arachidonic Acid Metabolites

- Arachidonic acid can be generated from fatty acids within cell membranes by phospholipases. These phospholipases can be activated by increases in cytoplasmic calcium.
- Arachidonic acid is metabolized into proinflammatory prostanoids (prostaglandins, prostacyclin, and thromboxanes) by cyclooxygenase (COX) (Fig. 19–6).
- These prostanoids mediate vascular permeability or resistance and platelet aggregation or adherence.
- COX is the enzyme targeted by nonsteroidal anti-inflammatory drugs (NSAIDs). Both COX-1 and COX-2 isoforms increase after blunt spinal cord injury.
- The involvement of COXs in the generation of these inflammatory mediators after spinal cord injury makes them a potential target for intervention because the pharmacologic means of inhibiting these enzymes are available and in widespread clinical use.

Tumor Necrosis Factor

- Tumor necrosis factor-alpha (TNFα) is perhaps the most extensively studied cytokine involved in secondary CNS injury.
- TNFα is expressed by neutrophils, macrophages, microglia, astrocytes, and T-cells; it accumulates quickly at the site of spinal cord injury.

Figure 19–5: Inflammatory and immunologic response to spinal cord injury.
The inflammatory and immunologic response to CNS injury involves a complex interaction between cellular and noncellular elements, both of which are implicated not only in the secondary damage but also in the native reparative response.

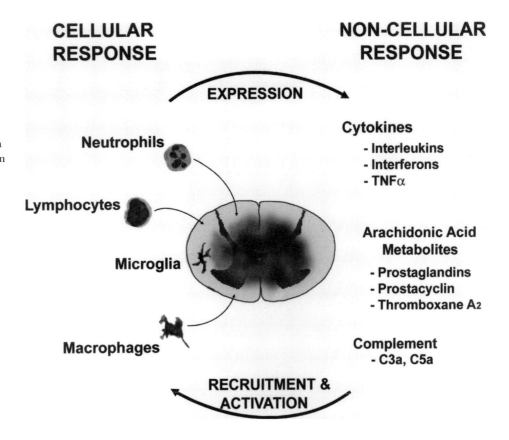

Figure 19–6: Arachidonic acid metabolism.
Phospholipases can mobilize arachidonic acid from the cell membrane. COX metabolism of arachidonic acid produces thromboxane, prostacyclin, and prostaglandins, all of which influence the inflammatory process. Prostacyclin has vasodilatory properties that promote vascular permeability and edema at sites of inflammation, and thromboxane A2 tends to worsen venous thrombosis and ischemia by promoting platelet aggregation and vasoconstriction.

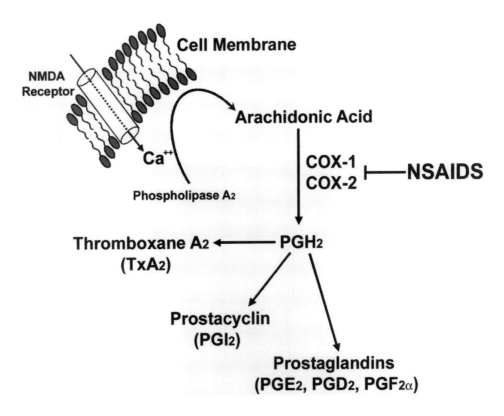

- Animal studies have shown TNFα to have both neuro-toxic and neuroprotective properties.

The Good and the Bad of Inflammation

- The conflicting actions of TNFα reflect a growing awareness that it is a gross oversimplification to view inflammation solely as a detrimental process.
- The inflammatory and immune response to injury is extremely complex, and inflammation is more appropriately considered a dual-edged sword, with both neurotoxic and neuroprotective properties after spinal cord injury (Bethea 2000) (Fig. 19–7).
- Some cytokines (e.g., the interleukins IL-2 and IL-3) are proinflammatory, and others (e.g., IL-10) are considered to have anti-inflammatory properties. The beneficial or deleterious effects of some of these cytokines, such as TNFα, probably depend on where and when they are expressed.
- IL-10 is an anti-inflammatory cytokine secreted by many of the same cells that produce TNFα. It has been shown to be neuroprotective after experimental spinal cord injury, possibly by inducing antiapoptotic genes.

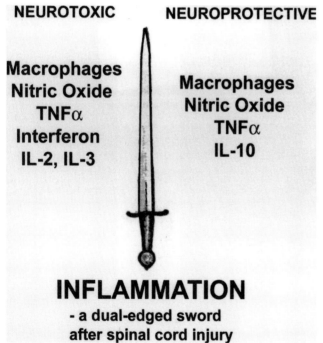

Figure 19–7: Neuroprotective and neurotoxic elements of the inflammatory response. **The inflammatory response can be considered a dual-edged sword with both neurotoxic and neuroprotective properties. Notice that some of the inflammatory elements, such as TNFα, macrophages, and nitric oxide, have both beneficial and detrimental effects—likely related to when they are expressed after spinal cord injury and on which cells they act.**

- Phagocytic macrophages have traditionally been thought to further destroy neural tissue. It was suggested recently that they are an important part of the reparative response after CNS injury. This prompted a human clinical trial in which macrophages were implanted into the spinal cords of acutely injured patients—representing quite a different view of the role of macrophages from what has been adhered to for many years.
- A better understanding of which aspects of inflammation are beneficial and which are detrimental will be required to develop strategies that target these responses.

Necrotic and Apoptotic Cell Death

- The manner in which cells die during normal development and aging and in response to injury can take on different morphologic appearances. These have been described as **apoptosis** and **necrosis**. (Table 19–1)
- Both necrosis and apoptosis are initiated by many of the same insults, such as ischemia, oxidative stress, and excitotoxicity. *In general, the greater the severity of the insult, the more likely the cell will be overwhelmed, lose its energy or ATP stores, and undergo necrosis.*
- Addressing the secondary injury processes will likely prevent both necrotic and apoptotic death after spinal cord injury. However, the pathways activated during apoptotic cell death represent another potential target for therapeutic intervention once apoptosis has been initiated.
- In the setting of spinal cord injury, it is generally thought that cells at the "epicenter" of injury will frequently undergo rapid necrotic death, whereas cells in the surrounding area are susceptible to both necrotic and apoptotic death.
- Both necrotic and apoptotic cell death are known to occur after human spinal cord injury (Emery et al. 1998).
- Apoptotic cell death can occur for weeks after injury remote from the point of mechanical impact (Crowe et al. 1997, Emery et al. 1998).
- Oligodendrocytes in particular appear quite vulnerable to apoptotic cell death. The death of these oligodendrocytes can result in the demyelination of otherwise spared axons, thus worsening neurologic function.
- Because the cell undergoing apoptosis must synthesize new proteins, one strategy to inhibit apoptotic death uses protein synthesis inhibitors such as cycloheximide. In animal models, this has been shown to inhibit apoptosis, reduce secondary damage, and improve functional outcome after experimental spinal cord injury.
- Other strategies to prevent apoptosis involve pharmacologic caspase inhibitors and the application of genes for proteins that influence their state of caspase activation, such as B-cell lymphoma-2.
- Strategies to inhibit apoptosis after spinal cord injury are in the very early stages of development and have not been tested in humans.

Table 19–1: Some Differences Between Necrotic and Apoptotic Cell Death*

	NECROSIS (CELLULAR HOMICIDE)	APOPTOSIS (CELLULAR SUICIDE)
Cellular and nuclear morphology	Swelling and bursting	Shrinkage and fragmentation
Gross organelle damage	Present	Absent
ATP and energy state §	Rapid loss of ATP	Requires ATP and protein synthesis
Death mechanism	Inability to maintain ionic gradients across membrane leads to swelling and bursting	Activation of caspases that target cytoskeletal and nuclear proteins, dismantling the cell
Inflammatory response induced by death	Present	Absent

* From a practical point of view, the most important difference between necrotic and apoptotic cell death is that we may be able to therapeutically intervene in the latter by inhibiting the activation, the function, or both of caspases, the enzymes that dismantle the cell.
§ *ATP,* adenosine 5′-triphosphate.

Pharmacologic Interventions for Acute Spinal Cord Injury

Corticosteroids

- The applicability of corticosteroids for acute spinal cord injury has been investigated for more than 30 years.
- Although many animal studies have supported the administration of steroids in experimental spinal cord injury, it is important to realize that not all have demonstrated a beneficial effect.
- Corticosteroids are thought to provide neuroprotection in a several ways (Young 2000) (Box 19–5).
- The inhibition of lipid peroxidation has been hypothesized to be the most important neuroprotective property of glucocorticoids. Methylprednisolone appears to be particularly effective in preventing lipid peroxidation when compared with other glucocorticoids (Braughler 1985).

The Rationale for Methylprednisolone after Acute Spinal Cord Injury

- The clinical practice of administering high doses of methylprednisolone to patients with acute spinal cord injury originated from three large, prospective, randomized, double-blinded, and multicentered clinical trials—the National Acute Spinal Cord Injury Studies (NASCIS) 1, 2, and 3—which were reported in several publications in the 1980s and 1990s (Box 19–6).

Box 19–5: Potential Mechanisms of Action for Corticosteroids after Central Nervous System Injury

- Inhibition of lipid peroxidation
- Improved microvascular perfusion
- Prevention of calcium influx into cells
- Suppression of proinflammatory cytokine expression
- Attenuation of the effects of inflammatory cytokines
- Inhibition of nitric oxide production
- Inhibition of apoptosis

Box 19–6: Chronological Bibliography of the NASCIS Trials

[AU7]**NASCIS 1**

- Bracken MB, Collins WF, Freeman DF et al. (1984) Efficacy of methylprednisolone in acute spinal cord injury. JAMA 251(1): 45-52.
- Bracken MB, Shepard MJ, Hellenbrand KG et al. (1985) Methylprednisolone and neurological function 1 year after spinal cord injury (Results of the National Acute Spinal Cord Injury Study). J Neurosurg 63(5): 704-713.

NASCIS 2

- Bracken MB, Shepard MJ, Collins WF et al. (1990) A randomized, controlled trial of methylprednisolone or naloxone in the treatment of acute spinal cord injury (Results of the second National Acute Spinal Cord Injury Study). N Engl J Med 322: 1405-1411.
- Bracken MB, Shepard MJ, Holford TR et al. (1992) Methylprednisolone or naloxone treatment after acute spinal cord injury: One-year follow-up data (Results of the second National Acute Spinal Cord Injury Study). J Neurosurg 76(1): 23-31.
- Bracken MB, Holford TR. (1993) Effects of timing of methylprednisolone or naloxone administration on recovery of segmental and long-tract neurological function in NASCIS 2. J Neurosurg 79: 500-507.

NASCIS 3

- Bracken MB, Shepard MJ, Holford TR et al. (1997) Administration of methylprednisolone for 24 or 48 hours or tirilazad mesylate for 48 hours in the treatment of acute spinal cord injury (Results of the third national acute spinal cord injury randomized controlled trial, National Acute Spinal Cord Injury Study). JAMA 277(20): 1597-1604.
- Bracken MB, Shepard MJ, Holford TR et al. (1998) Methylprednisolone or tirilazad mesylate administration after acute spinal cord injury: One-year follow-up (Results of the third national acute spinal cord injury randomized controlled trial). J Neurosurg 89(5): 699-706.

- The NASCIS treatment arms and findings are summarized in Box 19–7.
- NASCIS 1 evaluated two relatively low doses of methylprednisolone within 48 hours of spinal cord injury and found no difference between the two groups.
- NASCIS 2 evaluated a much higher dose of methylprednisolone (the currently employed 30 mg/kg bolus with a 5.4-mg/kg/hr infusion) against naloxone (an opioid receptor antagonist) and a placebo group in patients within 12 hours of spinal cord injury. This study reported a significant improvement in motor and sensory recovery with methylprednisolone in patients treated within 8 hours of injury. A subsequent analysis found that naloxone was also beneficial for incompletely injured patients.
- NASCIS 3 compared 24- and 48-hour infusions of the NASCIS 2 doses of methylprednisolone with tirilazad mesylate, an antioxidant developed to inhibit lipid peroxidation without stimulating glucocorticoid receptors, in patients treated within 8 hours of injury. This study reported that although a prolonged methylprednisolone infusion was of no benefit to those treated within 3 hours of injury, for patients in whom treatment was initiated between 3 and 8 hours after

injury, there appeared to be some benefit from extending the methylprednisolone infusion to 48 hours.

Criticisms of the NASCIS Trials

- Much criticism has been directed at the conduct, statistical analysis, interpretation, and conclusions of NASCIS, leading to its discontinuation in some centers.
- Several in-depth articles scrutinizing the NASCIS 2 and 3 have been published (Hurlbert 2001). The chief criticism is that in NASCIS 2 (upon which NASCIS 3 was subsequently based) the primary outcome analysis of motor and sensory recovery in all randomized patients was *negative* and that it was only after a post hoc analysis that a small yet statistically significant benefit was found in those patients receiving the steroids within 8 hours.
- The primary outcome measures of NASCIS 3 were also *negative*. However, a post hoc analysis determined that for those in whom treatment was started 3 hours after injury, there was some benefit from 48-hour methylprednisolone treatment.
- The administration of methylprednisolone was not benign in the NASCIS reports. Wound infection rates, pulmonary embolism, severe pneumonia, sepsis, and even death secondary to respiratory complications appeared to

---

Box 19–7:	**Summary of NASCIS Treatment Arms and Results**

NASCIS 1

- 330 patients randomized and treated **within 48 hours** of spinal cord injury
  1. Methylprednisolone—100-mg bolus, then 25 mg every 6 hours for 10 days
  2. Methylprednisolone—1000-mg bolus, then 250 mg every 6 hours for 10 days
- Findings:
  - No significant difference was found in neurologic recovery between the two groups at 6- and 12-month follow-up.

NASCIS 2

- 487 patients randomized and treated **within 12 hours** of spinal cord injury
  1. Methylprednisolone—30 mg/kg bolus then 5.4 mg/kg/hr for 23 hours
  2. Naloxone—5.4 mg/kg bolus then 4.5 mg/kg/hr for 23 hours
  3. Placebo
- Findings:
  - No significant difference was found in neurologic recovery among the three groups at 6 or 12 months after injury.
  - In patients receiving methylprednisolone within 8 hours of injury, significant motor and sensory improvement was observed at 6 months (Bracken et al. 1990) and at 12 months after injury (Bracken et al. 1992). Naloxone was not shown to be effective.
  - In patients with incomplete lesions, naloxone was subsequently shown to promote significant neurologic recovery (Bracken et al. 1993).

NASCIS 3

- 499 patients randomized and treated **within 8 hours** of spinal cord injury
  - 1. Methylprednisolone—30 mg/kg bolus then 5.4 mg/kg/hr for 23 hours
  - 2. Methylprednisolone—30 mg/kg bolus then 5.4 mg/kg/hr for 47 hours
  - 3. Tirilazad mesylate—2.5 mg/kg every 6 hours for 48 hours
- Findings:
  - No significant difference was found in neurologic recovery among the three groups at 6 or 12 months after injury.
  - If treatment was initiated 3-8 hours after injury, patients receiving methylprednisolone for 48 hours had significant recovery over those who received methylprednisolone for 24 hours; p=0.01 at 6 months after injury (Bracken et al. 1997); p=0.53 at 12 months after injury (Bracken et al. 1998). Neurologic recovery with tirilazad was equivalent to that observed with 24-hour methylprednisolone.

be higher with steroid use (in particular with the 48-hour methylprednisolone regimen of NASCIS 3). Although statistical significance was not achieved in these adverse outcomes, it is unlikely that either study was powered sufficiently to establish such significance.

- It has also been pointed out that despite the widespread use of methylprednisolone, the NASCIS 2 and 3 trials did not study pediatric spinal cord injuries, penetrating spinal cord injuries, and cauda equina injuries, leaving the applicability of the NASCIS results in these settings unsubstantiated.

Gangliosides

- Gangliosides are sialic acid–containing glycosphingolipids highly expressed on the outer surface of cell membranes within the CNS.
- The systemic administration of monosialotetrahexosylganglioside (GM1 or Sygen) has been neuroprotective in a variety of models of experimental CNS injury. Like corticosteroids, there are multiple potential mechanisms of action (Box 19–8).
- The results of a large-scale, multicenter, randomized trial of GM1 were published in December 2001 (Geisler et al. 2001).
- This trial randomized 797 patients between 1992 and 1997 to placebo, low-dose GM1 (a 300-mg loading dose then 100 mg/day for 56 days), or high-dose GM1 (a 600-mg loading dose then 200 mg/day for 56 days). All patients first received the NASCIS 2 methylprednisolone protocol; the GM1 therapy was initiated after its completion.
- The primary outcome measure of this large study was the proportion of patients who achieved marked recovery at 26 weeks after injury, defined as an improvement of at least two grades in a modified Benzel classification of motor and sensory function over their baseline American Spinal Injury Association (ASIA) score.
- GM1 treatment did not significantly increase the proportion of patients with marked recovery at 26 weeks compared with those who received the placebo. Hence, the primary outcome analysis for this trial was negative.
- There did appear to be a more rapid rate of recovery in patients treated with GM1, and many parameters, including motor and sensory scores, and bowel and bladder

function showed trends of improvement in GM1 treatment over placebo, particularly in incomplete patients.

Opioid Antagonists

- Naloxone is a nonspecific opioid receptor antagonist. It was intensively evaluated in the early 1980s because of its observed ability to reverse spinal shock. Naloxone was also observed to improve spinal cord blood flow and enhance recovery from spinal cord injury in animal models. It was thought to antagonize the effects of the endogenous opiates observed to increase after spinal cord injury.
- Naloxone was included as one of three treatment arms in NASCIS 2. Patients received a 5.4 mg/kg intravenous bolus then a 4-mg/kg infusion for 23 hours, although it was later suggested that this represented a subtherapeutic dose.
- The initial NASCIS 2 results indicated that naloxone was no better than placebo (Bracken et al. 1990).
- A subsequent reexamination of this data by two of the NASCIS 2 authors suggested that for incompletely injured patients, naloxone did promote motor and sensory recovery (Bracken et al. 1993).
- Large-scale clinical evaluations of naloxone or other more specific opioid receptor antagonists have not been performed since those trials.

Glutamate Receptor Antagonists

- Pharmacologic antagonism of NMDA receptors has been studied extensively in an effort to antagonize excitotoxicity. However, because glutamate and its receptors are distributed widely throughout the CNS, it is difficult to avoid significant side effects with systemically administered treatment.
- NMDA receptor antagonists such as MK801 and gacyclidine (GK11) have been promising in animal studies of spinal cord injury (Gaviria et al. 2000).
- Gacyclidine has been evaluated in France in a phase 2 double-blinded, randomized study of 280 spinal cord–injured patients. This study apparently failed to show significant improvement in ASIA scores compared with placebo treatment.

Calcium Channel Blockers

- Calcium channel blockers appear to work mainly by modulating the tone of vascular smooth muscle rather than by altering calcium movement across neuronal and glial membranes.
- Nimodipine is a calcium channel blocker observed to enhance spinal cord blood flow and reverse hypo-perfusion in experimental spinal cord injury.
- Nimodipine was evaluated in a French study of acute spinal cord injury. In this prospective trial, 106 patients were randomized to one of four arms within 8 hours of injury: methylprednisolone according to the NASCIS 2 recommendations, nimodipine at 0.15 mg/kg/hr for 2 hours then at 0.03 mg/kg/hr for 7 days, both

Box 19–8:	**Potential Mechanisms of Action for GM1 after Central Nervous System Injury**

- Inhibition of lipid peroxidation
- Mimicking or potentiating of the effects of neurotrophic factors, thus promoting neuronal survival and axonal sprouting
- Attenuation of excitotoxicity
- Inhibition of apoptosis

methylprednisolone and nimodipine, or placebo (Pointillart et al. 2000).

- In this study, no treatment arm, including nimodipine alone, was found to promote neurologic recovery over placebo, although it likely suffered from being underpowered.
- A potential hazard from the use of calcium channel blockers in acute spinal cord injury is the promotion of systemic hypotension, which could exacerbate spinal cord ischemia, particularly with the loss of autoregulation.

Sodium Channel Blockers

- To antagonize the pathologic influx of sodium into axons after spinal cord injury, tetrodotoxin, a potent inhibitor of voltage-gated sodium channels, has been injected into the spinal cord after injury in animal models. This has provided significant protection to axons within the white matter and improved functional outcomes (Rosenberg et al. 1999).
- Riluzole, another sodium channel blocker, has also been shown to have neuroprotective effects after a clip compression injury to a rodent spinal cord, with spared white and gray matter and improved locomotor function (Schwartz et al. 2001).
- Riluzole has received Food and Drug Administration approval for the treatment of amyotrophic lateral sclerosis. Therefore, many pharmacokinetic and toxicity issues have been addressed. We lack human studies of its application in spinal cord injury.

Other Novel Potential Pharmacologic Interventions

- Several other pharmacologic agents have shown promise in animal studies, and because they are in clinical use for other applications, they may be candidates for human trials in the near future.
- These include COX inhibitors, the tetracycline antibiotic minocycline, the immunosuppressants FK506 (Tacrolimus) and cyclosporin, and the hematopoietic agent erythropoietin.
- We should recognize that virtually every drug that has undergone human clinical trials has demonstrated substantially more convincing neuroprotection in animal models than in clinical practice. Clearly, strategies with early promise require vigorous testing before being subjected to human trials.

Cyclooxygenase Inhibitors

- The expression of the COX-2 enzyme isoform has been observed to increase in the rat spinal cord after contusion injury, and the specific pharmacologic inhibition of the COX-2 isoform was shown to improve functional outcome in moderately severe injuries (Hains et al. 2001).

- Ibuprofen and meclofenamate, two commonly used NSAIDs, have been shown to maintain spinal cord blood flow after spinal cord injury in cats.

Minocycline

- Minocycline has been shown to inhibit excitotoxicity and provide neuroprotection in models of Parkinson's disease, autoimmune encephalomyelitis, amyotrophic lateral sclerosis, and adult and neonatal brain ischemia.
- It is thought to work by inhibiting the activation of microglia (resident phagocytic cells within the CNS) after ischemia and traumatic injury.
- Minocycline is under investigation in animal models of contusive spinal cord injury. Preliminary results suggest that it provides significant neuroprotection and improves locomotor function after spinal cord injury in rats (Arnold et al. 2001).

FK506 and Cyclosporine

- These immunosuppressants have demonstrated some beneficial effects in the setting of peripheral nerve injury.
- Cyclosporin has been shown to promote tissue sparing and inhibit lipid peroxidation in models of brain and spinal cord injury (Diaz-Ruiz et al. 2000).
- FK506 has been shown to promote axonal regeneration within the CNS and functional recovery after experimental spinal cord injury (Wang et al. 1999).

Erythropoietin

- Erythropoietin is thought to have anti-inflammatory, antioxidant, and antiapoptotic properties.
- Erythropoietin has been neuroprotective in the setting of experimental brain injury and has been shown to prevent motor neuron apoptosis and improve neurologic function in a global ischemia model of spinal cord injury in rabbits (Celik et al. 2002).

Conclusions

- The pathophysiological processes initiated acutely after spinal cord injury are extremely complex.
- The extent to which we understand the acute pathophysiology of spinal cord injury is reflected in the limited number of neuroprotective strategies available. Even the efficacy of the one widely used pharmacologic agent—methylprednisolone—is being hotly contested.
- Promising research is nevertheless being done to further delineate the aspects of vascular dysregulation, inflammation, lipid peroxidation, and apoptotic cell death that may be amenable to pharmacologic intervention.
- Several drugs have demonstrated efficacy in animal models of spinal cord injury and may become appropriate for testing in the human setting in the near future.

References

Arnold PM, Ameenuddin S, Citron BA et al. (2001) Systemic administration of minocycline improves functional recovery and morphometric analysis after spinal cord injury. Soc Neurosci abstract 769.4.

These authors administered minocycline (90 mg/kg) 1 hour after a contusion spinal cord injury in rats and found increased tissue sparing at the site of injury, reduced numbers of cells undergoing apoptotic death, and improved locomotor function compared with control animals treated with tetracycline.

Bethea JR (2000) Spinal cord injury-induced inflammation: A dual-edged sword. Prog Brain Res 128: 33-42.

This is an excellent review of the inflammatory processes that occur in response to spinal cord injury, demonstrating how certain aspects of inflammation are deleterious and others may be neuroprotective.

Bracken MB, Shepard MJ, Holford TR et al. (1992) Methylprednisolone or naloxone treatment after acute spinal cord injury: One-year follow-up data (Results of the second National Acute Spinal Cord Injury Study). J Neurosurg 76(1):23-31.

Bracken MB, Shepard MJ, Holford TR et al. (1997) Administration of methylprednisolone for 24 or 48 hours or tirilazad mesylate for 48 hours in the treatment of acute spinal cord injury (Results of the third national acute spinal cord injury randomized controlled trial, National Acute Spinal Cord Injury Study). JAMA 277(20): 1597-1604.

Bracken MB, Shepard MJ, Holford TR et al. (1998) Methylprednisolone or tirilazad mesylate administration after acute spinal cord injury: One-year follow-up (Results of the third national acute spinal cord injury randomized controlled trial). J Neurosurg 89(5): 699-706.

[AU4]Bracken MB, Holford TR. (1993) Effects of timing of methylprednisolone or naloxone administration on recovery of segmental and long-tract neurological function in NASCIS 2. J Neurosurg 79: 500-507.

This report of patients in the NASCIS 2 study suggested that methylprednisolone administered within 8 hours of injury was associated with improvement in distal motor function (in addition to some local segmental root recovery). This study also indicated that although naloxone had been deemed ineffective in the previous reports of NASCIS 2, it did appear to be beneficial in the subset of patients with incomplete spinal cord injuries.

Bracken MB, Shepard MJ, Collins WF et al. (1990) A randomized, controlled trial of methylprednisolone or naloxone in the treatment of acute spinal cord injury (Results of the second National Acute Spinal Cord Injury Study). N Engl J Med 322: 1405-1411.

This was the report of the 6-month follow-up results from patients enrolled in NASCIS 2, demonstrating that although there were no significant differences between the groups as a whole, for those in whom methylprednisolone treatment was initiated within 8 hours after injury, there was a statistically significant motor and sensory improvement compared with those who received the placebo.

Braughler JM (1985) Lipid peroxidation-induced inhibition of gamma-aminobutyric acid uptake in rat brain synaptosomes: Protection by glucocorticoids. J Neurochem 44: 1282-1288.

This in vitro study suggested that, among the various glucocorticoids, methylprednisolone was comparatively very effective in its ability to prevent lipid peroxidation.

Celik M, Gokmen N, Erbayraktar S et al.(2002) Erythropoietin prevents motor neuron apoptosis and neurologic disability in experimental spinal cord ischemic injury. Proc Natl Acad Sci USA 99: 2258-2263.

These authors induced a global spinal ischemia injury to rabbits by occluding the aorta for 20 minutes then administered erythropoietin or saline intravenously. They observed a decrease in apoptotic cell death of motor neurons with erythropoietin treatment, and this was associated with improved neurologic function.

Crowe MJ, Bresnahan JC, Shuman SL et al. (1997) Apoptosis and delayed degeneration after spinal cord injury in rats and monkeys. Nat Med 3: 73-76.

This landmark study demonstrated in animal models that apoptotic cell death was occurring after spinal cord injury, particularly in oligodendrocytes (the loss of which could lead to demyelination). They also found apoptotic death to be occurring for up to 3 weeks after injury, suggesting that there was a temporal window of opportunity to intervene in this secondary damage.

Diaz-Ruiz A, Rios C, Duarte I et al. (2000) Lipid peroxidation inhibition in spinal cord injury: Cyclosporin A vs. methylprednisolone. Neuroreport 11: 1765-1767.

These authors demonstrated that cyclosporin A was as effective as methylprednisolone in reducing lipid peroxidation after contusion spinal cord injuries in rats, and survival rates were better with cyclosporin A.

Emery E, Aldana P, Bunge MB et al. (1998) Apoptosis after traumatic human spinal cord injury. J Neurosurg 89: 911-920.

This important study from the Miami Project examined 15 human patients who died between 3 hours and 2 months after sustaining a spinal cord injury. They observed that the apoptotic death of oligodendrocytes in particular was occurring in the spinal cords of almost all patients, again confirming that a window of opportunity exists during which this apoptotic death might be prevented.

Gaviria M, Privat A, d'Arbigny P et al. (2000) Neuroprotective effects of a novel NMDA antagonist, gacyclidine, after experimental contusive spinal cord injury in adult rats. Brain Res 874: 200-209.

This study evaluated gacyclidine (an NMDA receptor antagonist) administered at 10, 30, 60, or 120 minutes after contusion spinal cord injury in rats. It found that gacyclidine administered 10 minutes after injury provided significant tissue sparing and better locomotor function than placebo-treated animals. Of note, a human trial of this drug has been performed in France and apparently failed to demonstrate a significant benefit for acute spinal cord injury.

Geisler FH, Coleman WP, Grieco G et al. (2001) The Sygen multicenter acute spinal cord injury study. Spine 26: S87-S98.

This is the report of the main results from the prospective, randomized, multicentered clinical trial of GM1 ganglioside treatment of acute spinal cord injury, published in the 2001 focus edition of Spine on spinal cord injuries. The authors report that GM1 ganglioside did not increase the percentage of patients who achieved significant recovery at 26 weeks after injury as compared with placebo. However, recovery did occur more rapidly with GM1 ganglioside treatment, and there appeared to be some benefit for incomplete spinal cord injuries.

Hains BC, Yucra JA, Hulsebosch CE (2001) Reduction of pathological and behavioral deficits following spinal cord contusion injury with the selective cyclooxygenase-2 inhibitor NS-398. J Neurotrauma 18: 409-423.

This is a proof-of-principle study that demonstrated that the selective pharmacologic inhibition of COX-2 in the setting of a contusion spinal cord injury in rats reduced secondary damage, improved locomotor function, and diminished pain behavior patterns. The clinical applicability of this strategy requires further study because the authors of this paper administered the COX-2 inhibitor 15 minutes before the spinal cord injury.

Hurlbert RJ (2001) The role of steroids in acute spinal cord injury: An evidence-based analysis. Spine 26: S39-S46.

The author is one of several clinicians who have published detailed critiques on the methodology, statistical analysis, and interpretation of the NASCIS 2 and 3 trials. Concerns regarding the validity of the NASCIS trials as the basis for the widespread use of methylprednisolone have led to its discontinuation in the Canadian province of Alberta from which the author hails. This article provides a review of NASCIS and other human studies that have evaluated steroids in acute spinal cord injury.

Pointillart V, Petitjean ME, Wiart L et al. (2000) Pharmacological therapy of spinal cord injury during the acute phase. Spinal Cord 38: 71-76.

This is a report of a prospective, randomized clinical trial comparing nimodipine (a calcium channel blocker), methylprednisolone, nimodipine and methylprednisolone, and placebo in 100 acute spinal cord injured patients. It showed no significant neurologic benefit for any of the treatments over placebo, including methylprednisolone alone (given according to NASCIS 2 protocols).

Popovich PG, Wei P, Stokes BT (1997) Cellular inflammatory response after spinal cord injury in Sprague-Dawley and Lewis rats. J Comp Neurol 377: 443-464.

This study characterizes the invasion and activation of inflammatory cells after spinal cord injury in two strains of rats. The authors qualitatively and quantitatively describe the involvement of cells such as neutrophils, macrophages, and microglia at times up to 4 weeks after injury.

Rosenberg LJ, Teng YD, Wrathall JR (1999) Effects of the sodium channel blocker tetrodotoxin on acute white matter pathology after experimental contusive spinal cord injury. J Neurosci 19: 6122-6133.

These authors injected a potent sodium channel blocker (tetrodotoxin) into the spinal cord of rats 5 or 15 minutes after a contusion injury. They found this to have significant neuroprotective effects primarily in white matter, preserving axonal morphology and improving locomotor function.

Schwartz G, Fehlings MG (2001) Evaluation of the neuroprotective effects of sodium channel blockers after spinal cord injury: Improved behavioral and neuroanatomical recovery with riluzole. J Neurosurg 94: 245-256.

These authors performed clip compression spinal cord injuries on rats and then systemically administered several sodium channel blockers, including riluzole, a sodium channel blocker tested in patients with amyotrophic lateral sclerosis (Lou Gehrig's disease). They found that the riluzole provided significant tissue sparing in both gray and white matter, and this was associated with improved locomotor function.

Tator CH, Fehlings MG (1991) Review of the secondary injury theory of acute spinal cord trauma with emphasis on vascular mechanisms. J Neurosurg 75: 15-26.

This paper reviews the concept that secondary damage is an important component of the neurologic dysfunction after spinal cord injury. It focuses on the role that ischemia and altered spinal cord blood flow plays both systemically (e.g., hypotension) and locally (e.g., loss of autoregulation) to potentially worsen the damage incurred by the spinal cord tissue that escapes the original mechanical injury.

Wang MS, Gold BG (1999) FK506 increases the regeneration of spinal cord axons in a predegenerated peripheral nerve autograft. J Spinal Cord Med 22: 287-296.

These authors evaluated the potential for FK506 (an immunosuppressant known to promote the regeneration of peripheral nerves) to promote the regeneration of axons within the spinal cord of rats. They transplanted a segment of peripheral nerve into the spinal cord to provide a permissive environment and found that FK506 treatment promoted the regeneration of rubrospinal axons (which control several motor functions in rats).

Young W (2000) Molecular and cellular mechanisms of spinal cord injury therapies. In: Neurobiology of Spinal Cord Injury (Kalb RG et al., eds.). Totowa: Humana Press, pp. 241-276.

This is an excellent review of the pathophysiology of spinal cord injury and in particular of the scientific rationale behind such pharmacologic strategies as methylprednisolone.

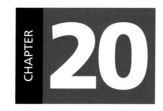

Spinal Cord Injury

Prehospital and Emergency Room Management, as well as Timing of Treatment

James S. Harrop★, Marco T. Silva★, Marc D. Fisicaro §, and Alexander R. Vaccaro †

★ M.D., Department of Neurosurgery, Jefferson Medical College, Thomas Jefferson University, Philadelphia, PA
§ B.A., Medical Student, Jefferson Medical College, Thomas Jefferson University, Philadelphia, PA
† M.D., Professor of Orthopaedic Surgery, Thomas Jefferson University and the Rothman Institute, Philadelphia, PA

Introduction

- Approximately 12,000–14,000 acute spinal cord injuries occur in North America annually; most affect adolescent males and are caused by motor vehicle collisions.
- Unfortunately, current medical knowledge and practices are not able to provide neurological tissue with the capability to regenerate neurons or facilitate neuronal growth.
- Over the last several decades, there have been significant advances in the overall treatment and management of spinal fractures and acute spinal cord injuries. The most dramatic advances have been in prehospital care, emergency room, and intensive care unit management.

Prehospital Evaluation Period

- The incidence of spinal cord injury has continually declined over the last several decades. This can be attributed to the following:
  1. Educating the medical community and general population about the prevention and early recognition of patients vulnerable to spinal fractures or spinal cord injury
  2. Advances in techniques and practices to protect the spinal column and spinal cord, such as improvements in automobile safety through the use of restraints and airbags
  3. Emergency rescue teams' increased awareness and prompt response to potential spinal cord injuries
- Care and management of any trauma patient begins with the complete immobilization of the spine at the scene of the injury, during transportation, and until radiographic documentation of the absence of a spinal fracture (Box 20–1).
- In the 1970s, at least 55% of patients visiting a regional spinal cord injury center had complete neurological injuries (absence of both motor and sensation below the injury). The majority of these injuries and neurological complications (27%) occurred during transport to a medical facility (Toscano 1988).
- During the 1980s, with improved adherence to spine immobilization techniques, hardboard transfers, and other spinal column protective strategies, there has been a dramatic decline in the reported patients with spinal cord injury (39%).
- Spinal cord resuscitation should be initiated at the scene of the injury, maintained during transportation, and continued in the emergency room.

Box 20–1:	Spine Stabilization

- Rigid cervical collar
- Hard backboard
- Lateral support devices
- Tape or straps

- The American College of Surgeons set forth guidelines for the initial in-field management of a trauma patient using the mnemonic ABCDE, where A stands for airway, B for breathing, C for circulation, D for disability or neurological status and E for exposure and environment (American College of Surgeons 1993) (Box 20–2).
- On a helmeted athlete such as a football player, the protective helmet and shoulder pads should not be removed until a controlled environment is established in which the patient's sagittal alignment is protected by immobilizing the patient's head and body in the same plane. Thereafter, the helmet and shoulder pads can be removed with the help of multiple assistants (Peris et al. 2002).
- Cervical spine immobilization should be maintained until the potential for injury is thoroughly evaluated and dismissed or confirmed as an injury.
- The American College of Surgeons recommends that trauma patients be immobilized with a rigid cervical orthosis and transferred using lateral bolsters to prevent head rotation. The patient should be placed on a long backboard and secured with tapes or straps to prevent patient movement (American College of Surgeons 1993) (Box 20–1). Beware of excessive skin pressure and the potential for the formation of decubiti if prolonged immobilization on a backboard is anticipated (>2 hours) in the insensate patient.
- Following adequate resuscitation and secure immobilization, the patient should be transported quickly to the nearest level 1 trauma or spinal cord injury center if possible.
- Transport priority should be as follows:
  - Ambulance—Hospital less than 50 miles from injury
  - Helicopter—Hospital between 50 and 150 miles from injury
  - Fixed-wing aircraft—Hospital greater than 150 miles from injury

Box 20–2:	Advanced Cardiac Life Support Mnemonic

- A—Airway
- B—Breathing
- C—Circulation
- D—Disability
- E—Exposure and environment

Emergency Room Care

- Particular care and attention should be given to the polytrauma patient, patients with an altered level of consciousness, or patients with injuries involving the head or neck. These patients are especially vulnerable to further worsening of their neurological injuries because they are less likely to "protect" their spinal cord through mechanisms such as muscle spasms, verbal notification of increased pain, or tenderness over an injured area.
- Once the ABCs have been examined and life-threatening injuries have been treated, a secondary survey should be performed. This includes a thorough but focused physical examination to assess the patient's neurological function and the presence of any injuries. The entire spinal column should be palpated for areas of increased tenderness or identification of a depression, or "step off," in the alignment of the spinous processes.
- The physical examination should proceed in a systematic manner, beginning at the patient's head and progressing caudally, such that each spinal segment or level is individually examined. All patients should be cared for with the assumption that a fracture or spinal instability exists. The assumption should be continued until the absence of a fracture is confirmed with radiographs.

Evaluation of Head Trauma

- The Glasgow coma scale grades a patient's neurological status based on the patient's response to external stimuli in three main areas: eye opening, verbal response, and motor response (Box 20–3). The score is tabulated, and the total score can range from 15 (normal responses to stimuli) to 3 (no response or comatose). This score is used as a baseline and provides physicians with a guide for appropriate treatment and for determining potential neurological recovery and rehabilitation strategies.

Box 20–3:	Glasgow Coma Scale

- Eye opening to the following:
  - Voice—3
  - Pain—2
  - None—1
- Verbal response
  - Oriented—4
  - Inappropriate—3
  - Incomprehensible—2
  - None—1
- Motor response
  - Obeys commands—5
  - Localizes pain—4
  - Withdraws from pain—3
  - Decorticate—2
  - Decerebrate—1

Table 20–1: Muscle and Sensation Grading

MUSCLE GRADING		SENSATION GRADING	
GRADE	DEFINITION	GRADE	DEFINITION
0	Absent	0	None
1	Palpable contraction	1	Impaired
2	Full ROM with gravity eliminated*	2	Normal
3	Full ROM with gravity present	NT	Not tested
4	Active movement with resistance		
5	Normal strength		
NT	Not tested		

* *ROM,* range of motion.

- On arrival to the emergency room, the patient's airway, vital signs, and hemodynamic stability should be reexamined and reassessed.

Evaluation of Airway and Breathing

- Patients that have severe head injuries or are unable to protect the airway because of a depressed level of consciousness (Glasgow coma score < 8) should be electively intubated.
- Patients with spinal cord injuries (particularly above C5) having difficulty with respiration because of fatigue of the accessory respiratory muscles, injury to the lung parenchyma, thoracic injury, or a combination of these should be considered for elective intubation.
- Vital capacity should be evaluated. If less than 300 ml, intubation should proceed because further decrease may jeopardize adequate ventilation and oxygenation.
- Manual in-line stabilization of the cervical spine during orotracheal intubation is a technique of intubation that minimizes motion of the unstable cervical spine (Gerling et al. 2000).

Neurological Examination

- The American Spinal Injury Association (ASIA) standard of neurological testing provides a concise and detailed method for evaluating spinal cord and peripheral nerve root function. It provides physicians with common nomenclature to document and follow each patient's neurological examination.
- Sensation is determined in all 28 dermatomes bilaterally by the patient's ability to detect the sharp end of a pin. It is recorded as absent (0), impaired (1), or normal (2) (Table 20–1).
- Motor function or strength is documented and graded 1–5 based on resistance to physical manipulation or gravity.
- Ten bilateral myotomes representing key spinal motor segments are identified and manually tested. These muscles are individually graded on a scale of 0–5 and combined such that the unimpaired patient has a score of 100 (Table 20–1).

- Based on both the motor and sensory examination, the patient is further classified or graded using the ASIA modification of the Frankel Neurological Classification System—from normal (ASIA E) to complete paralysis and no sensation (ASIA A) (Table 20–2).
- The presence or absence of rectal tone has a dramatic implication on prognosis regarding the potential for neurological recovery.
- Common variants of spinal cord and nerve root injury symptoms include anterior cord syndrome, Brown-Séquard's syndrome, central cord syndrome, posterior cord syndrome, and cauda equina syndrome.

Imaging Evaluation

- Initial radiographic examination includes standard anteroposterior and lateral plain x-ray films of the cervical, thoracic, and lumbosacral spine, including open-mouth odontoid view regions. Remember that 10%-15% of patients have noncontiguous spinal column fractures.
- Always visualize the alignment of the cervicothoracic junction (i.e., C7 and T1 vertebral bodies) (Fig. 20–1). It may be necessary to obtain an oblique or swimmer's view in patients with large shoulders, short necks, or those wearing shoulder pads.

Table 20–2: American Spinal Injury Association Impairment Scale

SCALE	INJURY SUBTYPE	MOTOR
A	Complete	No preservation
B	Incomplete	No preservation
C	Incomplete	More than one half of key muscles caudal to injury have strength graded **less** than 3
D	Incomplete	More than one half of key muscles caudal to injury have strength graded **greater** than 3
E	Normal	Normal or radicular loss

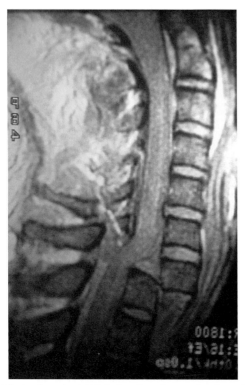

Figure 20–1: A sagittal MRI showing the cervicothoracic junction (C7 and T1 vertebral bodies). **It may be necessary to obtain an oblique or swimmer's view to visualize the junction in those with large shoulders, short necks, or those wearing shoulder pads.**

- Computed tomography (CT) scanning with coronal and sagittal reformatted images is useful to further define bony anatomy.
- Magnetic resonance imaging (MRI) is used an all cases of neurological compromise or to better visualize soft tissue anatomy—that is, neural compressive lesions such as disk herniations, epidural hematomas (Fig. 20–2), or traumatic ligamentous injuries (Figs. 20–3 and 20–4).
- Patients with ferromagnetic devices such as a pacemaker cannot undergo MRI. In these cases, a myelogram followed by a post-myelogram CT scan should be obtained to aid the identification of spinal cord or nerve root compression.

Timing of Treatment

- The initial or primary injury to the spinal cord results from direct mechanical compression or dispersion of this traumatic energy through the spinal cord.
- The severity of the initial impact on the spinal cord typically is reflected by the patient's initial neurological presentation.
- The extent of the patient's neurological recovery is not solely dependent on this primary injury. It is also influenced by the extent of the secondary injury to the spinal cord.

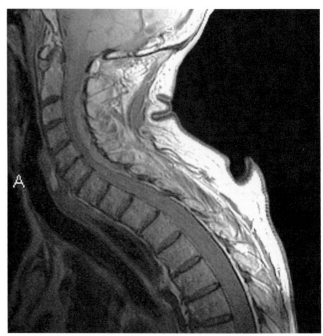

Figure 20–2: A sagittal MRI showing an epidural hematoma in the cervical region of the spinal cord. **An MRI may be necessary to visualize such lesions.**

- The secondary injury to the spinal cord results from a physiologic cascade involving initial hemorrhage followed by inflammation, membrane hydrolysis, ischemia, calcium influx, and cellular apoptosis or programmed cell death (Table 20–3).

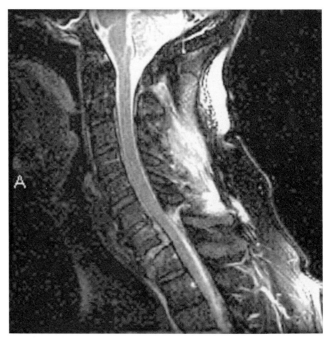

Figure 20–3: A sagittal MRI demonstrating a high-grade distraction–extension injury at the cervicothoracic junction. **This injury could be easily missed if imaging down to the T1 superior endplate is not done routinely.**

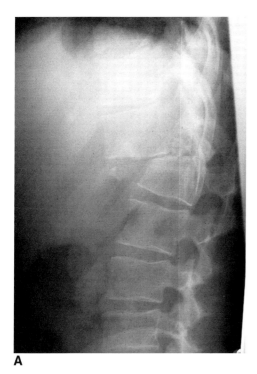

A

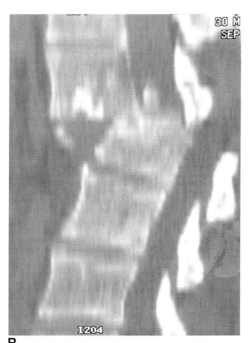

B

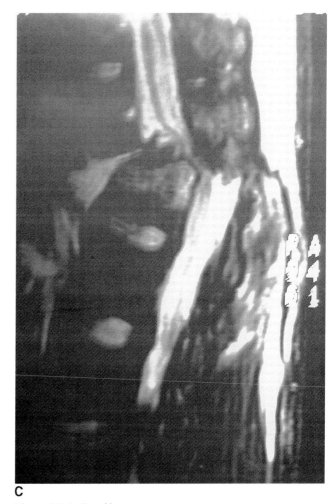

C

Figure 20–4: Cont'd

Figure 20–4: A, A lateral plain radiograph of a fracture dislocation at the T12 and L1 level. B, A CT scan with sagittal reconstruction further defining the bony details of the injury. C, A sagittal MRI demonstrating the details of the neural compression as a result of the fracture dislocation.

- There are no accepted clinical treatment strategies or algorithms that provide neurological regrowth or regeneration of the injured spinal cord.
- Treatment algorithms for the timing and method of treatment for traumatic spinal cord injury have not been standardized.

Table 20–3: Biology of Spinal Cord Injury	
TRAUMATIC ACTION	**RESULT**
Ischemia	Vessel thrombosis
	Impaired autoregulation
	Hemorrhage
	Vasoconstriction
Cell membrane dysfunction	Loss of sodium or potassium gradient
	Calcium influx
	Lipid peroxidation
Intracellular dysfunction	Free radical accumulation
	Loss of adenosine triphosphate
	Apoptosis

- Medical regimens to minimize the effects of the secondary cascade of injury include pharmacologic approaches or medical therapies aimed at increasing the spinal cord perfusion, membrane stabilization, and glial scar retardation.
- Physical treatment strategies aimed at improving neurological status range from closed reduction of dislocated vertebral segments to open surgical procedures to decompression of the neural elements.

Pharmacologic Intervention

- Pharmacologic agents used in the acute treatment of spinal cord injury are not uniformly accepted. Agents that have undergone the most laboratory and clinical evaluations are methylprednisolone; tirilazad mesylate; naloxone, an opioid receptor antagonist; nimodipine, a calcium channel blocker; and a GM1 ganglioside (Table 20–4).
- In animal experiments, these agents have been shown to improve the recovery of neurological function. However, these results are less conclusive in human clinical trials.
- In two multicentered, prospective, controlled, and randomized studies, methylprednisolone was shown to improve the motor scores in post-traumatic spinal cord injury patients when delivered more than 8 hours following injury (Bracken et al. 1990). However, the extent of recovery in terms of improved functional ability and the expense or risk to the individual has been extensively debated. Many clinicians believe there is insufficient evidence to support any pharmacologic therapies as a standard of care in the management of acute spinal cord injury.
- Gangliosides have both a neuroprotective and neuroregenerative effect in the laboratory and are abundantly present in the neuronal cell membrane (Geisler et al. 2001). Two clinical trials that evaluated the efficacy of this drug after spinal cord injury concluded that GM1 gangliosides enhanced neurological recovery after traumatic spinal cord injury. However, a recent larger, multicentered, double-blinded study with almost 800 patients found no statistical improvement in the neurological outcomes in treated patients. A secondary analysis did show the drug to be beneficial in terms of earlier recovery of motor function and improved sensory, bowel, and bladder function.

Timing of Surgery

- Data for the timing of surgical treatment of spinal cord injury, like pharmacologic agents, has not been shown conclusively to support either early or late intervention.
- Proponents of early surgical decompression advocate timely normalization of the intracellular environment and recovery of capillary perfusion by removing external pressure from the spinal cord and establishing spinal stability.
- Animal studies have found that early decompression consistently provides a better clinical and functional recovery.
- Data analysis documenting the beneficial effect of early surgery in humans has not been clearly elucidated.
- One reason is the numerous treatment factors that cannot be controlled in human trials unless a larger multicentered study is performed.
- There is substantial class 2 and 3 evidence (nonprospective, nonrandomized, and uncontrolled) that surgical decompression provides better outcomes than late or nonsurgical therapies.

Conclusion

- The timely recognition of spinal instability and spinal cord injury has improved the functional outcome of this disability through early immobilization, spinal cord resuscitation, and pharmacologic, surgical, or both types of intervention.
- Great strides have been made in the last two decades to elucidate the pathophysiology of spinal cord injury.
- Through multicentered collaborative investigations, issues such as the effectiveness of various pharmacologic agents and the timing and type of surgery can be better defined and instituted.

Table 20–4: **Pharmacologic Agents**		
NAME	**CLASS**	**MECHANISM**
Methylprednisolone	Steroid	Anti-inflammatory and antioxidant effect
Tirilazad mesylate	21-aminosteroid	Cell membrane stabilization and antioxidant effect
Nimodipine	Calcium channel antagonist	Prevents calcium influx into cell
4-aminopyridine	Potassium channel antagonist	Extends duration of action potentials
Sygen	GM1 ganglioside	Enhances nerve growth or sprouting
Naloxone	Mu-opioid receptor antagonist	Neuroprotective

References

American College of Surgeons Committee on Trauma. (1993) Advanced Trauma Life Support. Chicago: American College of Surgeons, pp. 201.

  Textbook describing the resuscitation, stabilization, immobilization, transportation, and treatment of patients who incur life-threatening trauma.

Bracken MB, Shepard MJ, Collins WF et al. (1990) A randomized, controlled trial of methylprednisolone or naloxone in the treatment of acute spinal cord injury: Results of the second National Acute Spinal Cord Injury Study. N Engl J Med 322: 1405-1411.

  Patients who were administered methylprednisolone or naloxone after incurring an acute spinal cord injury were evaluated at 6 weeks, 6 months, and 1 year after the event for sensory and motor loss and were compared with patients administered placebo. Patients who received steroids within 8 hours of injury had improved neurological scores compared with the scores of those receiving no steroids after 8 hours.

Bracken MB, Shepard MJ, Holford TR et al. (1997) Administration of methylprednisolone for 24 or 48 hours or tirilazad mesylate for 48 hours in the treatment of acute spinal cord injury: Results of the third National Acute Spinal Cord Injury Study. JAMA 277: 1597-1604.

  A double-blinded, randomized, clinical trial involving 16 trauma centers and 499 patients with acute spinal cord injury. Patients were administered either methylprednisolone or tirilazad mesylate 24 or 48 hours after their accident. The study compared the effects of the timing of the administration of drugs after injury. The study found that if steroids were given within 3 hours of injury, they should be continued for 24 hours. If they were given between 3 and 8 hours, they were recommended to be given for 48 hours.

Delamater RB, Sherman J, Carr JB. (1995) Pathophysiology of spinal cord injury: Recovery after immediate and delayed decompression. JBJS (Am) 77: 1042-1049.

  Study examining purebred dogs with 50% spinal cord compression for motor and sensory loss after increasing the amount of time until decompression.

Geisler FH, Coleman WP, Grieco G et al. (2001) The Sygen multicenter acute spinal injury study. Spine 26(suppl): S87-S98.

  Randomized, double-blinded, sequential, and multicentered clinical trial period comparing two doses of Sygen and placebo with acute spinal cord injury in 22 patients.

Gerling MC, Davis DP, Hamilton RS et al. (2000) Effects of cervical spine immobilization technique and laryngoscope blade selection on an unstable cervical spine in a cadaver model of intubation. Annals Emergency Med 36(4): 293-300.

  Randomized, crossover trial evaluating the effects of manual in-line stabilization and cervical collar immobilization with three laryngoscope blades on cervical spine movement during orotracheal intubation in a cadaver model.

Hadley MN, Walters BC, Grabb PA et al. (2002) Guidelines for the management of acute spine and spinal cord injuries. Neurosurgery 50(3): S63-S72.

  Clinical practice guidelines derived from a critical review of relevant literature that addresses 22 topics and tries to establish guidelines using an evidence-based approach.

Peris MD, Donaldson WF, Towers J et al. (2002) Helmet and shoulder pad removal in suspected cervical spine injury: Human control model. Spine 27(9): 995-998.

  Digital fluoroscopy was used to determine the amount of movement of the cervical spine during the removal of a football helmet and shoulder pads.

Tator CH, Rowed DW, Schwartz ML et al. (1984) Management of acute spinal cord injuries. Can J Surg 27: 289-294.

  Report describing the results of 144 patients with acute spinal cord injury admitted to Sunnybrook Medical Center, determining the advantage of regionalization and specialization in the field of acute spinal cord injury.

Toscano J. (1988) Prevention of neurological deterioration before admission to spinal cord injury unit. Paraplegia 26(3): 143-150.

  This study followed 123 patients with acute spinal cord injury admitted to Victorian Spinal Injury Unit and determined that neurological deficits caused between the time of injury and the time the patient was admitted to the hospital could be minimized by having an appropriate suspicion of a possible spinal cord injury and thereby initiating appropriate handling and immobilization as soon as possible.

CHAPTER 21

Cervical Spine Trauma

Arjun Saxena*, Jeff S. Silber §, and Alexander R. Vaccaro †

* B.S., Jefferson Medical College, Philadelphia, PA
§ M.D., Assistant Professor, Department of Orthopaedic Surgery, Long Island Jewish
Medical Center, North Shore University Hospital Center, Long Island, NY; Albert Einstein
University Hospital, Bronx, NY
† M.D., Professor of Orthopaedic Surgery, Thomas Jefferson University and the Rothman
Institute, Philadelphia, PA

Introduction

- Cervical trauma can result in an array of ailments, from minor neck pain to death.
- Each year, approximately half of the 50,000 reported spinal column or cord injuries involve the cervical spine; about one fourth of the spinal injuries result in some degree of neurological deficit (Lasfargues et al. 1995).
- Most spinal column or cord injuries occur in males between the ages of 15 and 24 (Kraus et al. 1975).
- There has also been an increase in spinal column or cord injuries in patients older than 55 (Kraus et al. 1975).
- The most common mechanisms of injury in adults are motor vehicle accidents (40%-56%), falls (20%-30%), violence such as gunshots (12%-21%), and sports (6%-13%) (Vaccaro 1999).
- Other associated systemic injuries are usually present and must be evaluated and managed.
- Historically, many patients who sustain cervical spine injuries had poor outcomes, but in recent years, early cervical immobilization, rapid and safe transport to a spinal cord trauma center, administration of appropriate pharmacologic agents, and methods of in-hospital management have contributed to improve long-term prognosis.

Initial Treatment and Examination

- Initial stages of management include evaluation, resuscitation, immobilization, extrication, and transport.
- Early recognition of injury begins in the field. A collar is placed and a spine board is applied. The patient is then transferred to a facility familiar with spinal trauma (Slucky et al. 1994).
- On arrival at the emergency ward, a trauma resuscitation team evaluates airway competency, breathing, and circulation.
- Anterior–posterior and lateral x-ray films of the entire spine are obtained.
- Noncontiguous spinal injuries are seen in 7.5%-10% of spine injured patients (Vaccaro et al. 1992) (Table 21–1).

In-hospital Management

- An initial respiratory and hemodynamic evaluation should be performed.
- Patients should be kept at arterial partial pressure of oxygen (PaO_2) of 100 torr and arterial partial pressure of carbon dioxide ($PaCO_2$) less than 45 torr to reduce the negative effects of ischemia on neuronal function (Vaccaro et al. 1997).

Table 21–1: Initial Stages of Management	
STAGE	
Evaluation	Primary and secondary survey
	ABCs—Airway, breathing, circulation
	A patient with neck pain, extremity weakness, altered sensation, spine tenderness to palpation, or soft-tissue bruises to the neck or trunk should be suspected to have a spinal injury.
	An unconscious or intoxicated patient should be assumed to have a spinal injury until proven otherwise.
	Follow the advanced trauma life support protocol.
	Avoid the "chin lift" method of the securing airway—it may decrease space available for spinal cord.
Resuscitation	Adequate oxygenation is imperative to maximize spinal cord function.
	In an alert patient, airway can be maintained by using a standard cutoff oral airway or an oropharyngeal, nasopharyngeal, or nasotracheal airway.
	An unconscious patient can be ventilated with an orotracheal airway.
	No differences in safety among airway methods have been identified as long as in-line manual cervical immobilization is maintained.
	Sufficient circulation must be maintained.
	Direct pressure should be applied to open bleeding wounds.
	Foreign penetrating objects should not be removed from the patient until arrival at an emergency room.
Immobilization	In-line manual traction should be performed before moving the patient to the spine board.
	Patient should be placed on a spine board in a neutral supine position.
	Use occipital padding for an adult and an occipital recess for a child younger than 8.
	A hard cervical collar with an opening in front is preferred.
Extrication	Extrication may be necessary when the patient is in a confined area.
	It must be organized to prevent further injuries.
	Considerations include the patient's medical status, accessibility to patient, and conditions of the proximate environment.
	Helmets should be left on; facemasks can be removed.
	A scoop style stretcher is safest.
Transport	Once stabilized, the patient should be transported to a level 1 trauma center if possible.
	Patient should be placed in the Trendelenburg position.
	Methods of transport include ambulance, helicopter, or fixed-wing aircraft.
	Long journeys may necessitate a nasogastric tube, intravenous lines, and a urinary catheter.

- Endotracheal intubation should be used for patients who cannot sustain $PaO_2/PaCO_2$ ratio of 0.75 or vital capacity > 10.0 ml/kg.
- Use the Trendelenburg position with intravenous fluids as initial treatment for hemorrhagic shock.
- Neurogenic shock should be treated judiciously with fluids and vasopressors (Table 21–2).
- Neurological examination should include the assessment of cranial nerves, motor and sensory function, reflexes, and rectal tone.
- The level of neurological function is graded according to the American Spinal Injury Association (ASIA) classification (Table 21–3).

Pharmacologic Therapy

- Acute spinal cord injury is treated with the administration of high-dose methylprednisolone:

commence with 30 mg/kg over 15 minutes. Then give 5.4 mg/kg/hr for the duration listed in Table 21–4.
- Contraindications to steroid administration are penetrating wounds, pregnancy, patients younger than 13 years, a gun shot wound, the presence of a significant infection, or unstable diabetes.
- Other drugs under investigation for modifying spinal cord injury are 21-aminosteroids, antioxidants, gangliosides, opioid antagonists, thyrotropin–releasing hormone, prostacyclin analogs, and calcium channel blockers (Vaccaro et al. 1997, Feuerstein et al. 1993, Zeidman et al. 1996).

Instability and Imaging Studies

- Instability is determined from data gathered from the physical examination, plain x-ray films, computed

Table 21–2: Differential Diagnosis of Shock				
TYPE OF SHOCK	**CHANGE TO BLOOD PRESSURE**	**CHANGE TO HEART RATE**	**CAUSE**	**TREATMENT**
Hemorrhagic	↓	↑	Blood loss	IV fluids, identify cause of blood loss
Neurogenic	↓	↓	↓ in sympathetic tone → lack of vasoconstriction	Judicious use of fluids, vasopressors

Table 21–3: American Spinal Injury Association Scale

CLASSIFICATION OF SPINAL CORD INJURIES ACCORDING TO LEVEL OF IMPAIRMENT*		
GRADE	MOTOR SCORE §	SENSORY DEFICIT §
A	0:5	Complete
B	0:5	Incomplete
C	<3:5	Incomplete
D	>3:5	Incomplete
E	5:5	None

* (American Spinal Injury Association 1992.)
§ Caudal to injury level.

Table 21–4: Methylprednisolone Dosing*

TIME FROM INJURY	DOSE OF METHYLPREDNISOLONE	DURATION
<3 hours	5.4 mg/kg/hr	24 hours
3-8 hours	5.4 mg/kg/hr	48 hours
>8 hours	No treatment	No treatment

* (Slucky et al. 1994, Vaccaro et al. 1997.)

tomography (CT), and magnetic resonance imaging (MRI) (Fig. 21–1, Table 21–5).

Classification of Spinal Column or Cord Injury

- Cervical spine trauma is divided into two main categories: upper cervical trauma and subaxial cervical trauma.

Upper Cervical Trauma

Occipital Condyle Fracture (Fig. 21–2)

- This type of fracture is a rare injury.
- Approximately 33% of occipital condyle fractures occur in conjunction with atlanto-occipital dislocations (Goldstein et al. 1982).

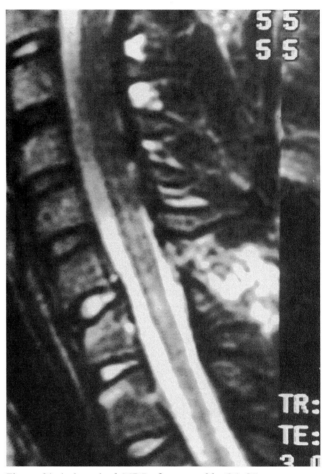

Figure 21–1: A sagittal MRI of an unstable C6–C7 flexion–distraction subaxial spine injury.

- They often are discovered on a head CT scan in an unconscious patient; cervical radiographs rarely show these fractures.
- Conscious patients complaining of an occipital headache should be suspected of having an occipital condyle fracture until proven otherwise.
- Though cranial nerves IX–XII are sometimes affected, neurological examination is often normal.

Table 21–5: Radiographic Findings Suggestive of Cervical Instability*

DIRECT EVIDENCE OF INSTABILITY	INDIRECT EVIDENCE OF INSTABILITY
Angulation > 11° between adjacent vertebral segments	Increased retropharyngeal soft-tissue shadow
Anteroposterior translation > 3.5 mm	Avulsion fractures at or near spinal ligament insertions §
Segmental spinous process widening on lateral view †	Presence of a cervical spinal cord injury
Facet joint widening ‡	Misalignment of spinous processes on an anteroposterior view
Rotation of facets on lateral view ‖	Lateral tilt of vertebral body on an anteroposterior view ‖

* Taken from Indications for Surgical Decompression and Stabilization by Benzel (Westurlund et al. 1999).
§ (Herkowitz et al. 1984, Mazur et al. 1983, Mori et al. 1983, Webb 1976.)
† (Daffner 1992.)
‡ (Woodring et al. 1982.)
‖ (Scher 1977.)

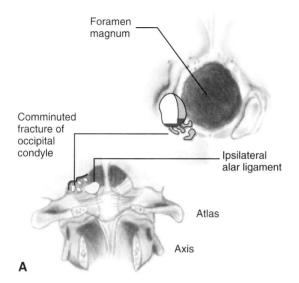

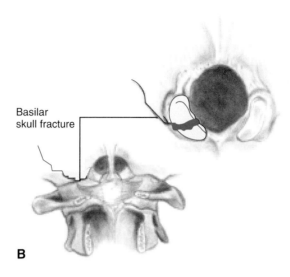

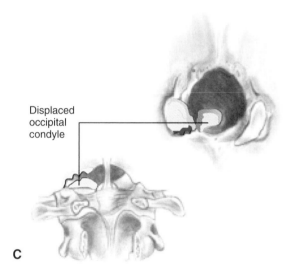

Figure 21–2: Anderson and Montesano classification of occipital condyle fractures. **A,** Type I—Comminuted and undisplaced fracture. **B,** Type II—Basilar skull fracture. **C,** Type III—Avulsion fracture at the attachment of the alar ligament. (Reprinted from Klein et al. 2003).

- Unstable injuries are often treated by posterior occipital–cervical arthrodesis (Westurlund et al. 1999) (Table 21–6).

Atlanto-occipital Dislocation (Figs. 21–3 through 21–5)

- Rare survivors usually have a neurological deficit, particularly with cranial nerves VII to X (Vaccaro 1999).
- Frequent diagnosis is at autopsies following death related to a spinal injury.
- High-resolution CT efficiently illustrates the injury (Table 21–7).
- Treatment includes closed reduction and surgical stabilization—often occiput to C2.

Fracture of Atlas (Figs. 21–6 and 21–7)

- This type of fracture is a relatively uncommon injury. It occurs as an isolated injury less than 50% of the time.
- Neurological injury is rare because of the wide spinal canal at that level, but cranial nerve injuries are frequently observed.
- An anteroposterior open-mouth view assesses the lateral masses of C1 relative to the lateral masses of C2. If the combined lateral masses of C1 are laterally displaced more than 6.9 mm relative to the C2 lateral masses, the transverse ligament may be disrupted, making it a potentially unstable injury.
- CT scan is the imaging modality of choice for diagnosis (Table 21–8).
- Most injuries can be treated conservatively with hard collar immobilization.

Table 21–6:		Anderson and Montesano Classification of Occipital Condyle Fractures*		
TYPE OF FRACTURE	STABLE?	DESCRIPTION OF FRACTURE		TREATMENT
I	Yes	Comminuted, undisplaced because of axial impact with the lateral mass of C1		Cervical orthosis
II	Yes	Linear—Part of the basilar skull fracture		Cervical orthosis
III	No	Avulsion at the attachment site of the alar ligament		Halo vest immobilization or surgical stabilization

* (Anderson et al. 1988.)

- Rarely, surgical intervention is selected following traction reduction. This can involve a Magerl C2 and C1 transfacet screw fixation technique with only [AU1]bone grafting (Vaccaro 1999).

Atlantoaxial Rotatory Subluxation (Fig. 21–8)

- This subluxation is more common in children than in adults.
- Common complaints are neck pain with evidence of torticollis, suboccipital pain, and limited cervical rotation (Westurlund et al. 1999).

- Lateral radiographs are helpful in determining the presence of retropharyngeal soft tissue swelling (Vaccaro 1999).
- Radiographic diagnosis includes open-mouth odontoid view, lateral cervical spine with or without flexion–extension views, dynamic (rotation to the right then the left) CT scan, and MRI. Dynamic CT scan confirms the injury; MRI rules in or out the possibility of a transverse ligament disruption (Table 21–9).
- Nonsurgical treatment methods include cervical orthosis, halo vest immobilization or halter, and skeletal traction reduction.
- Surgical treatment involves a C1-C2 fusion.

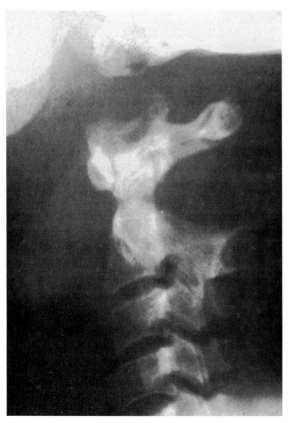

Figure 21–3: A lateral plain radiograph of an atlanto-occipital dislocation.

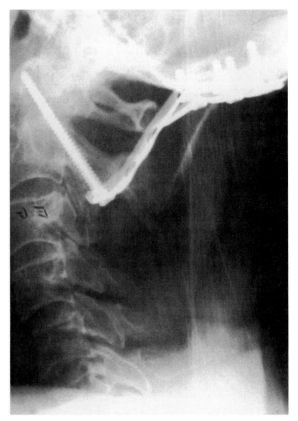

Figure 21–4: A lateral plain radiograph following a posterior occipital–cervical fusion.

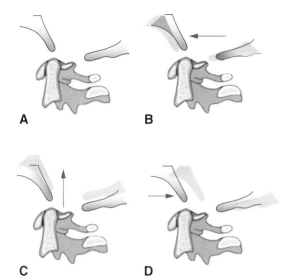

Figure 21–5: Traynelis et al. classification of atlanto-occipital injuries. **A,** A normal atlanto-occipital joint. **B,** Type I—Longitudinal dislocation. **C,** Type II—Axial-distraction injury. **D,** Type III—Posterior displacement. (Reprinted from Klein et al. 2003).

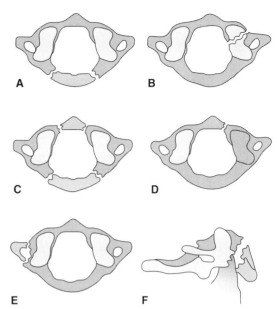

Figure 21–6: Levine and Edwards classification of atlas fractures. **A,** Type I Posterior arch fracture. **B,** Type II Lateral mass fracture. **C,** Type III Classic Jefferson's or burst fracture. **D,** Unilateral anterior arch fracture. **E,** Transverse process fracture. **F,** Avulsion fracture of the anterior arch. (Reprinted from Klein et al. 2003).

Odontoid Fracture (Figs. 21–9 and 21–10, Table 21–10)

- Type II fractures—Factors that correlate with increased risk of nonunion include greater than 6 mm of initial translation, failed reduction, age greater than 50, and angulation greater than 10°.

Traumatic Spondylolisthesis of the Axis

- The Effendi et al. classification of traumatic spondylolisthesis of the axis is presented in Fig. 21–11 and Table 21–11.

Axis Body Fractures

- Axis body fractures are inherently stable; nonoperative therapy is generally the initial treatment (Fujimura et al. 1996) (Table 21–12).

Subaxial Cervical Trauma

- Apply the Allen and Ferguson classification of subaxial cervical trauma (Allen et al. 1982).

- The classification system is based upon the mechanism of injury; there are six categories divided into stages.
- It provides probable biomechanical deficiencies of bony and ligamentous elements.
- The system guides treatment recommendations or approaches.

Table 21–7:	Traynelis et al. Classification of Atlanto-occipital Dislocations*	
TYPE OF FRACTURE	**DESCRIPTION**
I	Anterior displacement
II	Axial-distraction injury
III	Posterior displacement

* (Traynelis et al. 1986.)

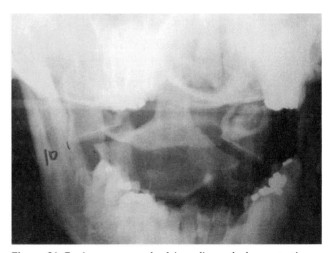

Figure 21–7: An open-mouth plain radiograph demonstrating overhang of the C1 lateral masses because of disruption of the transverse atlantal ligament in the setting of a C1 burst fracture.

Table 21–8:	Levine and Edwards Classification of Atlas Fractures*
TYPE OF FRACTURE	**DESCRIPTION OF FRACTURE**
I	Posterior arch fracture
II	Lateral mass fracture
III	Classic Jefferson's or burst fracture

* (Levine et al. 1991.)

Compression–Flexion (Figs. 21–12 through 21–14)

- Failure → anterior column compression—posterior column distraction
- Five Allen and Ferguson stages (Allen et al. 1982)
  - I—Blunting of the anterior–superior vertebral body
  - II—Progression to vertebral body beaking
  - III—Beak fracture
  - IV—Cephalad vertebral body retrolisthesis < 3 mm
  - V—Retrolisthesis > 3 mm (Table 21–13)

Vertical Compression (Figs. 21–15 and 21–16)

- Three Allen and Ferguson stages of increasing severity (Allen et al. 1982)
  - I—Cupping of the superior or inferior vertebral endplate

Table 21–9:	Fielding and Hawkins Classification of Atlantoaxial Rotatory Subluxations*
TYPE OF FRACTURE	**DESCRIPTION OF FRACTURE**
I (most common)	Simple rotatory displacement without anterior shift (subluxation)
II	Rotatory displacement with anterior displacement of 3-5 mm
III	Rotatory displacement with anterior displacement > 5 mm
IV	Rotatory displacement with posterior translation

* (Fielding et al. 1977.)

- II—Cupping and fracture of the vertebral endplates and minimal displacement
- III—Vertebral fragmentation or displacement (Table 21–14)

Distraction–Flexion

- See Figs. 21–17 through 21–19 and Table 21–15 for examples and classifications of distraction–flexion injuries.

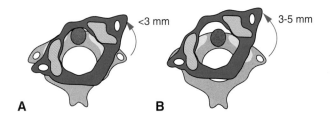
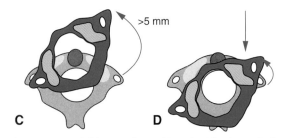

Figure 21–8: Fielding and Hawkins classification of atlantoaxial rotatory subluxation. **A**, Type I—Rotatory displacement without subluxation. **B**, Type II—Rotatory displacement with C1 anterior displacement of 3-5 mm. **C**, Type III—Rotatory displacement with anterior displacement of C1 greater than 5 mm. **D**, Type IV— Rotatory displacement with posterior translation. (Reprinted from Klein et al. 2003).

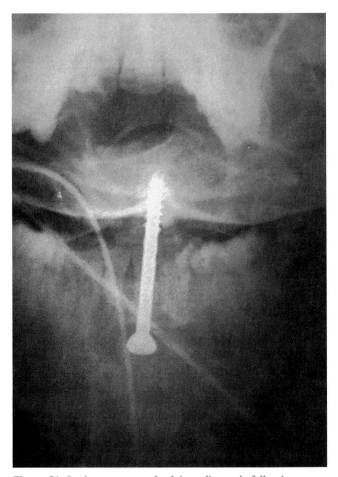

Figure 21–9: An open-mouth plain radiograph following odontoid screw fixation of a type II odontoid fracture.

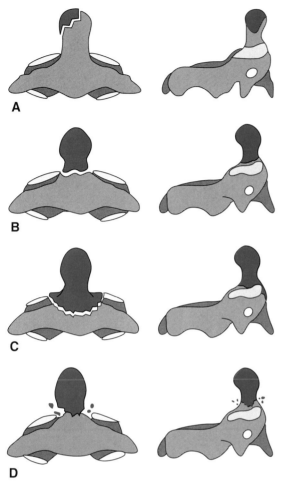

Figure 21–10: Anderson and D'Alonzo classification of odontoid fractures.
A, Type I—Odontoid tip avulsion. **B,** Type II—Fracture at the base of the dens. **C,** Type III—Fracture within the body of C2. (Reprinted from Klein et al. 2003). **D,** Hadley Type IIa odontoid fracture.

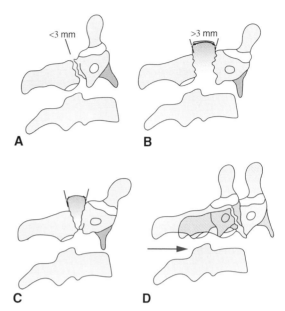

Figure 21–11: Effendi et al. classification of hangman's fracture.
A, Type I—Nondisplaced fracture (<3 mm displacement). **B,** Type II—Fracture with at least 3 mm of translation, significant angulation, and C3 anterior–superior endplate compression. **C,** Type IIA—No translation, significant angulation, anterior longitudinal ligament intact, posterior longitudinal ligament, and C2-C3 disk disrupted. **D,** Type III—Anterior C2-C3 displacement, angulation, and unilateral or bilateral facet dislocation of C2 on C3. (Reprinted from Klein et al. 2003).

Table 21–10:	Anderson and D'Alonzo Classification of Odontoid Fractures*	
TYPE OF FRACTURE	DESCRIPTION OF FRACTURE	TREATMENT
I	Odontoid tip avulsion	Cervical orthosis for 3 months
II	Most common; at the base of the dens	Nondisplaced or displaced <5 mm—Skeletal traction reduction followed by halo vest immobilization Displaced > 5 mm—Possible surgery
IIa Hadley§	At base of dens with significant comminution	Consider surgical intervention
III	Body of C2	Cervical orthosis or halo vest immobilization

* (Anderson et al. 1974.)
§ (Hadley et al. 1988.)

Table 21–11:	Effendi et al. Classification of Traumatic Spondylolisthesis of the Axis*	
TYPE	DESCRIPTION OF FRACTURE	TREATMENT
I	<3-mm displacement No angulation	Cervical orthosis or halo vest immobilization
II	3-mm translation Significant angulation C3 anterior superior endplate compression	Traction or halo vest immobilization
IIA	No translation Significant angulation Anterior longitudinal ligament intact Posterior longitudinal ligament, C2-C3 disk disrupted	Reduction in extension followed by halo vest immobilization (no traction)
III	Anterior C2-C3 displacement Angulation Unilateral or bilateral facet dislocation of C2 on C3	Attempted closed skeletal reduction followed by open stabilization with cervical orthosis or halo vest immobilization

* (Effendi et al. 1981, Levine et al. 1989.)

Table 21–12:	Fujimura et al. Classification of Axis Body Fractures*	
TYPE	**DESCRIPTION OF FRACTURE**
I	Avulsion fracture at the anteroinferior axis body
II	Transverse fracture through the central part of the axis body
III	Burst fracture to the body
IV	Sagittal plane fracture to the body

* (Fujimura et al. 1996.)

Treatment

- Reduction is appropriate for all four stages.
- Treatment may proceed with closed reduction before an MRI evaluation in an awake, alert, and cooperative patient.
- Prereduction MRI is recommended in any of the following clinical situations: neurological deterioration, a failed attempted closed reduction, or an unreliable examination (i.e., an unconscious, sedated, or intoxicated patient) (Fig. 21–20)

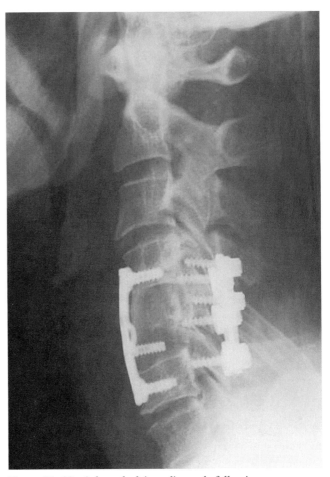

Figure 21–13: A lateral plain radiograph following an anterior–posterior decompression and fusion with stabilization for a high-grade subaxial compression–flexion cervical spine injury.

Compression–Extension

- Failure → posterior column compression—anterior column distraction
- See Figs. 21–21 and 21–22 and Table 21–16 for examples and classifications of compression–extension injuries.

Distraction–Extension

- See Figs. 21–23 and 21–24 and Table 21–17 for examples and classifications of distraction–extension injuries.

Lateral Flexion

- See Figs. 21–25 and 21–26 and Table 21–18 for examples and classifications of lateral flexion injuries.

Conclusions

- Appropriate, organized prehospital management and aggressive emergency resuscitation are paramount for optimal spinal cord function.

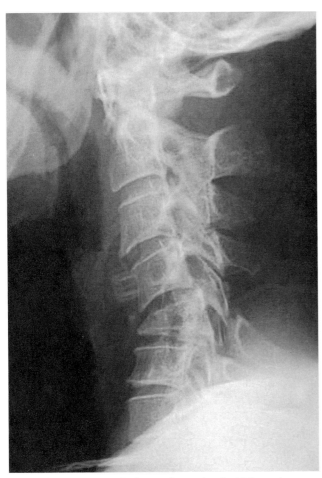

Figure 21–12: A lateral plain radiograph of a high-grade subaxial cervical compression–flexion injury.

Figure 21–14: Allen and Ferguson classification of compression–flexion injuries.
A, Normal. **B,** Stage I—Blunting of the anterior–superior vertebral body. **C,** Stage II—Progression to vertebral body beaking. **D,** Stage III—Beak fracture. **E,** Stage IV—Cephalad vertebral body retrolisthesis less than 3 mm. **F,** Stage V—Retrolisthesis greater than 3 mm.
(Reprinted from Klein et al. 2003).

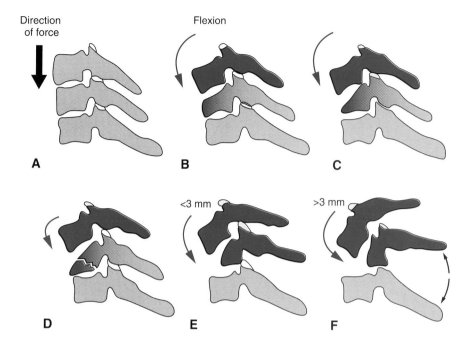

- Pharmacologic treatment (high-dose steroids) is effective according to several peer-reviewed articles if given within 8 hours of injury.
- A thorough understanding of the mechanism of injury and pathoanatomy is necessary for the safest and most efficient means of treatment.
- Timing of advanced imaging studies (e.g., MRI) before definitive treatment is dependent on the cooperativeness of the patient.
- If surgical intervention is necessary, a full appreciation of contemporary internal fixation methods should be mastered before undertaking this form of fracture management.

Table 21–13:	Treatment of Compression–Flexion Injuries
STAGE	**TREATMENT**
I and II	Cervical orthosis or halo vest immobilization, rarely surgery
III and IV (with limited kyphosis)	Halo vest immobilization or anterior decompression and reconstruction or posterior cervical fusion
III and IV (with kyphosis)	Anterior decompression and reconstruction or posterior cervical fusion
V	Anterior decompression and reconstruction, anterior or posterior fusion, or both

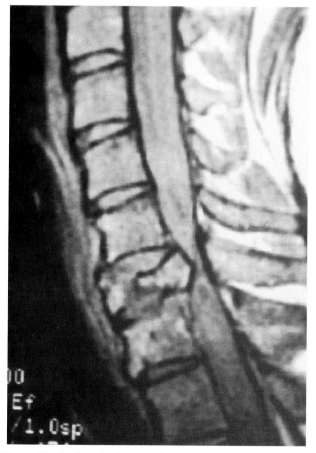

Figure 21–15: A sagittal MRI of a subaxial, cervical, vertical compression injury.

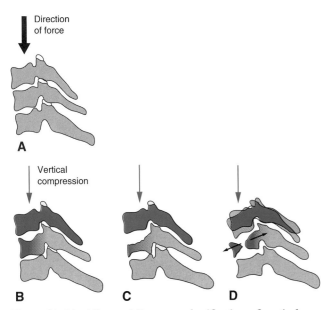

Figure 21–16: Allen and Ferguson classification of vertical compression injuries.
A, Normal. **B,** Stage I—Cupping of superior or inferior vertebral endplate. **C,** Stage II—Cupping and fracture of vertebral endplates and minimal displacement. **D,** Stage III—Vertebral fragmentation or displacement into spinal canal. (Reprinted from Klein et al. 2003).

Table 21-14:	Treatment of Vertical Compression Injuries
STAGE	**TREATMENT**
I and II	Cervical orthosis or halo vest immobilization
III	Halo vest immobilization or surgery (anterior decompression, reconstruction)

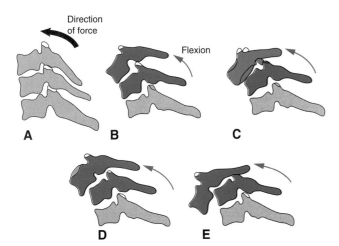

Figure 21–17: Allen and Ferguson classification of distraction–flexion injuries.
A, Normal. **B,** Stage I—Less than 25% subluxation of facets. **C,** Stage II—Unilateral facet dislocation. **D,** Stage III—Bilateral facet dislocation. **E,** Stage IV—Bilateral facet dislocation with displacement of the full vertebral width. (Reprinted from Klein et al. 2003).

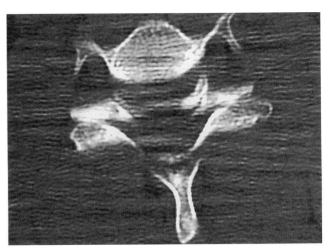

Figure 21–18: A CT scan of a distraction–flexion bilateral facet dislocation.

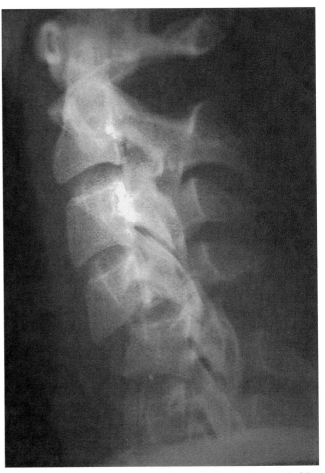

Figure 21–19: A lateral plain radiograph illustrating a C4-C5 bilateral facet dislocation.

Table 21–15: Allen and Ferguson Classification of Distraction–Flexion Fractures*

STAGE	DESCRIPTION OF FRACTURE
I	<25% subluxation of facets
II	Unilateral facet dislocation
III	Bilateral facet dislocation
IV	Bilateral dislocation with displacement of the full vertebral width

* (Allen et al. 1982.)

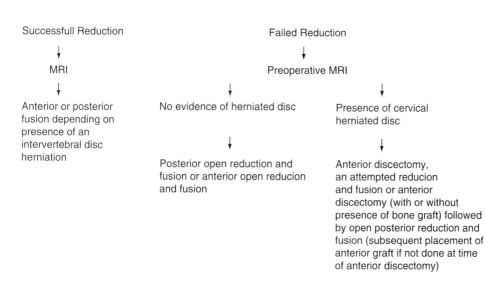

Successfull Reduction
↓
MRI
↓
Anterior or posterior fusion depending on presence of an intervertebral disc herniation

Failed Reduction
↓
Preoperative MRI
↓

No evidence of herniated disc
↓
Posterior open reduction and fusion or anterior open reducion and fusion

Presence of cervical herniated disc
↓
Anterior discectomy, an attempted reducion and fusion or anterior discectomy (with or without presence of bone graft) followed by open posterior reduction and fusion (subsequent placement of anterior graft if not done at time of anterior discectomy)

Figure 21–20: Algorithm for MRI use in reduction of compression–flexion injuries.

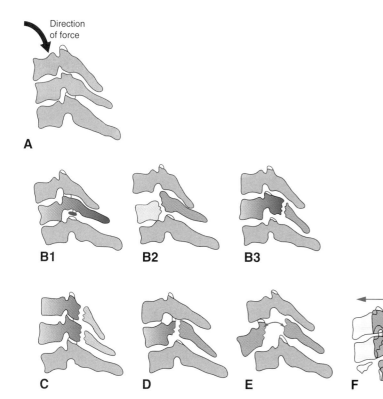

Figure 21–21: Allen and Ferguson classification of compression–extension injuries.
A, Normal. **B,** Stage I—Unilateral laminar fracture. **C,** Stage II—Bilateral laminar fracture. **D,** Stage III—Bilateral, nondisplaced fracture. **E,** Stage IV—Bilateral, partially displaced fracture. **F,** Stage V—Full displacement.
(Reprinted from Klein et al. 2003).

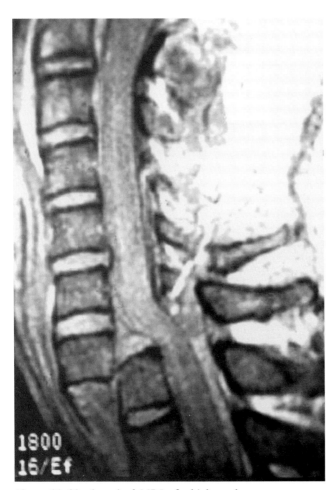

Figure 21–22: A sagittal MRI of a high-grade compression–extension injury.

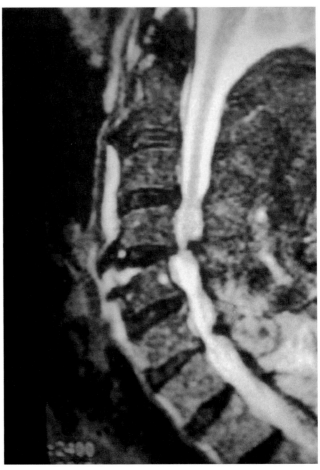

Figure 21–23: A sagittal MRI of a distraction–extension injury at the C4-C5 level.

Table 21–16: Allen and Ferguson Classification and Treatment of Compression–Extension Injuries*		
STAGES	**DESCRIPTION OF FRACTURE**	**TREATMENT**
I	Unilateral laminar	Cervical orthosis or halo vest immobilization
II	Bilateral laminar—Multiple levels	Cervical orthosis or halo vest immobilization
III	Bilateral, nondisplaced	Cervical orthosis or halo vest immobilization
IV	Bilateral, partially displaced	Posterior cervical fusion
V	Full displacement	Posterior cervical fusion

* (Allen et al. 1982.)

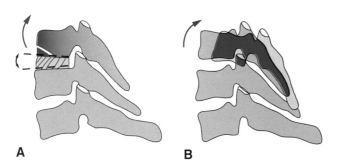

A   **B**

Figure 21–24: Allen and Ferguson classification of distraction–extension injuries.
A, Stage I—Anterior longitudinal ligament disruption and possible transverse body fractures. **B,** Stage II—Displacement and injury to the posterior column.
(Reprinted from Klein et al. 2003).

Table 21–17: Allen and Ferguson Classification and Treatment of Distraction–Extension Injuries*

STAGE	DESCRIPTION OF FRACTURE	TREATMENT
I	Anterior longitudinal ligament disruption, transverse fracture of body	Halo vest immobilization
II	Displacement—Injury to the posterior column	Anterior decompression or fusion

* (Allen et al. 1982.)

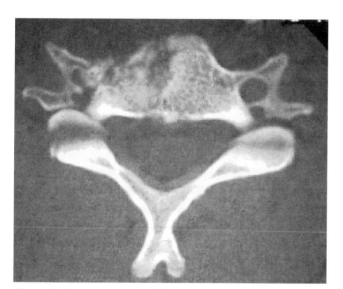

Figure 21–25: A transaxial CT of a lateral flexion injury.

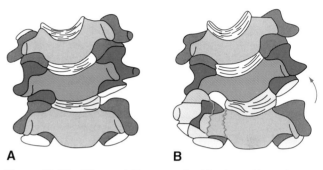

Figure 21–26: Allen and Ferguson classification of lateral flexion injuries.
A, Stage I—Asymmetric centrum and unilateral arch. B, Stage II—Displacement and contralateral ligamentous failure. (Reprinted from Klein et al. 2003).

Table 21–18: Allen and Ferguson Classification and Treatment of Lateral Flexion Injuries*

STAGE	DESCRIPTION OF FRACTURE	TREATMENT
I	Asymmetric centrum, unilateral arch	Cervical orthosis
II	Displacement, contralateral ligamentous failure	Posterior cervical fusion

* (Allen et al. 1982.)

References

Allen BL, Ferguson RL, Lehman TR et al. (1982) A mechanistic classification of closed, indirect fractures and dislocations of the lower cervical spine. Spine 7: 1-27.

   In this article, 165 cases of lower cervical spinal trauma are categorized into six groups, each with multiple stages.

American Spinal Injury Association. (1992) Standards for Neurological and Functional Classification of Spinal Cord Injury, revised edition. Chicago: American Spinal Injury Association.

   ASIA's classification of spinal cord injuries according to level of impairment.

Anderson PA, D'Alonzo RT. (1974) Fractures of the odontoid process of the axis. J Bone Joint Surg 56A(8): 1663-1674.

   The authors present a classification system for odontoid fractures. Three types of fractures are described with a proposed management protocol.

Anderson PA, Montesano PX. (1988) Morphology and treatment of occipital condyle fractures. Spine 13(7): 731-736.

   The authors present a classification system and suggest treatments for this rare injury.

Daffner RH. (1992) Evaluation of cervical vertebral injuries. Semin Reontgenol 27: 239-253.

   Patients who are suspected of cervical spine trauma should undergo specific imaging studies such as CT, polydirectional tomography, and MRI to confirm the initial impression based on plain radiographic findings. Cervical injuries may be diagnosed, looking for irregularities of spinal alignment in regards to the bony anatomy, cartilage or joint spaces, and changes in soft tissue measurements.

Effendi B, Roy D, Cornish B et al. (1981) Fractures of the ring of the axis—A classification based on the analysis of 131 cases. J Bone Joint Surg 63B: 319-327.

The authors reviewed 131 patients with an axis injury. The data was then analyzed for the creation of a classification system. In addition, management recommendations are presented.

Feuerstein G, Rabinovici R. (1993) Recent advances in the pharmacology of spinal cord injury. Traum Quart 9: 5-64.
This article explains the pharmacologic management of spinal cord injuries.

Fielding JW, Hawkins RJ. (1977) Atlantoaxial rotatory fixation (fixed rotatory subluxation of the atlantoaxial joint). J Bone Joint Surg 59A(1): 37-44.
The authors developed a classification system for atlantoaxial rotatory fixation. They explain the management principles of this disorder. All 13 patients were treated with skeletal traction followed by atlantoaxial arthrodesis (successful in 11 of 13 patients).

Fujimura Y, Nishi Y, Kobayaski K. (1996) Classification and treatment of axis body fractures. J Orthop Trauma 10(8): 536-540.
The authors describe the classification and treatment of axis body fractures using data from 31 patients.

Goldstein SJ, Woodring JH, Young AB. (1982) Occipital condyle fracture associated with cervical spine injury. Surg Neurol 17: 350-352.
The authors report a case of this extremely rare injury and review the literature.

Hadley MN, Browner CM, Lui SS, Sonntag VK. (1998) New subtype of acute odontoid fractures (type IIa). Neurosurgery 22 (1 pt 1): 67-71.

Herkowitz HN, Rothman RH. (1984) Subacute instability of the cervical spine. Spine 9: 348-357.
Subacute instability of the cervical spine manifested itself 3 weeks following injury. The authors recommend collar immobilization during the period of cervical spasm followed by delayed dynamic plain radiography to assess occult instability.

Klein GR, Vaccaro AR. (2003) Cervical spine trauma: Upper and lower. In: Principles and Practice of Spine Surgery (Vaccaro AR et al., eds.). Philadelphia: Mosby.

Kraus JF, Franti CE, Riggins RS et al. (1975) Incidence of traumatic spinal cord lesions. J Chron Dis 28: 471-492.
This article describes the frequency and demographics of spinal column and cord injuries.

Lasfargues JE, Custis D, Morrone F et al. (1995) A model for estimating spinal cord injury prevalence in the United States. Paraplegia 33: 62-68.
After reviewing the data on incidence, mortality, and prevalence of spinal cord injuries in the United States, a model was designed to show trends in populations of people with spinal cord injuries at the national and state level. The information garnered from this model is essential in planning and allocating resources for spinal trauma.

Levine AM, Edwards CC. (1989) Traumatic lesions of the occipito–atlantoaxial complex. Clin Orthop 239: 53-68.

This article describes the incidence, diagnostic criteria, and treatment methods used in the management of injuries to the occipito–atlantoaxial complex.

Levine AM, Edwards CC. (1991) Fractures of the atlas. J Bone Joint Surg 73A: 680-691.
The authors studied 34 patients studied for an average of 4.5 years after their atlas fractures. The authors grouped the 34 injuries into five main fracture categories.

Mazur JM, Stauffer ES. (1983) Unrecognized spinal instability associated with seemingly simple cervical compression fractures. Spine 8: 687-692.
Here, 27 patients with cervical compression fractures were treated with a cervical orthosis. None of the patients were managed with a halo vest or with surgery. Of the patients, 20 healed without incident; the other 7 developed a spinal deformity or instability. Most of the patients with instability underwent surgery. The paper demonstrates the need for better assessment of potential spinal instability and the need for close follow-up in the peritrauma period.

Mori S, Nobuhiro O, Ojima T et al. (1983) Observation of "tear drop" fracture dislocation of the cervical spine by CT. J Jpn Orthop Assoc 57: 373-378.
Five cases of tear-drop fracture dislocations of the cervical spine were studied using CT and conventional radiographs. Conventional radiographs were insensitive in detailing the degree of spinal canal narrowing and vertebral comminution. The CT imaging was effective in illustrating the nature and severity of the injury.

Scher AT. (1977) Unilateral locked facet in cervical spine injuries. AJR 129: 45-48.
A unilateral facet dislocation is easy to miss radiographically because often there is little vertebral displacement. Rotational misalignment of one vertebra in relation to another usually identifies the injury.

Slucky V, Eismont FJ. (1994) Treatment of acute injury of the cervical spine. J Bone Joint Surgery 76-A: 1882-1896.
This article outlines the protocol for treating an acute injury to the cervical spine. Initial management, pharmacologic therapy, nonsurgical, and surgical treatments are described.

Traynelis VC, Marano GD, Dunker RO et al. (1986) Traumatic atlanto-occipital dislocation. J Neurosurg 65: 863-870.
The article covers a system for classification for this decreasingly fatal injury. Radiographic criteria and rationale for treatment are proposed.

Vaccaro AR. (1999) Cervical spine trauma. In: Orthopaedic Knowledge Update (Beaty JH, ed.). Rosemont, IL: American Academy of Orthopaedic Surgeons.
A contemporary review of the natural history, diagnosis, and nonoperative and operative management principles in regards to cervical trauma.

Vaccaro AR, An HS, Betz RR et al. (1997) The management of acute spinal trauma—Prehospital and in-hospital emergency care. Instr Course Lec 46: 113-125.

A detailed protocol outlining the prehospital and in-hospital management of a patient with a cervical spinal column or cord injury.

Vaccaro AR, An HS, Lin S et al. (1992) Noncontiguous injuries of the spine. J Spinal Disord 5(3): 320-329.
Of the 372 consecutive spinal injury patients evaluated at the Regional Spinal Cord Injury Center of Delaware Valley, 39 patients (10.5%) were found to have noncontiguous spinal column injuries.

Vaccaro AR, Zlotlow DA. (2001) Fractures and dislocations of the lower cervical spine. In: Rockwood and Green's Fractures in Adults (Bucholz RW et al., eds.). Philadelphia: JB Lippincott Co.
A contemporary book chapter covering all of the aspects of lower cervical spine injury management including its natural history and nonoperative and operative management.

Webb JH. (1976) Hidden flexion injury of the cervical spine. J Bone Joint Surg 55B: 322-327.
This paper describes clinical and radiological features of cervical flexion injuries and explains the importance of appropriate and timely management.

Westurlund LE, Dafner S, Vaccaro AR. (1999) Cervical spine trauma—Indications for surgical decompression and stabilization In: Spine Surgery—Techniques, Complication Avoidance, and Management (Benzel EC, ed.). Philadelphia: Churchill Livingstone.
A concise treatise on the indications for surgical intervention in the management of cervical spine trauma.

Woodring JH, Goldstein SJ. (1982) Fractures of the articular processes of the cervical spine. Am J Radiol 139: 341-344.
Of 77 patients with cervical spine fractures, 16 (20.8%) had fractures of the articular processes of the cervical spine. CT imaging identified all of these fractures; plain films identified only 2. CT scanning should be considered in selected cases to evaluate for articular process fractures in patients following cervical trauma who develop a radiculopathy.

Zeidman SM, Ling GS, Ducker TB et al. (1996) Clinical applications of pharmacologic therapies for spinal cord injury. J Spinal Disord 9: 367-380.
The literature on the effects of glucocorticosteroids, tirilazad, and GM1 ganglioside on spinal cord injuries is reviewed and critiqued and recommendations are made for the pharmacologic management of a spinal cord injury patient.

CHAPTER 22

Thoracic and Lumbar Spine Trauma

Kern Singh★, Arjun Saxena §, and Alexander R. Vaccaro †

★ M.D., Assistant Professor, Department of Orthopedic Surgery, Rush University Medical Center, Chicago, IL
§ B.S., Thomas Jefferson Medical College, Philadelphia, PA
† M.D., Professor of Orthopaedic Surgery, Thomas Jefferson University and the Rothman Institute, Philadelphia, PA

Introduction

- The thoracolumbar spine is the most common site of spinal injuries.
- Most of these injuries occur in males (15-29 years) usually as the result of a significant-force impact, such as a motor vehicle accident or fall (Gertzbein 1992).
- Most injuries (52%) occur between T11 and L1 followed by L1 through L5 (32%) and T1 through T10 (16%) (Gertzbein 1994, Gertzbein 1992, Kraus et al. 1975).
- Depending on the type of fracture, associated injuries occur in up to 50% of patients mainly as a result of a distraction force.
- Associated injuries include intra-abdominal bleeding from liver and splenic injuries, vessel disruption, and pulmonary injuries (20% of patients).
- Contiguous and noncontiguous spine injuries are present in 6% to 15% of patients (Box 22–1).

Initial Treatment and Examination

- Initial evaluation should begin with the "ABCs" (airway, breathing, and circulation) of trauma care (Fig. 22–1).
- It has been found that 30% of patients with persistent localized tenderness after trauma to the thoracolumbar spine and absence of an obvious radiographic deformity may have an occult spinal fracture (Chapman et al. 1994).
- The neurological examination should include motor testing, dermatomal sensory testing, lumbar sacral root motor evaluation, and an examination of reflexes.
- "Spinal shock" refers to flaccid paralysis because of a physiologic disruption of all spinal cord function.
- The presence of the bulbocavernosus reflex heralds the end of spinal shock and allows an accurate assessment of

> ### Box 22–1: Thoracolumbar Anatomy
>
> - The thoracic spinal cord is protected from injury by the surrounding paraspinal musculature, the vertebral elements, and the thoracic rib cage.
> - The thoracolumbar junction is a transitional region between the less mobile thoracic spine and the more flexible lumbar spine.
> - Decreasing the spinal canal diameter to spinal cord ratio, particularly between T2 and T10, makes this region more susceptible to spinal cord injury.
> - Physiologic kyphosis of the thoracic spine may predispose it to flexion-axial load–type injuries.
> - Spinal injuries in this region are associated with a high incidence of neurological injury.
> - Thoracic vertebral bodies are not as large as the lumbar vertebral bodies; thus, they are less able to resist deformity following specific load applications.

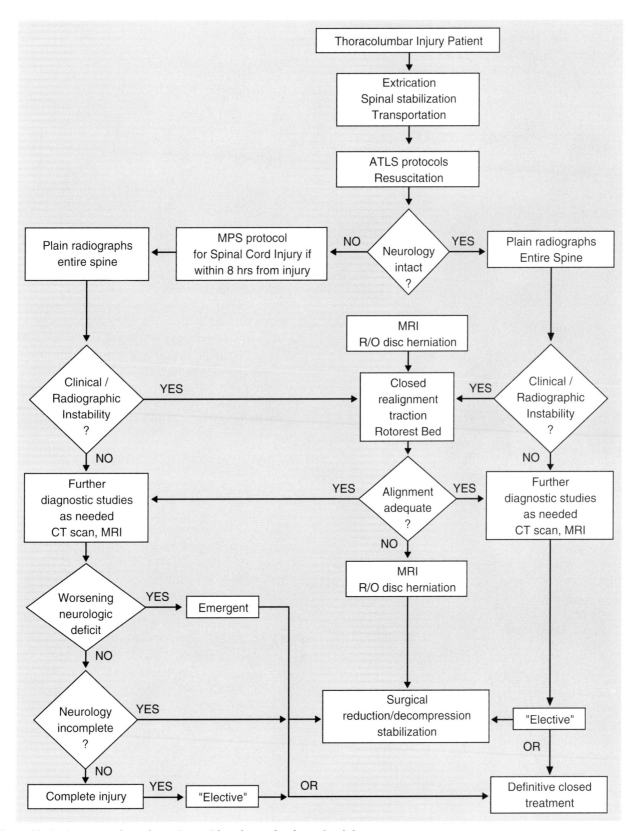

Figure 22–1: An approach to the patient with a thoracolumbar spine injury.
(*ATLS,* advanced trauma life support.)

the patient's neurological status typically 48 hours after the injury (Figs. 22–2 through 22–4).

- A "complete" neurological injury is marked by an absence of sensory and motor function below the anatomic level of injury in the absence of spinal shock (Fig. 22–5).

- In an incomplete lesion, residual spinal cord function, nerve root function, or both exist below the anatomic level of injury.

- An incomplete spinal cord lesion may manifest as one of four syndromes (Fig. 22–6, Table 22–1; also see Fig. 5–1).

- Hypotension secondary to neurogenic or hemorrhagic shock must be reversed through fluid replacement, blood replacement or both with or without the use of vasopressors.

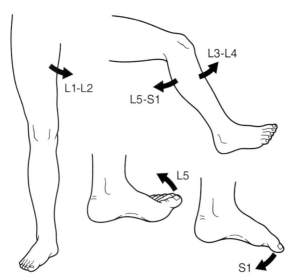

Figure 22–2: A schematic of a lower extremity examination with the corresponding nerve root innervations.

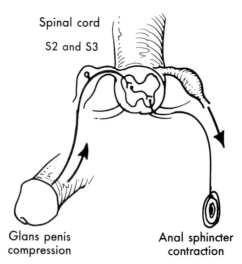

Figure 22–3: A schematic of the bulbocavernosus reflex. (Reprinted from Leventhal 2003).

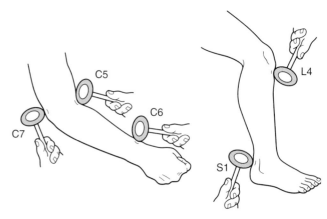

Figure 22–4: Reflex testing of the lower extremity with the corresponding nerve root innervations.

- Intravenous methylprednisolone is routinely administered within 8 hours of a spinal cord injury in the absence of specific contraindications (Table 22–2).

- Deep venous thrombosis prophylaxis is paramount. The use of intermittent external pneumatic compression devices, static compression stockings, and—in select patients—subcutaneous (5000 units subcutaneously every 12 hours) or intravenous low-molecular weight heparin helps to minimize potentially fatal pulmonary emboli.

Radiologic Evaluation

- All patients who have injuries suspicious for spinal trauma should undergo plain radiographic imaging (anteroposterior or lateral) of all vertebral levels.

- Plain x-ray film is the initial screening modality with computed tomography (CT) scanning or magnetic resonance imaging (MRI) used as an adjunct depending upon whether the surgeon needs to further evaluate bony or soft tissue anatomy (Table 22–3).

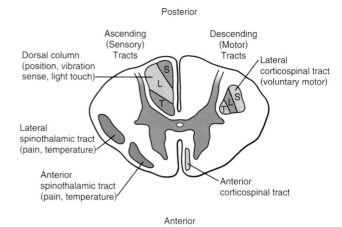

Figure 22–5: Schematic of a transverse section of the spinal cord at the thoracic level, showing the anatomic organization of the corticospinal tract and posterior column. (*L*, lumbar; *S*, sacral; *T*, thoracic).

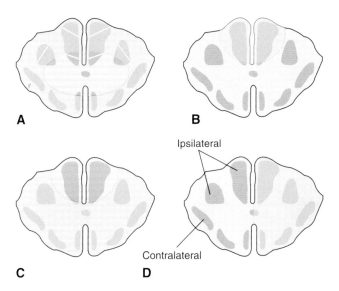

Ipsilateral

Contralateral

Figure 22–6: Types of spinal cord injury (shaded zones) that produce the four main incomplete injury patterns seen clinically.
A, Central cord syndrome. **B,** Anterior cord syndrome. **C,** Posterior cord syndrome. **D,** Brown-Séquard's syndrome. (Reprinted from Klein et al. 2003).

Classification Methods

- The three-column theory of spinal instability by Denis is commonly used to define vertebral column injuries (Denis et al. 1992, Denis 1983) (Fig. 22–7).
- Denis divided thoracic and lumbar spinal injuries into minor and major injures.
  - Fractures of the spinous and transverse processes, the pars interarticularis, and the facet articulations were categorized as minor injuries.
  - Major spinal injuries were divided into compression fractures, burst fractures, flexion–distraction injuries, and fracture dislocations.
- Ferguson and Allen presented a mechanistic classification of thoracolumbar injuries, describing seven injury

patterns: compressive flexion, distractive flexion, lateral flexion, translational, torsional flexion, vertical compression, and distractive extension injuries (Ferguson et al. 1984) (Table 22–4).

Surgical Decision Making

- The goals of surgical management include maximizing patient function, facilitating nursing care, preventing deformity and instability, and possibly improving neurological function.
- Surgery is often determined by the integrity of the posterior osteoligamentous complex (Box 22–2).
- The choice of surgical approach is dictated by the spinal level, the degree and nature of canal compromise, and the experience of the surgeon.
- Multiple variations on the approach to the thoracolumbar spine exist based upon three methods of decompressing the thecal sac: anterior, posterior, and posterolateral (Table 22–5).

Spinal Instrumentation

- Since the introduction of Harrington rod internal fixation, there has been progressive development of various spinal fixation systems based on segmental fixation of the spine.
- The choice of spinal implant is determined by the nature, degree, or biomechanics of the existing instability, the quality (bone density) of the spinal elements, and the medical condition of the patient (Box 22–3).

Anterior Instrumentation

- Of the axial load transmitted through the spine, 80% is through the intact anterior and middle spinal column.
- A functional posterior osteoligamentous complex is critical to the success of healing of an anterior spinal fusion (Figs. 22–8 and 22–9).

Table 22–1:	**Spinal Cord Injury Syndromes**	
SYNDROME	**CHARACTERISTICS**	**PROGNOSIS**
Central	Most common Upper extremity > lower extremity Motor and sensory loss	Fair
Anterior	Loss of motor function with possible sparing of proprioception and pressure sensation	Poor
Posterior	Rare Loss of proprioception and pressure sensation No motor loss	Good
Brown-Séquard	Ipsilateral motor loss and contralateral pain and temperature loss	Good

Table 22–2:	**Methylprednisolone Dosing***	
TIME FROM INJURY	**DOSE OF METHYLPREDNISOLONE**	**DURATION**
<3 hours	5.4 mg/kg/hr	24 hours
3-8 hours	5.4 mg/kg/hr	48 hours
>8 hours	No treatment	No treatment

* All patients should receive an initial 30-mg/kg bolus followed by the listed dosage regimen.

Posterior Instrumentation

• See Box 22–4 and Fig. 22–10.

Fracture Subtypes

• Spinal injuries can be divided into several categories based upon their biomechanical and anatomic characteristics and the patient's neurological status (Table 22–6).

Compression Fractures

• Of compression fractures, 85% are caused by primary osteopenia.
• In North America, $14.7 billion dollars are spent annually as a result of medical complications associated with compression fractures.
• Potential indications for surgical intervention in the setting of a compression fracture include the following:
    • 25-30° of initial kyphosis (significant posterior osteoligamentous disruption)

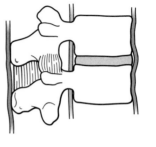

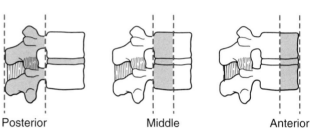

Posterior   Middle   Anterior

Figure 22–7: A schematic of the three columns of the spine.

• >50% loss of anterior vertebral body height (potential for significant posterior osteoligamentous disruption) (Figs. 22–11 and 22–12)

Burst Fractures

• Burst fractures involve disruption of the anterior and middle spinal columns.
• No definitive evidence correlates the degree of neural impingement with the severity of neurological deficit following a thoracolumbar burst fracture (Figs. 22–13 through 22–16).

Table 22–3:	**Diagnostic Imaging Modalities**		
IMAGING MODALITY	**ADVANTAGES**	**DISADVANTAGES**	**OTHER**
Plain radiograph	Inexpensive Quick	Poor visualization of middle spinal column disruption and canal involvement	Assess posterior vertebral body line on lateral radiograph (disruption suggestive of burst fracture)
CT	Excellent visualization of bony anatomy, particularly the middle spinal column Excellent assessment of spinal canal shape and patency	Poor visualization of soft tissues	
MRI	Excellent visualization of soft tissues including ligaments, disk, and spinal cord	Poor visualization of detailed bony anatomy	Hematoma has decreased T2 signal Adjacent edema appears as an increased signal on a T2-weighted image. Edema extending more than two vertebral levels and the presence of hematoma within the spinal cord are considered poor prognostic signs

Table 22–4:   Ferguson and Allen Classification System for Spinal Fractures

| | | TYPE OF FRACTURE | |
COLUMN	ANTERIOR	MIDDLE	POSTERIOR
Compressive flexion			
Type I	Compression	None	None
Type II	Compression	None	Tension
Type III	Compression	Blown out*	Tension
Distractive flexion	Tension	Tension	Tension
Lateral flexion			
Type I	Unilateral compression	Unilateral compression	None
Type II	Unilateral compression	Unilateral compression	Ipsilateral compression or contralateral tension
Translational	Shear	Shear	Shear
Torsional flexion	Compression or rotation	Disrupted	Tension or rotations
Vertical compression	Compression	Bony compression	Bony involvement
Distractive extension	Tension		Compression

* Blown out—Evidence of a middle column bone rotated into the neural canal between pedicles.

Box 22–2:   Instability and Outcomes

- Denis defined instability as a disruption of two or more of the three spinal columns.
  - Mechanical—Posterior osteoligamentous elements disrupted in distraction with obvious kyphosis
  - Neurological—Neurological deficit in a setting of spinal fracture
  - Combined
- A study performed on patients with a cervical spinal cord injury found no significant difference in functional neurological recovery when patients were operated on either early (<3 days) or late (>5 days) (Vaccaro et al. 1997).
- No studies have found a direct correlation between the percentage of canal occlusion radiographically and the severity of neurological deficit following burst fractures (Gertzbein 1994).
- Late decompression, even several years following injury, may enhance neurological recovery of the spinal cord, the conus medullaris, and the cauda equina.

Distraction–Flexion Injuries

- Specific variants are also known as seat belt injuries (Chance fracture). This injury type may involve bone, ligaments, or both (Figs. 22–17 and 22–18).
- Bone-only injuries in children may be successfully reduced in a closed fashion and immobilized in an extension cast.
- Surgery is often indicated in the presence of a soft tissue variant of this injury regardless of the patient's age.

Fracture Dislocations

- These are often high-energy injuries and are frequently associated with severe neurological compromise.
- These injuries usually require a posterior or a circumferential spinal stabilization procedure (Figs. 22–19 through 22–27).

Distraction–Extension Injuries

- These are commonly referred to as lumberjack injuries.

Table 22–5:   Surgical Approaches to Spinal Decompression

APPROACH	ADVANTAGES	COMMENTS
Anterior	Easier access to retropulsed vertebral bone and discal material	Anterolateral approach—Transthoracic T4-T9, thoracoabdominal T10-L1, retroperitoneal T12-L5
	Direct visualization of compressed neural tissue	Right-sided approach above T10 to avoid great vessels
	Minimal manipulation of the spinal cord	
Posterior	Effective when using distractive instrumentation to reduce retropulsed bone fragments	Posterior indirect reduction through ligamentotaxis more efficient if done within 2-3 days of injury
Posterolateral	Instrumentation without the need for a second anterior staged procedure	Access to the thecal sac through the pedicle
		Difficult anterior column reconstruction
	Advantageous in lower lumbar fractures and lateralized nerve root entrapment	Increased risk of neural injury secondary to neural manipulation

Box 22–3: Interbody Grafts

- Interbody spacers inserted in an intracolumnar position act as load-sharing devices restoring axial stability until arthrodesis is obtained.
- The most commonly used interbody spacer is an autologous tricortical iliac crest.
  - It has a faster rate of bony incorporation than allograft strut grafts because of its biocompatibility.
- An allograft strut graft is able to withstand greater physiologic loads than an autologous iliac crest in the erect spine in the early reconstruction and healing period (White et al. 1978).
  - Allograft sources such as a tibial shaft, femoral shaft, or metallic mesh cages are gaining popularity.

- There is a high association with metabolic bone disease and a preexisting spinal deformity.
  - Ankylosing spondylitis
  - Diffuse idiopathic skeletal hyperostosis (Figs. 22–24 through 22–27)

Conclusions

- Despite the advancements in spinal implants and radiographic imaging, controversy continues to exist over the indications for surgical intervention, the timing of such intervention, and the approach with which to correct any existing spinal deformity.
- The basic tenets of trauma surgery should be strictly adhered to in the management of thoracolumbar spine trauma.
- Once the patient is medically stabilized, a detailed neurological examination and a careful radiographic evaluation should be performed.
- The surgeon should be aware of the biomechanics of the thoracolumbar spine, the mechanism of injury, and the various implants available for treatment.
- Most thoracolumbar injuries, in the absence of a neurological deficit, are stable and can be treated successfully nonoperatively.
- For the rare unstable spinal fracture, with or without a neurological deficit, surgical treatment is often beneficial in improving patient mobilization and an early functional return to society.
- The goals in managing thoracolumbar injuries are to maximize neurological recovery and to expeditiously stabilize the spine for early rehabilitation and an early return to a productive lifestyle.

Text continued on p. 303

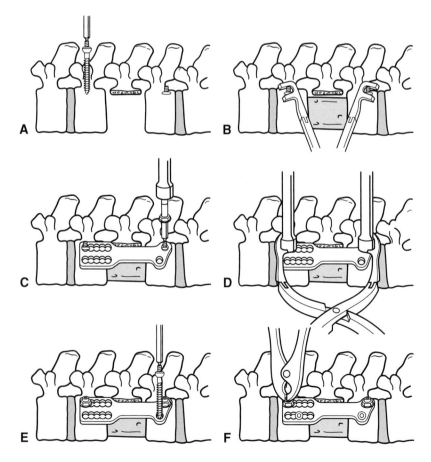

Figure 22–8: An illustration of the technique for anterior spinal instrumentation following corpectomy. A, Insertion of vertebral body screws. B. Use of vertebral body screws to distract corpectomy site. C, Placement of anterior vertebral body plate. D, Compression of graft through the vertebral body screws. E, F, Securing the plate with addition vertebral body

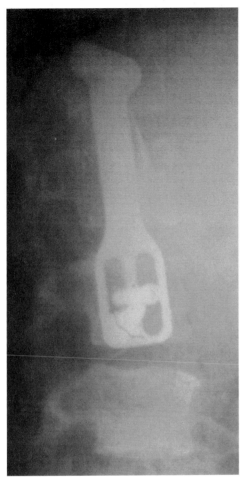

Figure 22–9: A postoperative lateral radiograph following the completion of an anterior thoracolumbar decompression and a stabilization procedure using a titanium mesh cage and an anterior thoracolumbar plate.

Box 22–4:   Fixation

- Biomechanically, a longer application of a longitudinal component (rod) reduces the risk of terminal implant cutout or dislodgement.
  - However, this may contribute to increased global spinal stiffness and subsequent junctional degeneration.
- Shortcomings of distraction rod–hook techniques for fracture reduction and stabilization include the following:
  - Hook dislodgement
  - Overdistraction, possibly leading to iatrogenic loss of lumbar lordosis (flatback deformity) or excessive thoracic kyphosis
- Pedicle screw anchors provide three-column bony fixation.
  - They allow potentially shorter posterior fixation lengths yet confer adequate spinal stability (Lim et al. 1997).
- The best candidates for posterior short-segment pedicle screw fixation (one level above and one level below the fracture level) are as follows:
  - Flexion–distraction injuries
  - Lower lumbar burst fractures in which the weight bearing line is posterior to the posterior vertebral body wall

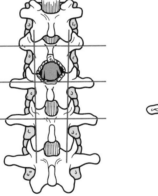
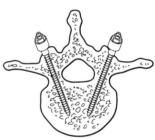

Figure 22–10: Schematic of pedicle screw insertion sites and placement of pedicle screws within the vertebral body.

Table 22–6: Management of Thoracolumbar Fractures

TYPE	NONSURGICAL MANAGEMENT	SURGICAL INDICATIONS	OTHER
Minor injuries	TLSO Fracture below L3—Add unilateral thigh extension	At follow-up obtain flexion or extension plain x-ray films to rule out occult instability	Transverse, spinous, or articular process fractures
Compression fractures	Extension TLSO cast or orthosis Early ambulation If fracture proximal to T7—add a cervical extension to brace or cast	>20-30° of initial kyphosis (significant posterior osteoligamentous disruption) >50% loss of anterior vertebral body height	Nonsegmental hook–rod construct applying distraction–lordosis force vectors for reduction Short segment pedicle screw construct followed by immobilization in a custom-molded hyperextension orthosis or body cast for a minimum of 3 months Recent reports of percutaneous cement augmentation in symptomatic osteopenic compression fractures (vertebroplasty with or without balloon elevation of the vertebral endplates)*
Burst fracture	Bed rest until resolution of constitutional symptoms Progressive ambulation in a full contact orthosis or cast for 12-24 weeks with or without a unilateral thigh extension (fracture L3 or lower) for the initial 6 weeks of treatment	Neurologically intact Kyphosis > 20° Facet subluxation or spreading of the interspinous process distance >50% loss of anterior vertebral body height Neurologically compromised Surgical decompression with imaging documentation of significant neural compression	No definitive evidence that correlates the degree of neural impingement with the severity of neurologic deficit following thoracolumbar trauma
Distraction–flexion injury	Rarely indicated in an adult patient because of the unpredictable nature of healing of this injury subtype	Posterior compression force vector to reduce the injury deformity; take care not to cause iatrogenic retropulsion of bone or discal material into the canal	Anterior longitudinal ligament serves as a tension band with this injury Look for associated intra-abdominal viscus injury with this injury mechanism
Fracture dislocations	Rarely indicated because of the significant degree of instability and deformity associated with this injury subtype	Posterior facet fracture dislocation, rotational instability, or a translational shear injury in the absence of a neurological deficit, requiring an initial posterior segmental reduction and stabilization procedure before considering the need for an anterior decompressive and stabilization procedure	Awake intubation may minimize neurologic injury associated with positioning
Distraction–extension injury	Consider an attempt to reproduce the preinjury sagittal profile of the patient regardless of neurological status through bedding supplements or skeletal traction	Consider initial surgical stabilization with segmental internal fixation initially through a posterior approach Consider a staged anterior stabilization procedure if a significant anterior column defect is present	High association with metabolic bone disease and a preexisting spinal deformity (e.g., ankylosing spondylitis and diffuse idiopathic skeletal hyperostosis)

* (Verlaan et al. 2002.)
§ *TSLO*, thoracolumbosacral orthosis.

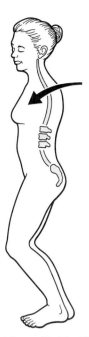

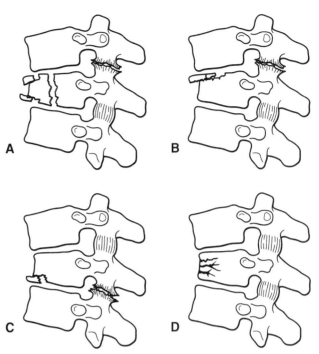

Figure 22–11: Flexion forces cause anterior compression of the vertebral bodies and disks and tension in the posterior elements.

Figure 22–12: Denis classification of thoracolumbar compression injuries. These fractures may involve both endplates (**A**, type A), the superior endplate only (**B**, type B), the inferior endplate only (**C**, type C), or a buckling of the anterior cortex with both endplates intact (**D**, type D).

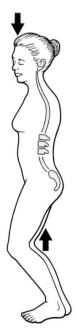

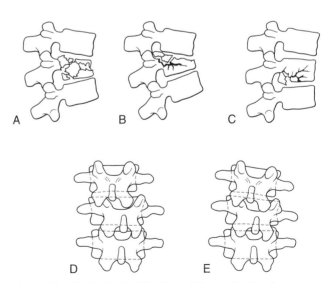

Figure 22–13: Axial compression forces across the straight thoracolumbar region result in pure compressive loading of the vertebral body, most often resulting in a thoracolumbar burst fracture.

Figure 22–14: Denis classification of thoracolumbar burst fractures. **A-C**, Types A, B, and C represent fractures of both endplates, the superior endplate, and the inferior endplate, respectively. **D**, A type D fracture is a type A burst fracture with rotation, which is best appreciated on an anteroposterior radiograph. The superior endplate, inferior endplate, or both may be involved with this fracture.

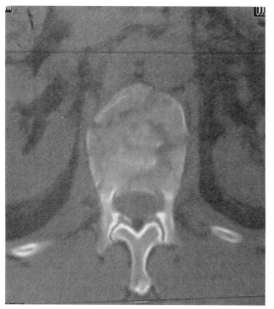

Figure 22–15: An axial CT image of a T12 burst fracture demonstrating middle column failure with approximately 30% canal occlusion.

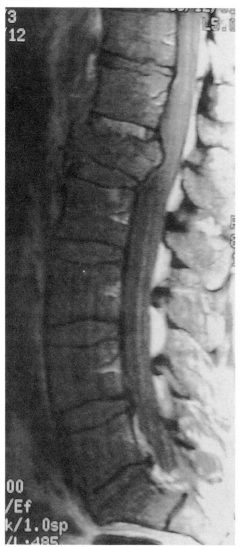

Figure 22–16: A sagittal MRI of a 34-year-old male who sustained a burst fracture to the T12 vertebral body. Note the retropulsion of the posterior vertebral body with compression of the anterior thecal sac.

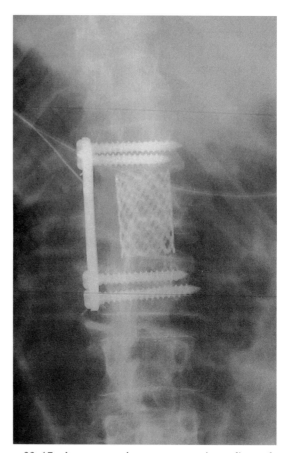

Figure 22–17: A postoperative anteroposterior radiograph following an anterior L1 corpectomy and fusion using a titanium Harms mesh cage and an anterior plate and screw construct.

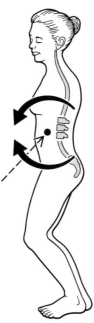

Figure 22–18: Flexion–distraction forces across the thoracolumbar spine frequently produce the typical seat belt injury.

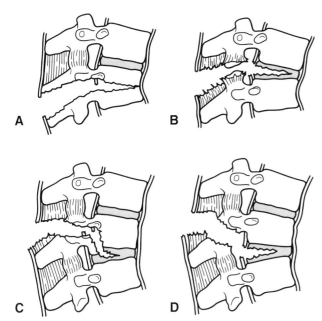

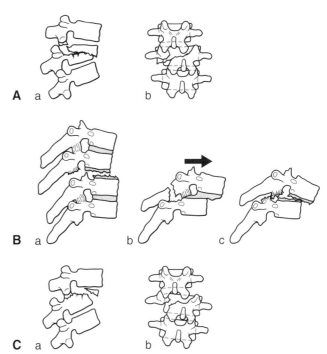

Figure 22–19: Denis classification of flexion–distraction injuries. These may occur at one level through the bone (**A**), at one level through the ligaments and disk (**B**), at two levels with the middle column injured through the bone (**C**), or at two levels with the middle column injured through the ligament and disk (**D**).

Figure 22–21: Denis classification of fracture dislocations. These may occur at one level through the bone (**A**), at one level through the ligaments and disk (**B**), at two levels with the middle column injured through the bone (**C**), or at two levels with the middle column injured through the ligament and disk (**D**).

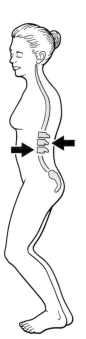

Figure 22–20: Shearing requires forces from opposing directions to pass through the spine at slightly different levels, resulting in a fracture dislocation.

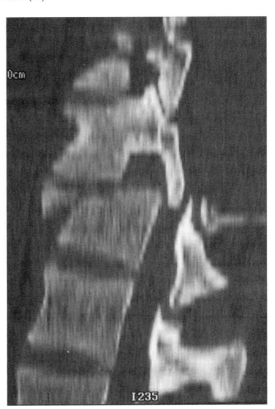

Figure 22–22: A sagittal CT reconstruction of a fracture dislocation of the thoracolumbar spine demonstrating marked vertebral body displacement and canal narrowing.

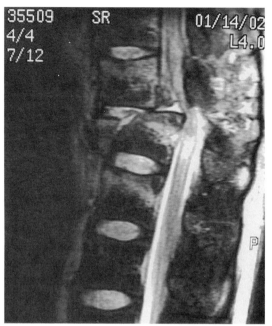

Figure 22–23: A sagittal MRI of the thoracolumbar spine of the patient in Fig. 22–22, demonstrating marked canal narrowing. Note the draping of the spinal cord over the posterosuperior edge of the caudal thoracic vertebrae.

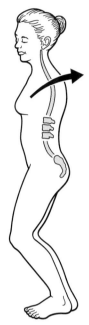

Figure 22–25: Extension forces occur when the upper trunk is thrust posteriorly, resulting in an anterior tension and posterior compression force complex.

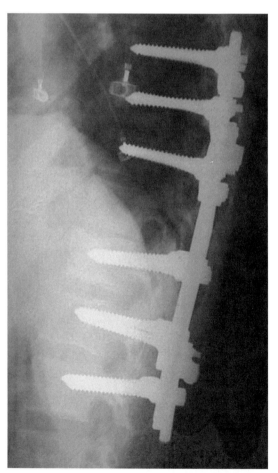

Figure 22–24: A postoperative lateral radiograph of the patient in Fig. 22–22, demonstrating reduction of the spinal deformity followed by a fusion and stabilization with segmental pedicle screw anchors spanning three levels above and below the level of injury.

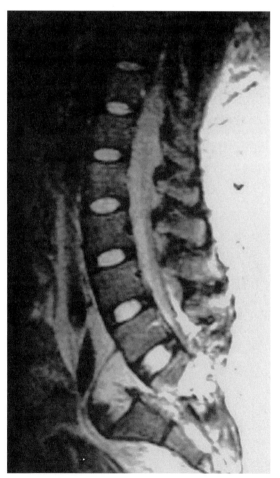

Figure 22–26: A sagittal T2-weighted MRI demonstrating a complete fracture–displacement through the L5 vertebral body because of a distraction–extension injury mechanism.

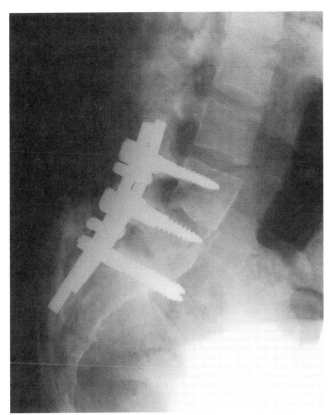

Figure 22–27: A lateral postoperative radiograph of the lumbosacral spine following reduction of the fracture–displacement and stabilization with pedicle screw instrumentation from L4-S1.

References

Abe E, Sato K, Shimada Y et al. (1997) Thoracolumbar burst fracture with horizontal fracture of the posterior column. Spine 22(1): 83-87.

Nine patients with a burst fracture and a horizontal fracture of the posterior column were successfully treated conservatively except for one patient that required posterior spinal fusion secondary to a worsening kyphotic deformity.

Alanay A, Acaroglu E, Yazici M et al. 2001 Short-segment pedicle instrumentation of thoracolumbar burst fractures—Does transpedicular intracorporeal grafting prevent early failure? Spine 26(2): 213-217.

This paper demonstrates that transpedicular intracorporeal grafting in the treatment of burst fractures does not have a detectable effect on the rate of reconstruction of the canal area or on remodeling. Spinal canal remodeling was observed in all patients regardless of grafting.

Bohlman HH, Kirkpatrick JS, Delamarter RB. (1994) Anterior decompression for late pain and paralysis after fractures of the thoracolumbar spine. Clin Orthop Rel Res 300: 24-29.

Anterior decompression of the thoracolumbar spine for chronic pain after thoracolumbar fractures is a safe and effective treatment for patients even as long as 5 years after the initial injury.

Bracken MB, Holford TR. (1993) Effects of timing of methylprednisolone or naloxone administration on recovery of segmented and long-tract neurological function in NASCIS 2. J Neurosurg 79: 500-507.

This analysis demonstrates that the greatest proportion of all neurological recovery and of recovery because of treatment with very high doses of methylprednisolone within 8 hours of injury occurs below the lesion.

Bracken MB, Shephard MJ, Collins W.F. (1990) A randomized, controlled trial of methylprednisolone or naloxone in the treatment of acute spinal cord injury—Results of the second National Acute Spinal Cord Study. N Engl J Med 322: 1405-1411.

The first controlled trial of methylprednisolone evaluating its effect on neurological recovery in acute spinal cord injury patients.

Bradford DS, McBride GG. (1987) Surgical management of thoracolumbar spine fractures with incomplete neurological deficits. Clin Orthop Rel Res 218: 201-216.

The authors note that neurological recovery was greater with anterior decompression mainly as a result of improved canal clearance.

Carlson GD, Minato Y, Okada A. (1997) Early time-dependent decompression for spinal cord injury—Vascular mechanisms of recovery. J Neurotrauma 14(12): 951-962.

The authors found that a critical window of 1-3 hours after the initial spinal injury exists before an electrophysiological decline of evoked potentials of the spinal cord begins.

Chapman JR, Anderson PA. (1994) Thoracolumbar spine fractures and neurological deficits (review). Orthop Clin North Am 25: 595-612.

A comprehensive review of thoracolumbar fractures and the appropriate management of these injuries.

Daffner RH, Deeb ZL, Rothfus WE. (1987) Thoracic fractures and dislocations in motorcyclists. Skeletal Radiol 16: 280-284.

A radiological evaluation and illustration of various thoracic spinal injuries sustained in high-energy trauma patients.

Denis F. (1983) The three column spine and its significance in the classification of acute thoracolumbar spinal injuries. Spine 8(8): 817-831.

The original paper describing the division of the vertebral column into three columns to help assess spinal stability.

Denis F, Burkus JK. (1992) Shear fracture dislocations of the thoracic and lumbar spine associated with forceful hyperextension (lumberjack paraplegia). Spine 17: 152.

A description of the unusual fracture dislocation associated with a distractive extension–type injury mechanism.

Ferguson RL, Allen BL Jr. (1984) A mechanistic classification of thoracolumbar spine fractures. Clin Orthop 189: 77-88.

The authors categorize spinal injury as a result of the mechanism of injury with various grades according to the severity.

Flanders AE. (1999) Thoracolumbar trauma imaging overview. Instruct Course Lect 48: 429-431.

A review of the various thoracic imaging modalities available to the spine surgeon.

Gertzbein SD. (1994) Neurological deterioration in patients with thoracic and lumbar fractures after admission to the hospital. Spine 19: 1723-1725.

The authors describe the potential for neurological worsening from misdiagnosis and improper immobilization of patients with thoracolumbar injuries.

Gertzbein SD. (1992) Scoliosis Research Society—Multicenter spine fracture study. Spine 17: 528-540.

A comprehensive review of the incidence, demographics, and etiology of spine fractures in the American population.

Klein GR, Vaccaro AR. (2003) Cervical spine trauma: Upper and lower. In: Principles and Practice of Spine Surgery (Vaccaro AR et al., eds.). Philadelphia: Mosby pp. 198–202.

Kraus JF, Franti CE, Biggin RS et al. (1975) Incidence of traumatic spinal cord lesions. J Chronic Dis 28: 471-492.

An evaluation of the incidence of incomplete and complete neurological injuries in the spinal cord injury patient.

Leventhal MR. (2003) Fractures, dislocations, and fracture dislocations of spine. In: Campbell's Operative Orthopaedics, 10th edition (Canale ST, ed.). Philadelphia: Mosby pp. 687–693.

Lim TH, An HS, Hong JH et al. (1997) Biomechanical evaluation of anterior and posterior fixations in an unstable calf spine model. Spine 22(3): 261-266.

A short, transpedicular instrumentation provided less rigid fixation in flexion and extension without the anterior structural graft.

McAfee PC, Yuan HA, Fredrickson BE et al. (1983) The value of computed tomography in thoracolumbar fractures—An analysis of one hundred cases and a new classification. J Bone Joint Surg 65A: 461-473.

A categorization of thoracolumbar injuries based upon CT.

Oskouian RJ, Johnson JP. (2002) Vascular complications in anterior thoracolumbar spinal reconstruction. J Neurosurg 96 (1 Suppl): 1-5.

The authors describe the potential complications, including vascular injury to the great vessels, deep venous thrombosis, and pulmonary embolism.

Saboe LA, Reid DC, Davis LA et al. (1991) Spine trauma and associated injuries. J Trauma 31: 43-48.

The authors describe the importance of evaluating for other injuries commonly associated with spinal cord injury patients, such as intra-abdominal and pleural injuries.

Saifuddin A, Noordeen H, Taylor BA et al. (1996) The role of imaging in the diagnosis and management of thoracolumbar burst fractures—Current concepts and a review of the literature. Skel Radiol 25(7): 603-613.

This review article describes the use of radiological imaging in diagnosing and guiding the management of thoracolumbar burst fractures.

Singh K, DeWald CJ, Hammerberg KW et al. (2002) Long structural allografts in the treatment of anterior spinal column defects. Clin Orthop 394: 121-129.

The authors retrospectively reviewed the use of long segment allografts in the face of anterior column reconstruction secondary to tumor, trauma, and infection.

Vaccaro AR, Daugherty RJ, Sheehan TP. (1997) Neurological outcome of early versus late surgery for cervical spinal cord injury. Spine 22(22): 2609-2613.

No significant benefit was found when cervical spinal cord decompression after trauma was performed less than 72 hours after injury as opposed to waiting longer than 5 days.

Verlaan JJ, van Helden WH, Oner FC et al. (2002) Balloon vertebroplasty with calcium phosphate cement augmentation for direct restoration of traumatic thoracolumbar vertebral fractures. Spine 27(5): 543-548.

The authors suggest that balloon vertebroplasty may be a safe and feasible procedure for the restoration of traumatic thoracolumbar vertebral fractures.

White AA, Panjabi MM. (1978) Clinical Biomechanics of the Spine. Philadelphia: J.B. Lippincott pp. 19–37.

One of the original descriptions and analyses of spinal biomechanics, describing the anatomy and the relationship to injury and instability.

Willen J, Lindahl S, Nordwall A. (1985) Unstable thoracolumbar fractures. Spine 10(2): 111-122.

A description of the treatment with fixation options for unstable thoracolumbar fractures, particularly burst fractures.

Index

Page numbers followed by "f" denotes figures; "b" denote boxes; and "t" denote tables.